# Physical Culture and the Body Beautiful

## Purposive Exercise In the Lives of American Women 1800–1870

Jan Todd, Ph.D.

Mercer University Press
Macon, Georgia 31210

ISBN 0-86554-561-8

©1998 All rights reserved
Mercer University Press
6316 Peake Road
Macon, Georgia 31210

First edition.

∞The paper used in this publication meets the mini-
mum requirements of the American National
Standard for Information Sciences—Permanence of
Paper for Printed Library Materials, ANSI Z39.48-
1984.

Library of Congress Cataloging-in-Publication Data

Todd, Jan.
Physical Culture and the body beautiful: purposive exercise in the
lives of American women, 1800-1870 / Janice Suffolk Todd.
p. cm.
Includes bibliographical references and index.
ISBN 0-86554-561-8 (alk. paper)
1. Physical education for women—United States—History—19th century.
2. Exercise for women—United States—History—19th century. 3.
Feminine beauty (Aesthetics)—United States—19th century. 4. Popular
culture—United States—History—19th. I. Title.
GV439.T63 1997
613.7'045—dc21
97-42876
CIP

# Contents

Acknowledgments ............................................................................ix

Introduction ....................................................................................1

*Chapter 1*
Majestic Womanhood vs. "Baby Faced Dolls": ...................................11
The Debate Over Women's Exercise

*Chapter 2*
"Souls of Fire in Iron Hearts": ..........................................................31
The 1820s Gymnastics Revolution

*Chapter 3*
William Fowle's Monitorial School for Girls: ....................................71
The First American Gymnastics Experiment

*Chapter 4*
The Literature of Calisthenics ..........................................................89

*Chapter 5*
"I Practice Calisthenics Every Day and Like It Quite Well": ............119
Mary Lyon, Mount Holyoke, and American Calisthenics

*Chapter 6*
Becoming Catharine Beecher: ........................................................137
Antebellum Proponent of Women's Exercise

*Chapter 7*
Bigger Bodies—Better Brains: ........................................................173
Phrenology and the Health Lift

*Chapter 8*
Dio Lewis and the New Gymnastics: ...............................................211
Birth of a System

*Chapter 9*
Textbooks for Majestic Womanhood: ...............................................239
The Literary Legacy of Dio Lewis

*Chapter 10*
The Influence of Dio Lewis: .............................................................263
"Courage and Strength to Take Up the Battle"

*Chapter 11*
"Reaping the Reward":.....................................................................281
The Quest for Health by Lizzie Morley and Her Sisters

Methodology ...................................................................................301

Bibliography ...................................................................................305

Index ..............................................................................................355

For Terry,
who likes big things

# Acknowledgments

Many people have provided support and encouragement during the preparation of this book. Special thanks are due to Dr. William H. Goetzmann of the American Civilization Program at the University of Texas at Austin. Throughout my graduate work in the American Civilization Program, Dr. Goetzmann supported my intellectual interest in women, exercise, and body ideology and proved to be an exceptional mentor. I would also like to acknowledge Dr. Desley Deacon, whose friendship and intellectual support during my years in graduate school and during the preparation of this manuscript means more than she can ever know. I am likewise indebted to Dr. Mary Lou LeCompte, now retired from the Department of Kinesiology and Health Education at the University of Texas at Austin. It was Dr. LeCompte who first piqued my curiosity about Dio Lewis with her gift of several issues of *Dio Lewis's Gymnastic Monthly and Journal of Physical Culture.* I am especially grateful to Dr. LeCompte for introducing me to the North American Society for Sport History and for her guidance and criticism of my work as a sport historian. I would also like to thank my good friend and colleague Kim Beckwith for her numerous contributions to this project. There isn't enough space to mention all of Kim's favors over the past several years but her decision to create this book's index leaves me deeply in her debt. I am also grateful to the Roy J. McLean Fellowship at the University of Texas which provided financial assistance for my research during several summers. I would also like to thank my family, especially my mother, Wilma White, for her constant love and encouragement.

And I am grateful to my husband, Dr. Terry Todd, for his seemingly endless faith in my ability to do whatever I set my mind to. Terry's involvement with my research for this volume, however, goes well beyond the boundaries of traditional spousal support. For one thing, he made it possible for me to have my own library. Largely through his efforts and imagination, the Todd-McLean Physical Culture Collection at the University of Texas became a reality. He garnered support from the College of Education, the Barker Center for the Study of American History, and the Department of Kinesiology and Health Education; he convinced many private individuals to donate materials and money; and he gradually assembled what is considered to be the world's largest archive of materials in the English language in the field of physical culture. This collection provided me with an enviable base for my research into the history of nineteenth-century exercise.

Yet even the largest of collections is never totally complete, and so I would like to thank the indefatigable staff of the Interlibrary Loan Service of the University of Texas at Austin, as well as library director Jerry Davis and archivist Mary Jane Sabinski-Smith at Springfield College and Patricia Albright at Mount Holyoke, for their assistance. I am also grateful to the expert staffs of the Institute Archives at Cal Tech, the Massachusetts Historical Society, the Schlesinger Library at Radcliffe, the Boston Public Library, the Smith College Archives, the Harvard University Archives, and the University Archives at Wellesley College.

Several colleagues from the North American Society for Sport History should also be thanked, especially Dr. Jack Berryman, University of Washington; Dr. Patricia Vertinsky, University of Vancouver; and Dr. Ron Smith, Penn State University.

Finally, but certainly not least importantly, I would like to acknowledge an intellectual and emotional debt to retired English professor Dr. Al Thomas of Kutztown University. From the early 1970s through the mid-1980s, Dr. Thomas wrote for *Iron Man,* the most respected weight training magazine of that era. In each of his approximately eighty articles, Thomas dealt with some aspect of the conjunction of strength, femininity, and culturally approved womanhood. Some articles featured women athletes who chose to defy the societal conventions of the 1970s by pursuing muscularity and strength, while some articles were philosophical essays in which Thomas attempted to examine and eradicate our society's aversion to strong, muscular women. As a neophyte to lifting who was having a hard time reconciling an internal conflict about the issue of strength and womanhood, I found Thomas' articles to be invaluable. They allowed me to see over the walls of a narrow, somewhat sheltered garden into a rich, limitless meadow of possibility. Thomas was uncompromising; he accepted no barriers to womanhood. As Dio Lewis had done in the 1860s, Thomas challenged modern women to become the physical and intellectual equals of men. Most American women in the 1970s came to feminism through reading Gloria Steinem and Betty Friedan, but I came to feminism through reading and talking to Al Thomas. By daring to practice what Thomas preached, I discovered untapped reservoirs of physical strength and a growing antipathy for those aspects of our culture that have in countless ways denied women access to this important part of themselves. His articles freed me to give full expression to my gift of physical power and helped me understand the political nature of that power. These insights enabled me to make history as an athlete and to want to write history as a professional.

# Introduction

In 1968, in a secondhand bookstore in Plant City, Florida, I discovered copies of Alice B. Stockham's *Tokology: A Book for Every Woman* and William A. Alcott's *The Young Woman's Guide*. I can't explain why, at age sixteen, in the midst of my longings for the Beatles and Bobby Kennedy, I felt drawn to those two nineteenth-century women's advice books. At fifty cents apiece, however, the books were an affordable lark, and I bought them both. As a teenager, I found Stockham's quaint approach to maternity and Alcott's insistence on spiritual purity very amusing, and I read both books completely through during the next couple of weeks. Although many of Stockham's and Alcott's pronouncements made me smile, what delighted me most were their discussions of appropriate exercise for women, especially Stockham's suggestion that rolling over and over in bed could be regarded as healthful exercise. Through the years my other memories of Stockham's and Alcott's teachings gradually faded, but the image of those nineteenth-century mothers-to-be rolling around on their beds in search of exercise remained sharp and never failed to produce a chuckle.[1]

Since that day in 1968, much of my life has been spent dealing in one way or another with the question of appropriate exercise for women. Following college graduation, I spent more than a decade involved in powerlifting, a type of competitive weight lifting. During those years I had to confront personally my intellectual and emotional feelings about the relationship of strength to femininity, and I had to reconcile my interest in strength with the general societal belief that my sport was not only masculine but possibly dangerous for women. On the other hand, I began to understand that the regular physical training I did as part of my athletic life made me feel differently about my body and my sense of life's possibilities. To use a newly chic term, the heavy exercise empowered me, and I wondered if other women's lives had been similarly changed.

My interest in nineteenth-century women's exercise evolved from my discovery that a surprisingly large number of women had worked as professional strongwomen in the circus and vaudeville at the turn of the century. Those women, whom I considered my athletic

foremothers, seemed anomalous to me at first. Physically large and frequently muscular, those early strength athletes were nevertheless often
described as beautiful and feminine in the newspaper reports of their
public exhibitions. Furthermore, their lives seemed to contradict
everything I knew about womanhood in Victorian America. Why, I
began to wonder, were music hall athletes such as Minerva, Athleta,
and Belle Gordon—who seemed to defy every tenet of women's proper
place in Victorian society—so popular with late nineteenth-century
audiences? Why did men and women pay to see these women swing
Indian clubs and lift cannons? If *fin de siecle* America viewed these
women as freaks, then why did the sporting press describe them so
positively? Was it possible that some segments of Victorian society val-
ued size and strength in women?[2]

As I struggled to understand the meaning of these professional
strongwomen, I began to search for their antecedents in the early nineteenth century. I did not expect it to be easy to trace the evolution of
these public entertainers, and it was not. It proved equally difficult to
trace the dumbbell drills, Indian club routines, and other types of purposive movements that constituted women's exercise. No one, it turned
out, had ever written a book dealing solely with the early history of
women's exercise in America.

The academic specialization we now call "women's sport history"
can be said to have begun officially with the formation of the North
American Society for Sport History in 1973. During the past two
decades a considerable number of scholars have contributed to the
ongoing analysis of the complex world of competitive women's sports.
Thanks to the efforts of these pioneering historians, we now know a
great deal about the origins of intercollegiate sport for women; the
workings of many women's team sports; the lives and personal relationships of the heroines of the modern Olympic Games; and school
physical education programs for women. Although no one in the field
would call women's sport history well documented at this point, historians of women's sport can, nonetheless, point with pride to an
extensive body of monographs, dissertations, journal articles, and
essays dealing with the American sportswoman.[3]

I found, however, that few historians have taken an interest in the
fascinating story of purposive exercise, which differs significantly from
competitive sports and leisure activities. While purposive exercise is
often fun, it lacks the "play impulse" that characterizes true games.[4]
Furthermore, although women's participation in sport is at times

associated with specific hygienic and behavioral goals, much of sport remains joyous and, in a positive sense, irrational. Purposive exercise is always rational; its regimens are undertaken to meet specific physiological and philosophical goals. While women's sport relates primarily to play and relaxation, purposive exercise is about change—about creating a new vision of the body. Nineteenth-century women picked up dumbbells, took long walks, and joined together in calisthenics and gymnastics classes for basically the same reasons women exercise today: the implicit promise of improved appearance, the quest for better health, and a desire to feel stronger and more competent.

It is my personal conviction that purposive exercise has had as much influence on the lives of American women as competitive sport has had. And yet, we still know very little about women's personal relationships to exercise. Dio Lewis' New Gymnastics, Walter Camp's Daily Dozen, and Jane Fonda and her many imitators had an impact on the lives of millions American women, yet historians have paid little attention to these exercise regimens or to how women felt about this aspect of their lives.

Although research on school physical education programs touches some of these issues, much of the historical scholarship on physical education has concerned itself with the struggle to control women's participation in sport and with organizational issues of power within physical education associations. These studies have not featured as their primary focus an analysis of the exercises performed by the women in their programs or an analysis of how the participants in the programs—the women themselves—felt about their physical training experiences.

There are, of course, some exceptions to this generalization, the most notable of which is the scholarship of Canadian historian Patricia Vertinsky. Using feminist analysis, in her persuasive book *The Eternally Wounded Woman: Women, Exercise and Doctors in the Late Nineteenth Century*, Vertinsky carefully examined the late nineteenth-century medical community's dicta regarding appropriate exercise for women.[5] Another exception is professor Roberta Park, who has written several important essays on nineteenth-century exercise, the most valuable of which, in this context, is her 1978 article, "'Embodied Selves': The Rise and Development of Concern for Physical Education, Active Games and Recreation for American Women, 1776–1865."[6] Historian Martha Verbrugge has also contributed to our knowledge about issues of personal health for women through her well-regarded book, *Able Bodied*

*Womanhood: Personal Health and Social Change in Nineteenth-Century Boston.*[7] But Verbrugge and Vertinsky deal primarily with the last half of the nineteenth century; and Park's essay, although richly detailed, tells only part of the tale.[8] To find the story of women's exercise in the first half of the nineteenth century, one can only turn to general histories of sport and physical education. There, for the most part, discussions of antebellum women's exercise consist of a few scant paragraphs describing calisthenics and the influence of Catharine Beecher.[9]

Throughout the antebellum era, however, at least two competing ideals struggled to control the course of women's purposive exercise. Jean Jacques Rousseau's philosophical heirs argued that women were physiologically different from men and thus required nonvigorous, distinctly feminine exercises such as light calisthenics. Feminist philosopher Mary Wollstonecraft, on the other hand, initiated an ideological movement that argued women had as much right to physical strength, muscularity, and robust health as men did. In examining the course of this debate in the first decades of the nineteenth century, I have reached several conclusions.

First, a much more diverse spectrum of women's exercise existed in the antebellum era than is currently described in modern historical texts. Second, several exercise systems had significant links to an ideal of womanhood—called in this text Majestic Womanhood—that directly competed with the prevailing constructs of the cult of True Womanhood first described by historian Barbara Welter. Third, purposive training mattered in the lives of American women. It influenced them physically, intellectually, and emotionally, and, in many instances, empowered them to step beyond the confines of their separate sphere of domestic duty and involve themselves in the world outside their homes.

In this attempt to fill some of the gaps in our knowledge of women's exercise history, I have placed special emphasis on examining the physiological effects of the various exercise systems. Scholars have been too quick to categorize all antebellum women's exercise as "light calisthenics." Upon examination, several systems actually required high levels of strength and endurance. Devotees of these latter systems— Wollstonecraft's ideological heirs—also adopted a stronger, larger, more robust ideal of femininity, an ideal made possible by the grafting of phrenology, neoclassicism, and Lamarckianism to antebellum America's enthusiasm for physical culture. The phrenologist Orson Fowler played a major role in championing this ideal of Majestic

Womanhood. While phrenology's scientific claims and racist tendencies have been rejected, the pseudoscience nonetheless influenced people's lives at all levels of nineteenth-century American society in many ways. In particular, phrenology exerted a powerful influence on women's attitudes toward appropriate education, marriage relations, and the need for exercise. Bigger bodies led to better brains according to Fowler, and he used this maxim repeatedly to promote vigorous exercise for American women.

These conclusions about nineteenth-century exercise help corroborate the findings of University of Georgia historian Frances B. Cogan. Using primarily literary sources, Cogan's revisionist history, *All-American Girl: The Ideal of Real Womanhood in Mid-Nineteenth-Century America* (1989), argues that, at least in the northeastern United States, an ideal for femininity existed that competed with Welter's "Cult of True Womanhood." Historians Lois Banner, Carroll Smith-Rosenberg, and Catharine Clinton amplified our understanding of True Womanhood, while many contemporary historians, especially women's sport historians, have employed True Womanhood as a one-dimensional lens for viewing the lives of nineteenth-century women.[10] Cogan's book is based on an important question. She asks, "How could vast numbers of American middle-class women have clutched to their bosoms an ideal of the "submissive maiden" when that ideal was physically injurious, economically unworkable, legally contraindicated for survival within the restraints of marriage, and intellectually vacuous?"[11]

Cogan contends that many American women did not subscribe to this ideal. She documents convincingly that an alternative model of behavior existed—an ideal she calls Real Womanhood. Cogan argues that Real Womanhood's foundation was not based on frailty, piety, and submissiveness—the three pillars supporting the pedestal of True Womanhood—but on the much more desirable qualities of strength, vitality, energy, and competence.

Majestic Womanhood differs only in degree from Cogan's ideal of Real Womanhood. Adherents of Majestic Womanhood, such as Wollstonecraft, the physician Elizabeth Blackwell, Orson Fowler, radical hydropath Harriet Austin, and exercise entrepreneur Dio Lewis subscribed to the basic tenets of Real Womanhood but then took the model even further by arguing that women should try to become the physical and intellectual equals of men. In particular, Majestic Womanhood proposed a new physical model for American womanhood—a model based on size, strength, and substance—that, theoretically, would allow women to be taken seriously as they pursued a professional life outside the home. Cogan's ideal of Real Womanhood, while similar in many respects, was neither physically nor socially as liberating.

The ultimate aim of this monograph, however, is not to become involved in feminist hairsplitting but to try to depict accurately the changing nature of purposive exercise in the early nineteenth century. Barbara Welter's Cult of True Womanhood also had links to purposive training that need to be documented and analyzed. True Womanhood's adherents, of course, imbued their systems with value-laden rhetoric supporting their vision of a domestic, submissive role for women in society. Catharine Beecher was a significant figure in this movement in purposive training but not its originator. Several other physical educators also made important contributions to the spread of both calisthenics and "domestic exercise," the two systems generally attributed to Beecher and to the Cult of True Womanhood.

*****

How these competing ideals manifested themselves in the lives of real women can be better understood by an examination of the life of Anna Elizabeth Morley, who became a patient of Dr. Dio Lewis in early 1866. Prior to her arrival at Lewis's movement cure sanitarium, Lizzie Morley endured five long years of ever-diminishing health and strength. The regimen Dio Lewis suggested to cure Morley's ill health was a potent combination of dress reform, diet, and purposive exercise. Morley's decision to try exercise was not unusual. Like most middle-class New Englanders, Morley grew up in an atmosphere of health reform and medical experimentation. At mid-century, medical treatment at the hands of regular physicians was still considered a gamble, at best. In response to those troubled hygienic times, a widespread, popular health movement developed. This quasi-religious movement encompassed such so-called hygienic therapies as vegetarianism, hydropathy, homeopathy, mesmerism, botanical therapy, phrenology, and, at times, purposive exercise. As increasing numbers of Americans sought remedies outside the traditional medical canon of bleeding and purging, a large body of didactic literature came into print describing alternative methods of maintaining health.[12] These books and journal articles preached that health was a moral duty and that every man—

and every woman—must take responsibility for his or her own physical destiny. Again and again, nineteenth-century Americans read that the truly moral person was vigorous, fit, and free of disease.

Several distinct systems of exercise became interwoven into the tapestry of the health reform movement. Some of these purposive exercise systems were incorporated into the curricula of America's early schools, while others were taught by private entrepreneurs at the new public gymnasia that opened in cities along the Eastern Seaboard—gyms that frequently served women as well as men. Regardless of their place of origination, these purposive exercise systems found many converts because, unlike some medical therapies, purposive exercise worked. Sedentary American women who began a regular program of calisthenics, or dared the even more difficult gymnastics, found themselves feeling vibrant and youthful. Superfluous flesh dropped away. Energy increased. Posture improved. Furthermore, many of these women found, as Lizzie Morley did, that their lives fundamentally changed.

I contend that, regardless of the system or its stated philosophical goals, these early nineteenth-century exercise regimens encouraged women to have a new relationship to their bodies—to view them as trainable and, more importantly, controllable. Feeling in control of one's body in a day when professional medical opinion frequently supported the notion that women were nervous, hysterical, and high-strung was a powerful tool. It was also a very modern concept. Historians such as Welter and Smith-Rosenburg have argued that woman's sphere was limited to the home because of her inability to control her own physiology. Hysteria, menstruation, neurasthenia, and other so-called common female disorders were associated with women's lack of bodily control and exemplified their physical and emotional instability. Women who exercised, however, discovered that the body obeyed commands, that it could change and grow stronger. Some women who exercised were not so easily reduced to hysterics or driven to their beds; they continued living and contributing to their families and society. Roberta Park has speculated that the feelings of empowerment enjoyed by the women who participated in these early exercise programs may even have served as a catalyst of the women's rights campaign of the mid-nineteenth century.[13] Although I am not able to completely corroborate Park's thesis, Lizzie Morley was not the only woman I discovered whose desire to be a "strong woman" turned out to be the pathway to doing something important with her life.

[1]Alice B. Stockham, M.D., *Tokology, A Book for Every Woman* (Chicago: Alice B. Stockham & Co, 1893); William A. Alcott, *The Young Woman's Guide* (Boston: Charles H. Pierce, 1847).

[2]See Jan Todd, "A Legacy of Strength: The Cultural Phenomenon of the Professional Strongwomen," paper presented at the North American Society for Sport History, Columbus OH, 1987; Jan Todd, "The Strong Lady in America: Professional Athletes and the *Police Gazette*," paper presented at the North American Society for Sport History, Clemson SC, 1989; Jan Todd, "Against All Odds: The Origins of Weight Training for Female Athletes in North America," *Iron Game History* 2 (April 1992): 4-14; and Jan Todd, "Minerva," Empress of Strength," *Iron Game History* 1 (April 1990): 14-15.

[3]At the 1992 annual meeting of the North American Society for Sport History, in a session entitled "Historiography and the Future," I presented a statistical analysis of women's sport history scholarship entitled, "Beyond the Ivy-Clad Walls: New Directions for Women's Sport History." For this project, I examined all the programs of the North American Society for Sport History's annual meetings and all the programs of the History Academy of the American Alliance for Health, Physical Education, Recreation, and Dance. In these programs I counted all the papers presented on women's topics and looked at the total number of women scholars. I also counted published articles by women and about women's topics in *The Journal of Sport History*, *The International Journal of Sport History*, the *Canadian Journal of the History of Sport*, the *Journal of Health, Physical Education, Recreation, and Dance* [*JOHPERD*], and the *Research Quarterly*. In a nutshell, I discovered that scholars of women's sport had primarily focused on associational and institutional histories and on competitive sport. For instance, I identified 115 papers by women historians on women's topics that were presented at the annual meetings of NASSH during 1973–1991. Sixty of these papers dealt primarily with institutional or associational topics, thirty-nine with competitive women's sports. Only eleven papers from this twenty-year time span examined issues of exercise and health. Male scholars, I discovered, shared this bias toward competitive sport and institutional history. Of the twenty-four papers on women's sport presented by men at NASSH, nine dealt with institutional histories, and seven with competitive sport. No male scholars examined women's exercise. I found the distribution of subject matter to be similar in published articles and in papers presented at the History Academy of AAHPERD.

[4]Allen Guttman, *From Ritual to Record: The Nature of Modern Sport* (New York: Columbia University Press, 1978), 3-5, argues that "play is non-utilitarian physical or intellectual activity pursued for its own sake . . . play is to work as process is to results . . . This definition rules out commonly accepted goals like better health, character development, improved motor skills, and peer group socialization."

[5]Patricia Vertinsky, *The Eternally Wounded Woman: Women, Exercise, and Doctors in the Late Nineteenth Century* (New York: Manchester University

Press, 1990). See, especially, the chapter on Charlotte Perkins Gilman, 204-33.

[6]Roberta J. Park, " 'Embodied Selves': The Rise and Development of Concern for Physical Education, Active Games and Recreation for American Women, 1776–1865," *Journal of Sport History* 5 (Summer 1978): 5-41. See also Roberta J. Park, "Physiologists, Physicians, and Physical Educators: Nineteenth-Century Biology and Exercise, Hygienic and Educative," *Journal of Sport History* 14 (Spring 1987): 28-60.

[7]Martha Verbrugge, *Able-Bodied Womanhood: Personal Health and Social Change in Nineteenth-Century Boston* (New York: Oxford University Press, 1988).

[8]There are also several excellent studies of women's sport and physical education in Great Britain that deal with the late Victorian era. See, for instance, June Kennard, "Women, Sport, and Society in Victorian England" (Ph.D. diss., University of North Carolina at Greensboro, 1974) and Kathleen McCrone, *Playing the Game: Sport and Physical Education of English Women: 1870–1914* (Lexington, KY: University Press of Kentucky, 1988).

[9]Betty Spears and Richard Swanson, *History of Sport and Physical Activity in the United States* (Dubuque, IA: William C. Brown, 1978), for instance, devote one paragraph (pp. 72-73) to "the early fitness movement," two paragraphs (pp. 78-80) to physical education in the early women's colleges, and deal with Beecher and Fowle in one paragraph of sixteen lines (p. 84). An earlier text, Deobold B. Van Dalen, Elmer D. Mitchell, and Bruce L. Bennett, *A World History of Physical Education* (Englewood Cliffs, NJ: Prentice-Hall, 1963), covers the first seventy years of the nineteenth century in six short paragraphs (pp. 376-77).

[10]Barbara Welter, "The Cult of True Womanhood: 1820–1860," *American Quarterly* 18 (Summer 1966): 151-74; Lois Banner, *American Beauty* (New York: Knopf, 1983); Catharine Clinton, *The Other Civil War: American Women in the Nineteenth Century* (New York: Hill and Wang, 1984); Carroll Smith-Rosenberg, "The Female Animal: Medical and Biological Views of Woman and Her Role in Nineteenth-Century America," *Journal of American History* 60 (September 1973): 332-56.

[11]Frances B. Cogan, *The All-American Girl: The Ideal of Real Womanhood in Mid-Nineteenth-Century America* (Athens, GA: The University of Georgia Press, 1989), 3-4.

[12]Between 1820 and 1852, the *Bibliotheca Americana* lists more advice books than any other genre. Quoted in Cogan, *All-American Girl*, 16.

[13]Park, "Embodied Selves," 5.

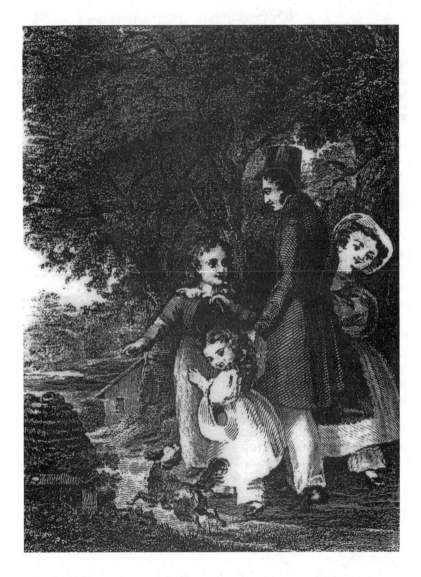

Frontpiece: "The morning is the most favorable season for exercising the frame as well as for making useful impressions on the mind and heart." Engraving entitled "An Early Walk," from *The Mother's Assistant and Young Lady's Friend* (September 1843).

# Chapter 1
## Majestic Womanhood vs. "Baby-Faced Dolls": The Debate Over Women's Exercise

Calvinist doctrine, which denigrated the body in favor of the soul, made physical activity seem frivolous and even ungodly.[1] In the eighteenth century, however, French philosopher Jean Jacques Rousseau provided a philosophical rallying point for exercise with his descriptions of the importance of outdoor athletics in the formation of manly, ideal men. Unfortunately, Rousseau did not advocate the same sorts—or the same intensity—of purposive exercise for women. As chief prophet of what might be called the eugenic school of womanhood, Rousseau did not want women to be truly weak, but he did want them to be fertile, submissive, nonambitious and content to stay at home. However, the very fact that Rousseau addressed the question of women's exercise in his influential essay *Emile* (1762) meant that other thoughtful, literate individuals also began to think seriously about woman's physical nature, woman's education, and woman's need for physical exercise. One of those individuals was British feminist Mary Wollstonecraft, whose influential essay, *A Vindication of the Rights of Woman* (1793), attacked Rousseau's fecund domestics and introduced an alternate ideal—predicated on competence, education, and physical fitness—called in this book "Majestic Womanhood."

As didactic literature aimed at women flourished during the early nineteenth century, Rousseau's and Wollstonecraft's original messages were repeated and reinterpreted endlessly. While the majority of the books printed in this era agreed with Rousseau's essential message regarding women, a few authors, such as the American Charles Brockden Brown, argued that exercise should be genderless. They believed that women had a right to health and physical strength and, furthermore, that the then-current educational system denied these inalienable rights to women. As one anonymous female correspondent explained the situation in a 1791 magazine article, women could not compare with men in bodily strength but, "this may be chiefly attributed to the exercise permitted and encouraged in their youth; but forbidden to us."[2]

As the number of women's schools increased in post-Revolutionary America, accommodations to include physical training began to be seen and discussed in the popular magazines of the day.

Although dance remained the finishing school exercise of choice, at least one school, Sarah Pierce's Litchfield Academy, adopted a more systematic approach to the question of physical fitness.

## Women Should Not Be Strong Like Men

It would be difficult to exaggerate the influence of Jean Jacques Rousseau's theories on physical education and the nature and status of women. Inspired by John Locke's powerful essay, *Some Thoughts Concerning Education* (1693), Rousseau produced several philosophical treatises in mid-century concerned with what he regarded as the evil, debilitating effects of civilization on the individual.[3]

In *Emile*, Rousseau argued for man's return to a natural or more primitive lifestyle. He believed that his century's methods of education emasculated young men and deprived them of their physical strength and vigor. To counter this, Rousseau suggested a radically different curriculum, one that placed strong emphasis on the physical aspects of human development. Boys should be educated like young animals, he argued, free of cares and concerns, and with long, daily bouts of physical exercise.[4]

Rousseau's ideas on women are discussed in Book Five of *Emile*, in which the education and growth of Sophie, Emile's future wife, is described. Although Rousseau urged "naturalness" for women as well as for men, Sophie's education was far less rigorous than Emile's, for Rousseau believed that men and women were innately different. "When once it is proved that men and women are and ought to be unlike in constitution and temperament, it follows that their education must be different," Rousseau explained.[5] Where Emile's physical training was expected to instill the desirable attributes of strength, autonomy, and independent thinking, Sophie exercised because it enhanced her physical appeal to Emile. The more attractive women were, Rousseau reasoned, the more men would wish to mate with them, and the stronger the family would be.[6] A eugenicist at heart, Rousseau claimed, "Women should not be strong like men, but for them, so that their sons may be strong."[7] From Rousseau's narrow perspective, woman's potential was limited to a sheltered, hidden life as man's companion and mate.

Although socially repressive in many ways, Rousseau's eugenic approach to women did result in a new consciousness regarding the need for women's exercise. Rousseau feared the exaggerated delicacy he saw developing among some upper-class women because he believed it would lead to effeminancy in their male offspring. He urged parents to send their daughters away from home for schooling because he believed girls would be less constrained regarding exercise in "Convents and boarding-schools, with their plain food and ample opportunities for amusements, races, and games in the open air and in the garden." According to Rousseau, most girls educated at home led unhealthy lives in which they were "without a moment's freedom to play or jump or run or shout."[8]

Few eighteenth-century intellectuals embraced wholeheartedly Rousseau's vision of the ideal man as a kind of noble savage striving to remain free of the corrupting influence of civilization.[9] A surprisingly large number of intellectuals and laymen did adopt Rousseau's limiting vision of woman's role in the social order, however.

### Majestic Womanhood

Mary Wollstonecraft led an unconventional life for an eighteenth-century woman. Born in 1759, in Hoxton, England, Mary claimed her independence and moved to London to begin a career as a writer in 1788. Although she later married philosopher William Godwin, her reputation never recovered from the scandal of an early romantic liaison that left her with an illegitimate child.[10] Wollstonecraft's tarnished past hampered her philosophical career and enabled some individuals to dismiss out-of-hand the ideas contained in *A Vindication of the Rights of Woman*, her powerful essay arguing for woman's rights. However, open-minded individuals, particularly many women, found much to admire in Wollstonecraft's plea for gender equity. According to historian Mary Beth Norton, a lively debate over the question of woman's rights erupted on both sides of the Atlantic following the essay's publication in 1792.[11] Sadly for Wollstonecraft, many of the criticisms of her essay resembled this *ad hominem* satire of a visiting female philosopher penned by American Timothy Dwight:

> Women . . . are entitled to all the rights, and are capable of all the energies of men. I do not mean merely mental energies . . . I intend bodily energies. They can naturally run as fast, leap as high, and as far, and wrestle, cuffle and box with as much success. . . . This is a mistake (said an old man just before her.) It is no mistake, (said the Female Philosopher.) Why then, (said the senior again) are women always feebler than men? Because (said Mary) they are educated to be feeble; and by indulgence . . . are made poor, puny, baby-faced dolls; instead of the *manly women,* they ought to be. *Manly women!*

(cried the wag) Wheu! a manly woman is a hoyden, a non descript. Am I a hoyden? (interrupted Mary with spirit.) You used to be a strumpet.[12]

Although painful, this passage succinctly sums up Wollstonecraft's argument for the rights of women. She believed that woman's subordinate role in eighteenth-century society resulted not from real, physiological inadequacies, but from woman's limited educational opportunities and the low expectations of her culture. "Let their faculties have room to unfold, and their virtues to gain strength," she protested to Rousseau and others, "and then determine where the whole sex must stand in the intellectual scale."[13]

A consistent theme throughout Wollstonecraft's essay is the importance of the strong, healthy body. The woman who "strengthens her body and exercises her mind," she wrote, "will . . . become the friend, and not the humble dependent of her husband."[14] Wollstonecraft did not, as Dwight suggests, believe that women could ever become as truly strong as men, but she did believe that they greatly undervalued this aspect of their nature, and wrote, "Should it be proved that woman is naturally weaker than man, whence does it follow that it is natural for her to labor to become still weaker than nature intended her to be?"[15]

Wollstonecraft found most offensive the developing upper-class ideals of physical frailty, indolence, and fashion-consciousness. She railed at those women whose confining dress meant that their "limbs and faculties are cramped with worse than Chinese bands," and argued that the "sedentary life which they are condemned to live . . . weakens the muscles and relaxes the nerves."[16] Wollstonecraft understood that woman's attitudes toward fashion and beauty developed at an early age, a fact that made education all the more important. By the time women reached adulthood, she argued, their indoctrination into the world of fashion was nearly complete. "Nor can it be expected," Wollstonecraft reasoned, "that a woman will resolutely endeavor to strengthen her constitution and abstain from enervating indulgences, if artificial notions of beauty, and false descriptions of sensibility, have been early with her motives of action." Though she would have liked to believe otherwise, Wollstonecraft finally concluded that "genteel women are, literally speaking, slaves to their bodies, and glory in their subjection."[17]

Wollstonecraft also chided genteel women for overplaying their weakness and ineptitude, a practice she felt degraded women and indicated the limitations of their childhood development. "I am fully

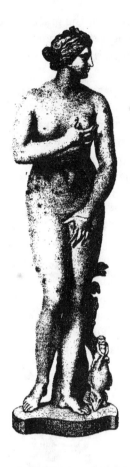

Figure 1: The Venus de Medici as drawn for Alexander Walker's *Beauty: Analysis and Classification of Beauty in Women* (1836).

persuaded that we should hear of none of these infantine airs," she wrote, "if girls were allowed to take sufficient exercise, and not confined in close rooms till their muscles are relaxed, and their powers of digestion destroyed."[18] Indeed, explained Wollstonecraft, the women she most admired, those who in her circle of acquaintances acted like rational creatures and showed vigor of intellect, "have been allowed to run wild" as children.[19]

Ultimately, Wollstonecraft did not want women to become men or to have power over men, "but [power] over themselves."[20] Responding to Rousseau and other critics of equality, Wollstonecraft wrote, "I know that libertines will exclaim that woman would be unsexed by acquiring strength of body and mind, and that beauty, soft bewitching beauty! would no longer adorn the daughters of men." On the contrary, Wollstonecraft wrote, "I think . . . we should see dignified beauty and true grace . . . Not relaxed beauty, it is true, or the graces of help-lessness; but such as appears to make us respect the human body as a majestic pile, fit to receive a noble inhabitant, in the relics of antiq-uity."[21]

Wollstonecraft's image of the ideal body as a majestic antiquity inhabited by a noble, independent intellect was not lost on the *fin-de-siecle* intellectuals who struggled with questions of woman's rights, woman's exercise, and woman's beauty. Although Wollstonecraft's ref-erence to Grecian beauty played only a small part in her essay, it emerged as one of her most important legacies. By evoking the classical ideal of womanhood, Wollstonecraft initiated the development of an alternate feminine ideal, called in this essay "Majestic Womanhood." Although physically modeled on the bodies of such ancient statues as the Venus de Milo and the Venus de Medici, the full expression of the ideal of Majestic Womanhood also embraced physical strength, educa-tion, intelligence, competence, and independence for women. While authors of nineteenth-century women's advice literature fell along Rousseauian and Wollstonecraftian party lines on questions related to women's intellect, physical capacities, and social standing, nearly all antebellum didactic authors agreed that the statuary of ancient Greece represented the ideal female body.

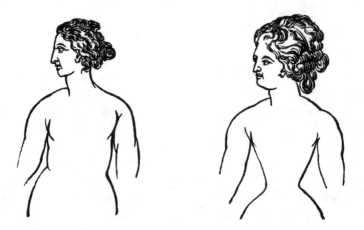

Figure 2. Comparative illustration of the classical ideal for womanhood, represented by the Venus de Medici, with that of a "deformed" fashion-conscious belle of the 1850s. From Catharine Beecher's *Letters to the People on Health and Happiness* (1856).

Large-limbed, broad-waisted, and somewhat athletic in appearance, the Venuses appeared throughout the didactic literature aimed at women published after Wollstonecraft's early lead. Shadrach Ricketson, for instance, argued against corset wearing by suggesting that "the Grecian form is justly preferred to all artificial shapes."[22] In the middle of the nineteenth century, educator Catharine Beecher compared illustrations of the Venus de Medici, which she described as "the most perfect model of a beautiful female form," with that of a woman whose body has been "deformed" by corset wearing.[23] Phrenologically-inspired health reformer Daniel H. Jacques told readers: "The Venus de Medici is considered the most perfect existing model of the female form, and has been the admiration of the world for ages."[24] Bestselling author and Scottish phrenologist George Combe said he had "recommended to my audience the study of the human figure in statuary and painting, not only as an interesting object of taste, but [so that] ... a mother, once familiar with those proportions, and convinced of their relationship to health, would watch, with increased attention, the habits, postures and nutrition of her children."[25]

As happens with most radical philosophical systems, the majority of late eighteenth- and early nineteenth-century Americans fixed on only part of Wollstonecraft's total message—the need for physical and intellectual education for women. Many Americans took a positive view of Wollstonecraft's plea for greater educational opportunities and her advocacy of a physical ideal based on classical art. Her larger message of the equality of the sexes was strongly criticized, however. Nonetheless, thanks to Mary Wollstonecraft, early nineteenth-century American women found the strength of their minds and the health and vigor of their bodies to be matters of widespread societal concern. By attacking Rousseau's belief that women should be weak, passive, and domestic, Wollstonecraft helped a number of women, and men, become more vocal in their demands for increased educational opportunities for women. Furthermore, and again because of Wollstonecraft, the seeds of the new ideal of Majestic Womanhood—an ideal based on size, physical strength, intelligence, and independence—had been sown on America's shores.

### The Push for Women's Education

There is little evidence to suggest that any widespread concern for purposive exercise existed in the pre-Revolutionary colonies for either men or women. Although Benjamin Franklin, physician Benjamin

Rush, and a few other American intellectuals commented on health and exercise issues, the large majority of pre-Revolutionary Americans apparently found ample exercise in the day-to-day exigencies of colonial life.[26] Following the Revolutionary War, however, as American men and women attempted to create, from the ground up, a workable system of government and a new social order, issues of public health and the nature of education repeatedly surfaced. At the center of many of these discussions was the question of the education, rights, responsibilities, and health of American women. Abigail Adams, for instance, bemoaned the "trifling, narrow and contracted education" that those few American women who were educated at all received.[27] "If we mean to have heroes, statesmen and philosophers," she wrote on another occasion, "we should have learned women."[28] Essayist Judith Sargeant Murray, writing under the pseudonym "Constantia," also contended that the current educational system lay at the heart of women's problems. Men are exalted by their education, Murray wrote, women depressed. "The one is taught to aspire, the other is early confined and limited. As their years increase, the sister must be wholly domesticated, while the brother is led by the hand through all the flowery paths of science."[29] Philadelphia physician Benjamin Rush pushed for female education "to concur in instructing their sons in the principles of liberty and government."[30]

This public outcry for the education of America's daughters did not go unheeded. Throughout New England, in the period between 1776 and 1820, dozens of schools for women students opened their doors for business. Although many of these schools were short-lived, and their curricula varied depending on the sense of propriety guiding the headmistress, many shared a desire to provide a more substantive education for young American women.[31] As these dame schools, academies, and seminaries proliferated, America's daughters could learn, for the first time, more than the rudiments of napkin folding and needlework. Furthermore, as word of the new European interest in philanthropic education became known among America's intellectual elite, the role of physical activity in the education for women assumed increasing importance.[32]

The German educator Johann Berhard Basedow is credited with beginning the philanthropic educational movement following his discovery of Rousseau's call for a simpler life. Basedow opened a school in 1774, called the *Philanthropinum,* in which the guiding principle was the idea that learning which imitated nature was best.[33] According to the prospectus for 1774, five hours in each day were to be allotted to study, three to recreation (riding, fencing, and dancing were favored), and two hours to manual labor. That Basedow intended for this system to be used by girls as well as boys can be inferred from the fact that his young daughter was an enrolled student.[34]

In America, although few schools wholeheartedly adopted the entire philanthropic model prior to 1820, some schools did begin setting aside time for physical exercise. Timothy Dwight, for instance, designated set recess periods at his school, Dummer Academy in Byfield, Massachusetts, and reportedly advised vigorous play activities for both the male and female students there.[35] Noah Webster spoke out on the need for physical training in 1790 and suggested that organized exercise be available through the schools.[36] Another early voice belonged to Charles Brockden Brown, who maintained in *Alcuin: A Dialogue* (1798) that the sexes should be educated together and that there must "be one best diet, regimen and type and amount of exercise to develop the human body regardless of the sex of the individual."[37]

### Litchfield Academy:
### A Forgotten Link in the History of Women's Physical Education

Most early women's schools were essentially finishing schools that focused on the social graces. In these institutions, dance was generally considered "an essential part of a good education," as it was regarded as socially useful, feminine, and was believed to correct any "awkwardness of gestures giving an easy and graceful motion to the body . . . perhaps even directing its grothe."[38] It comes as no surprise, then, that dance played a vital role in the life of the Litchfield Female Academy at the turn of the nineteenth century. Lucy Sheldon reported in her diary in 1803, for instance, "We danced all forenoon, and in the afternoon sewed and was examined in geography."[39] Fifteen-year-old Mary Bacon wrote in 1802, "School was dismissed at four, went to dansing [sic] school and Mama went with me . . ."[40] Although there were, apparently, numerous dances and balls at which the Litchfield law students, training under Judge Tappan Reeves, danced with headmistress Sarah Pierce's girls during the forty years of her school's existence, these are not of specific interest within the context of this study. It is significant, however, that in addition to dance, Sarah Pierce's female students also performed purposive exercise to aid their health and appearance.

Diminutive, blue-eyed Sarah Pierce was twenty-five years old when she opened a school in her dining room with only one student in 1792. Six years later, her classes had grown so large that the citizens of Litchfield raised funds to build a 30' x 70' schoolhouse.[41] At that time, the school was officially named the Litchfield Female Academy, and, until its closing in 1833, Sarah Pierce's academy was one of the most celebrated schools in America.[42] Averaging more than a hundred students a year, it attracted young women from as far away as Savannah, Georgia.[43]

Although Sarah Pierce prided herself on creating socially acceptable ladies, she also believed that women deserved the same educational opportunities as men.[44] Whether or not Pierce read Wollstonecraft's essay is unknown, but she certainly adopted several aspects of Wollstonecraft's plea for gender equity. In an 1818 address to her students, Pierce explained that her aim had been to "vindicate the equality of female intellect" by prescribing a course of study that would refute those who believed woman somehow to be man's inferior.[45] An educational innovator, she taught geography and history to her female students in the 1790s, and somewhere around 1800 began recommending regular physical training for her students.

Walking was by far the most popular form of purposive exercise the Litchfield girls practiced. E. D. Mansfield, who took his LL.D. at the Litchfield law school, remembered years later the daily walks the Litchfield girls took during the afternoons. He clearly recalled the first time he saw them. There was a "long procession of school girls," he remembered, "coming down North Street, walking under the lofty elms, and moving to the music of a flute and flageolet. The girls were gaily dressed and evidently enjoyed their evening parade . . ."[46] Several surviving student diaries also report on daily walks for exercise. In 1802, Mary Bacon wrote, "Sunday, the13 June: Arose at six 0clock walked in the garden came back and after breakfast went up stairs contemplating on the beauties of Nature . . ." The next morning, Bacon's journal reported, she rose at half past five and walked before breakfast. On Tuesday, June 15, she, "Arose at Six oClock after breakfasting took a walk . . ."[47] Caroline Chester of Hartford, Connecticut, was a student at Litchfield in 1816. Her detailed diary is filled with references to walking and exercise: "After school took a walk with Margaret Hopkins of Philadelphia," she reported early in January of that year. "Rose at an early hour and took a long but pleasant walk with Mary," she reported on another day.[48] "Took a long and pleasant walk with Miss Rockwell

& Spencer . . .," she wrote in the summer of 1816, "returned home quite fatigued . . ."[49]

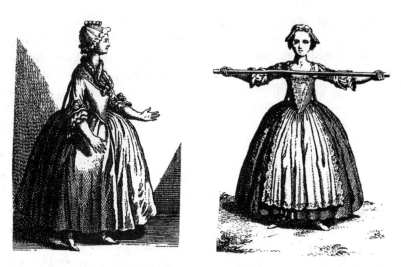

Figure 3: Illustrations from Nicholas Andry's *Orthopaedia* (1743). Left— walking with a powder-box upon the head to correct posture. Right— Andry believed that holding a wooden wand at arms length in front of the chest for extended periods of time would expand the chest and "make the Clavicles long and flat."

Sport historian Roxanne Albertson has suggested that Litchfield's physical education program included freehand exercises—which would be called calisthenics later in the century—and a one-mile walk each day.[50] Having examined Albertson's sources—Vanderpoel's extremely informative *Chronicles of a Pioneer School* and its companion volume, *More Chronicles of a Pioneer School*—it is not clear how Albertson concluded that calisthenics were performed by the Litchfield girls or that the desired distance for walking was one mile. In Caroline Chester's diary, for instance, there are days in which she refers to walking, and other days when she simply reports, "rose as usual early and exercised . . ."[51] On 20 May 1816, she noted in her journal, "rose earlier than usual exercised & performed the customary duties of the morning . . ."[52] On 30 May 1816, she noted again, "I rose early and exercised . . ."[53] Unfortunately, Chester never explained what she did in her exercise sessions if it was not walking. On another occasion, however, she reported that she had gone on an afternoon "walk for exercise with the girls and enjoyed myself very much," a statement that suggests, but does not prove, Chester differentiated in her own mind between exercise and walking.[54]

There were, of course, a fairly large number of exercise books available in English from which Pierce could have adopted exercises for women. Nicholas Andry's *Orthopaedia,* for instance, published in London in 1743, was available in the United States by this time, and, had she seen it, Sarah Pierce would have agreed with Andry's claim that specific exercises could remedy problems related to posture and body symmetry.[55] Lightweight wooden wands, Andry argued, could be used to stretch the arms, to produce large and well-shaped chests, and to lengthen and flatten too-prominent collarbones. For children whose shoulders were not square and even, Andry recommended standing on one leg on the side opposite the low, offending shoulder. Some people mistakenly place a lead weight on a shoulder that is too high, he explained, and try to depress it. A much better suggestion, he believed, was to carry a large book on the low side, which then caused the shoulder muscles to raise upward and correct the deformity.[56] He even described strengthening exercises using both large and small nine-pins, a precursor of one of the nineteenth century's favorite pieces of apparatus—the Indian club.[57]

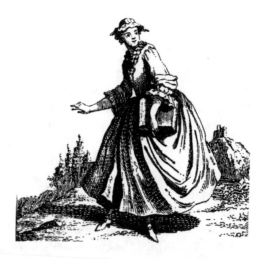

Figure 4: Spinal curvature and poor posture were matters of considerable concern in the eighteenth century. To correct uneven shoulders, Andry suggested carrying a weight, such as a heavy book, in the hand on the low side. From Andry, *Orthopaedia* (1743).

It is also possible that Pierce had heard of the several British girls' schools that, according to fashion historian Pierre Dufay, had instituted exercise programs by 1807, which were vigorous enough to necessitate the wearing of pantaloons. Again, the specifics of what sorts of exercises were done by the women in these early British schools has not survived.[58] However, further evidence that Pierce and the Litchfield girls probably differentiated between exercise and walking can be deduced from Lucy Sheldon's journal entry for Sunday, 5 February 1803: "Did not attend meeting, read very steady all day. In the afternoon was taken quite ill, but soon recovered after exercising some."[59] Had Sheldon gone for a walk, it seems she would simply have said so. Her use of "exercise" in this instance seems to suggest that she turned to some form of remedial or therapeutic exercise to help her feel better.

It seems a safe assumption that some sort of purposive training was done by Pierce's students in addition to walking and dance. Whether those exercises could be called calisthenics, however, is a different matter. Though we may never know precisely what the girls did, the exercise program at Litchfield Academy remained a regular part of school life. In 1821, the list of eighteen rules for students began with: "1st. You are expected to rise early and be drest neatly, to exercise before breakfast and to retire to rest when the family in which you reside desires you to . . ." The second rule read, "You are requested not only to exercise in the morning but also in the evening sufficiently for the preservation of health."[60] In 1825, the same two rules topped the list of desirable behavior for Litchfield girls.[61]

Pierce personally believed in the health-giving powers of exercise. Gideon Hollister, her good friend, wrote following her death at age eighty-five, "She was in the habit of practicing herself all the theories that she taught to her pupils, and, until physical infirmities confined her to her room, would take her accustomed walk in the face of the roughest March wind that ever blew across our hills."[62] Mrs. Asa Gray observed that even in old age, Pierce followed a strict regimen, "eating carefully, exercising faithfully indoors . . . [and] walking about sunset across her room so many times, until she had done certain proportions of a mile . . ."[63] Historian Alain White observed that Sarah Pierce never asked her students to "undertake any exercise which she was not ready to join in, nor to have any amusements which she did not lead."[64]

Although Pierce's decision to require physical training is historically significant in and of itself, its importance is considerably magnified by the fact that Litchfield Academy was the last school

Catharine Beecher attended as a student.[65] Beecher would go on to become one of America's more influential exercise proponents. (The story of her contributions to the advancement of women's physical education will be chronicled in Chapter Five.) Even if the Litchfield program was nothing more than regular walking, it provided early educators, such as Beecher, Zilpah Grant, and Mary Lyon with a model for the incorporation of physical training into the curricula of women's schools, a model they adopted as they opened their own women's academies during the next several decades.

Based on the scanty remains available to modern scholars, there is little evidence to suggest that many women's schools introduced systematic physical training prior to 1820 in the United States. This is not surprising when the total educational picture of this era is considered. Schools for women students were still rare in the early nineteenth century, and few teachers were lucky enough, as Sarah Pierce was, to have their own building. In many cases, girls attended classes only a few weeks at a time because their school "term" was held during the vacation periods of male students. Consequently, what little education women received generally came primarily at home from their mothers.

### Lamarckianism Enters the Debate

By 1820, four distinct rationales existed for the inclusion of exercise in a woman's life. First, exercise was believed to preserve a woman's health, increase her capacity for work, and add to her longevity. Second, certain exercises were considered medically therapeutic and were frequently recommended to ameliorate physical problems caused by confining dress, poor posture, and improper working and living conditions. Third, the neoclassical movement had advanced the belief that men and women had an obligation to look well, just as they did to function efficiently. Exercise, it came to be believed, could help a woman attain greater bodily symmetry and, thus, greater beauty.[66]

Finally, exercise advocates argued that purposive training by women could mean healthier and more intelligent children. For centuries, some writers had argued that physical and mental characteristics acquired during one's lifetime could be passed along to the next generation. In the first decade of the nineteenth century, however, the work of scientist J. B. Lamarck fostered widespread acceptance of this belief, a fact that dramatically influenced the push for women's physical training.[67] The popular interpretation of what came to be called Lamarckianism claimed that using the body resulted in develop-

ment, while disuse resulted in physical decline. As generations succeeded each other, the argument went, those parts of the body least
used would be correspondingly less well developed in the next generation.[68] As one Lamarckianism advocate, the physician L. B. Coles, put
it later in the century, women had a "sacred responsibility" to adopt an
exercise system that would "give expansion and strength to her whole
muscular system."[69]

As the first major physical fitness movement of the nineteenth century got underway in the 1820s, a few women had a chance to do
precisely what Coles suggested. For, during that decade, some women
participated in a new European fad: gymnastics, an exercise system that
philosophically was everything Mary Wollstonecraft could have wanted
it to be.

[1] Albert-Marie Schmidt, *John Calvin and the Calvinist Tradition*, trans.
Ronald Wallace (New York: Harper & Brothers, 1960), 133, 142.

[2] "On the Supposed Superiority of the Masculine Understanding, by a
Lady," *Columbian Magazine* 7 (July 1790): 47. Quoted in Mary Beth Norton,
*Liberty's Daughters: The Revolutionary Experience of American Women,
1750–1800* (Boston: Little, Brown and Co., 1980), 249.

[3] Written in part as a rebuttal of Calvinism's denigration of the body, John
Locke's *Some Thoughts Concerning Education*, argued that both men and
women had dual natures. Locke postulated that the mind began as a *tabula
rasa*, that it was a blank slate, ready to be written upon by the impressions
received through the body's senses and through intellectual reflection. The
body, therefore, had a definite importance. It served as the mind's conduit to
exploring and experiencing the world. By linking the body to the mind (or
soul), Locke implied that only the physically fit could accurately understand
the world and, by extension, God. In the late eighteenth and early nineteenth
centuries as Scottish Common Sense Philosophy came to dominate American
intellectual life, Locke's approach to the question of mind/body fundamentally changed the way many people viewed health and vigor. Possessing a
healthy body was no longer merely a matter of convenience or personal pride,
but a moral imperative. As historian James Whorton noted in his excellent
intellectual history, *Crusaders for Fitness: The History of American Health
Reformers*, a sort of "Physical Arminianism" broke out in America. People
came to believe that by doing good to the body, one opened the door to a
closer understanding of God as well as to a healthy, long life. John Locke, *Some
Thoughts Concerning Education* (Cambridge: University Press, [1693] 1913).
This book was written as a companion to Locke's 1690 *Essay Concerning
Human Understanding*. James C. Whorton, *Crusaders for Fitness: The History*

*of American Health Reformers* (Princeton: Princeton University Press, 1982), 15.

Jean Jacques Rousseau's philosophical works included *Emile*, in Linda A. Bell, ed., *Visions of Women* (Clifton, NJ: Humana Press, 1983); *Discourse on the Origin of Inequality* (1755); *Discourse on Political Economy* (1755); *Julie or The New Héloise* (1761); and *The Social Contract* (1762).

[4]Rousseau, *Emile*, in Bell, *Visions of Women*, 198.

[5]Ibid., 201.

[6]Ibid.

[7]Ibid., 203.

[8]Ibid., 203-204.

[9]Ellen Gerber, *Innovators and Institutions in Physical Education* (Philadelphia: Lea and Febiger, 1971), 36-39, 76-81. In fact, in Catholic France, Rousseau's ideas were considered so incendiary that *Emile* was banned by both the Church and the government in the year it was printed.

[10]See Roberta Park, "Concern for the Physical Education of the Female Sex from 1675 to 1800 in France, England, and Spain," *Research Quarterly* 45 (May 1974): 104-19, for insight into Wollstonecraft's life and contributions to the fight for female physical education.

[11]Though she had published *Thoughts on the Education of Daughters* in 1787, it was with *A Vindication of the Rights of Woman* that Wollstonecraft found a wide audience both in Great Britain and America for her views on equality. Historian Mary Beth Norton reported considerable evidence in the diaries and letters she examined for *Liberty's Daughters* that *Vindication* was read and discussed throughout the colonies. Mary Beth Norton, *Liberty's Daughters: The Revolutionary Experience of American Women, 1750–1800* (Boston: Little, Brown and Company, 1980), 251-53. Other evidence that Wollstonecraft's arguments made an impression on American women can be found in Emma Willard's "Address" in the *Ladies Magazine and Literary Gazette* 6 (May 1833): 236.

[12]*Mercury & New England Palladium,* 1 March 1802. Quoted in: Linda Kerber "The Republican Mother," *Women's America: Refocusing the Past,* 2nd ed., Linda Kerber and Jane DeHart-Matthews, eds. (New York: Oxford University Press, 1987), 87.

[13]Mary Wollstonecraft, *A Vindication of the Rights of Woman* (Girard, KS: Haldeman-Julius Publications, 1944 [1792]), 9.

[14]Ibid., 10.

[15]Ibid., 12.

[16]Ibid. The Chinese bands are a reference to footbinding, a practice many dress reformers of the eighteenth and nineteenth century used as an analogy for the fashion-conscious woman's tightly worn corset.

[17]Ibid., 13.

[18]Ibid., 18.

[19]Ibid., 13.

[20]Ibid., 18-19.

[21]Ibid., 39.

[22]Shadrach Ricketson, M.D., *Means of Preserving Health and Preventing Diseases: Founded Principally on an Attention to Air and Climate, Drink, Food, Sleep, Exercise, Clothing, Passions of the Mind, and Retentions and Excretions* (New York: printed by Collins, Perkins and Co., 1806), 181.

[23]Catharine E. Beecher, *Letters to the People on Health and Happiness* (New York: Harper & Brothers, 1856), 176-77.

[24]D[aniel]. H. Jacques, *Hints Toward Physical Perfection: Or the Philosophy of Human Beauty, Showing How to Acquire and Retain Bodily Symmetry, Health and Vigor, Secure Long Life and Avoid the Infirmities and Deformities of Age* (New York: Fowler & Wells, 1861), 7.

[25]George Combe, *Notes on the United States of America During a Phrenological Visit in 1838-39-40*, vol. 2 (Edinburgh: Maclachlan, Stewart, & Co., 1841), 191.

[26]For information on women's exercise in the eighteenth century, see Nancy L. Struna, "'Good Wives' and 'Gardeners,' 'Spinners and Fearless Riders': Middle and Upper-Rank Women in the Early American Sporting Culture," in J. A. Mangan and Roberta J. Park, eds., *From Fair Sex to Feminism: Sport and the Socialization of Women in the Industrial and Post-Industrial Eras* (London: Frank Cass and Company, 1987), 235-56. See also Nancy Struna, "Puritans and Sport, The Irretrievable Tide of Change," *Journal of Sport History* 4 (Spring 1977): 15-30; Jennie Holliman, *American Sports 1785-1835* (Durham, NC: The Seemen Press, 1931); C. W. Hackensmith, *History of Physical Education* (New York: Harper & Row, 1962), 311-27; and Betty Spears and Richard A. Swanson, *History of Sport and Physical Activity in the United States* (Dubuque, IA: William C. Brown, 1978), 43-57.

[27]Abigail Adams to John Adams, 30 June 1778, in Charles Francis Adams, ed., *Letters of Mrs. Adams, The Wife of John Adams. With an Introductory Memoir*, 4th ed. (Boston: Wilkins, Carter and Company, 1848), 98.

[28]Quoted in Gerda Lerner, *The Woman in American History* (Menlo Park, CA: Addison-Wesley Publishing Co., 1971), 39.

[29]Constantia [Judith Sargeant Murray], *The Gleaner* (Boston, 1798) III: 188-89. Quoted in Eleanor Flexnor, *Century of Struggle: The Woman's Rights Movement in the United States*, rev. ed. (Cambridge: Belknap Press of Harvard University Press, 1975), 16.

[30]Nathan G. Goodman, *Benjamin Rush: Physician and Citizen, 1746-1813* (Philadelphia: University of Pennsylvania Press, 1934), 313-14. Rush's views on exercise for men are contained in *Sermons to Gentlemen on Temperance and Exercise* (Philadelphia: by the author, 1772).

[31]For information on the growth of women's schools and academies, see Gladys Marilyn Haddad, "Social Roles and Advanced Education for Women in Nineteenth-Century America: A Study of Three Western Reserve Institutions" (Ph.D. diss., Case Western Reserve University, 1980). See also Dorothy

Ainsworth, *The History of Physical Education in Colleges for Women* (New York: A. S. Barnes and Company, 1930), 1-23; Norton, *Liberty's Daughters*, 263-94; and Nancy Woloch, *Women and the American Experience* (New York: Alfred A. Knopf, 1984), 91-94.

[32]An excellent discussion of the philanthropic educational movement appears in James C. Federle's "Bodies, Gardens, and Pedagogies in Late Eighteenth-Century Germany" (Ph.D. diss., University of California at Berkeley, 1991).

[33]Gerber, *Innovators*, 83-84.

[34]Fred Eugene Leonard, *A Guide to the History of Physical Education*, 2nd ed., R. Tait McKenzie, ed. (Philadelphia: Lea and Febiger, 1927), 68.

[35]Nehemiah Cleaveland, *The First Century of Dummer Academy* (Boston, 1865), 26-27, quoted in Roxanne Albertson, "Sports and Games in Eastern Schools, 1780–1880," *Sport in American Education: History and Perspective*, eds. Wayne M. Ladd and Angela Lumpkin, History of Sport and Physical Education Academy Symposia, 24 March 1977 and 6 April 1988 (Washington DC: American Alliance for Health, Physical Education, Recreation, and Dance, 1979), 21.

[36]Noah Webster, *Address to Yung [sic] Gentlemen* (1790) quoted in Arthur Weston, *The Making of American Physical Education* (New York: Appleton-Century-Crofts, 1962), 29.

[37]Quoted in Roberta Park, "'Embodied Selves,' the Rise and Development of Concern for Physical Education, Active Games and Recreation for American Women, 1776–1865," *Journal of Sport History* 5 (Summer 1978): 8.

[38]Mary Bacon, "A Composition Written at Litchfield," quoted in Emily Noyes Vanderpoel, *Chronicles of a Pioneer School from 1792 to 1833, Being the History of Miss Sarah Pierce and her Litchfield School* (Cambridge: Harvard University Press, 1903), 73.

[39]Quoted in Vanderpoel, *Chronicles*, 51.

[40]Quoted in Vanderpoel, *Chronicles*, 70.

[41]Catharine Beecher, quoted in *Autobiography of Lyman Beecher*, vol. 1, 226-28, reprinted in Vanderpoel, *Chronicles*, 179.

[42]From Gideon Hollister's *History of Connecticut*, quoted in Vanderpoel, *Chronicles*, 7.

[43]Vanderpoel, *Chronicles*, 402-404.

[44]Alain C. White, *The History of the Town of Litchfield, Connecticut: 1720–1920* (Litchfield: Enquirer Print, 1920), 112-13. Pierce was apparently the first American educator to teach history and geography to female students. She later added chemistry, botany, and astronomy to her curriculum, which also included the social graces of music, dance, drawing, singing, and embroidery.

[45]Sarah Pierce, "Address at the Close of School, October 29, 1818," quoted in Vanderpoel, *Chronicles*, 177.

[46]E. D. Mansfield, quoted in Vanderpoel, *Chronicles*, 258.

[47]Quoted in Vanderpoel, *Chronicles*, 67.

[48]Ibid., 153.

[49]Ibid., 178.

[50]Roxanne Albertson, "Sports and Games in Eastern Schools, 1780–1880," 21. See also Roxanne Albertson, "Physical Education in New England Schools and Academies from 1780 to 1860: Concepts and Practices" (Ph.D. diss., University of Oregon, 1974).

[51]Quoted in Vanderpoel, *Chronicles*, 152.

[52]Quoted in: Emily Noyes Vanderpoel, *More Chronicles of a Pioneer School from 1792–1833; Being Added History On The Litchfield Female Academy Kept By Miss Sarah Pierce and Her Nephew, John Pierce Brace* (New York: Cadmus Book Shop, 1927), 165.

[53]Ibid., 168.

[54]Ibid., 179.

[55]Nicolas Andry, *Orthopaedia: Or, The Art of Correcting and Preventing Deformities in Children: By such Means as may easily be put in practice by Parents themselves, and all such as are employed in Educating Children: To which is added, A Defence of the Orthopaedia, by way of Supplement, by the Author*, 2 vols. (London: A. Millar, 1743). Pierce could also have looked at Francis Fuller, *Medicina Gymnasticsa, Or a Treatise Concerning the Power of Exercise, with Respect to the Animal Oeconomy, and the Great Necessity of it, in the Cure of Several Distempers* (London: John Matthews, 1705); Ricketson, *Means of Preserving Health*; and at the *Encyclopedie*, ed. Denis Diderot. For information on the latter, and eighteenth-century health texts in general, see W. Coleman, "Health and Hygiene in the *Encyclopedie*: A Medical Doctrine for the Bourgeoisie," *Journal of the History of Medicine* 29 (1974): 399-421; and W. Coleman, "The People's Health: Medical Themes in Eighteenth-Century French Popular Literature," *Bulletin of the History of Medicine* 51 (1977): 55-74.

[56]Andry, *Orthopaedia*, 119.

[57]Ibid.

[58]Quoted in Anne Wood Murray, "The Bloomer Costume and Exercise Suits," *Waffen-und Kostumkunde* (Munich: Deutscher Kunstverlag, 1982), 113.

The two best sources on the early British schools are Peter C. McIntosh, *Physical Education in England Since 1800* (London: G. Bell & Sons, 1952), 75-104; and Shirley M. Reekie, "A History of Sport and Recreation for Women in Great Britain, 1700–1850" (Ph.D. diss., Ohio State University, 1982).

[59]Quoted in Vanderpoel, *Chronicles*, 52.

[60]Ibid., 231.

[61]Ibid., 255.

[62]White, *History of Litchfield*, 115. Also quoted in Vanderpoel, *Chronicles*, 7.

[63]Mrs. Asa Gray, "Sketch of Miss Sarah Pierce," quoted in Vanderpoel, *Chronicles*, 322.

[64]Vanderpoel, *Chronicles*, 113.

[65]Beecher attended Litchfield from 1810 to 1816. Kathryn Kish Sklar, *Catharine Beecher: A Study in American Domesticity* (New York: W. W. Norton & Co., 1973), 17.

[66]For information on the history of hygienic exercise, see Jack Berryman, "The Tradition of the Six Things Non-Natural: Exercise and Medicine from Hippocrates through Antebellum America," *Exercise and Sport Sciences Reviews* 17 (1989): 518-19; L. H. Joseph, "Physical Education in the Early Middle Ages," *Ciba Symposia* 10 (March-April 1949): 1030; Gerald F. Fletcher, "The History of Exercise in the Practice of Medicine," *Journal of the Medical Association of Georgia* 72 (January 1973): 35; and J. W. F. Blundell, *The Muscles and Their Story from the Earliest Times; Including the Whole Text of Mercurialis, and the Opinions of Other Writers, Ancient and Modern, on Mental and Bodily Development* (London: Chapman and Hall, 1864), 48.

[67]When, as we shall see in Chapter Seven, Lamarckianism was embraced by the pseudoscience of phrenology, even greater attention was paid to the physical condition of women. J. B. Lamarck, *Zoological Philosophy: An Exposition with Regard to the Natural History of Animals* (London: MacMillan, 1809).

[68]For information on Lamarck's impact on American intellectual history, see George W. Stocking, "Lamarckianism in American Social Science: 1890–1915," *Journal of the History of Ideas* 23 (1962): 239-59; and Conway Zirkle, "The Early History of the Idea of the Inheritance of Acquired Characters and of Pangenesis," *Transactions of the American Philosophical Society* 35 (Part Two, 1946): 110-21.

[69]L. B. Coles, M.D., *The Philosophy of Health; or Health Without Medicine; A Treatise on the Laws of the Human System*, 4th ed. (Boston: Ticknor & Company, 1848), 114-15.

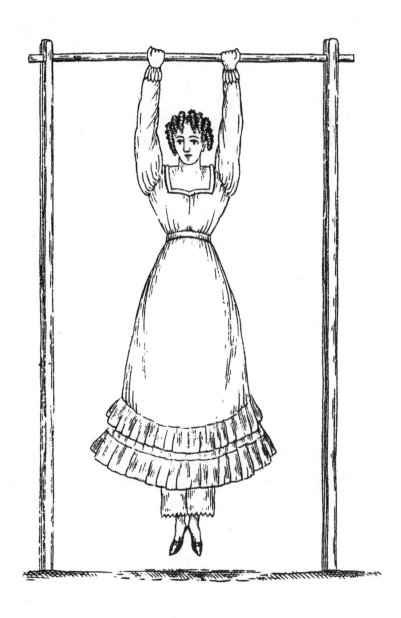

Figure 5: "To Raise the Body by Strength of the Arms on the Horizontal Bar."
Illustration from J. A. Beaujeu's *A Treatise on Gymnastic Exercises* (1828).

# Chapter Two
## "Souls of Fire in Iron Hearts:"
## The 1820s Gymnastics Revolution for Women

In 1845, in the *Common School Journal,* Horace Mann called the attention of his readers to a new establishment in Boston. A Mrs. Hawley, wrote Mann, known formerly as Madame Beaujeu, had recently opened an "excellent gymnastic school" on the corner of Bromfield and Tremont Streets. "The manners of this lady . . . her good sense as a guide, and her physiological knowledge, as an instructress, have entitled her to much more patronage than she has received." Parents who have not yet sent their daughters to take classes with Ms. Hawley because of the expense, he warned, "will hereafter have the bill to settle with the doctors."

Madame Beaujeu-Hawley is important to the history of women's exercise for several reasons. First, as a gymnasium owner in the 1840s, she was one of America's first exercise entrepreneurs of either sex. However, while this fact is quite significant in and of itself, Madame Beaujeu-Hawley also played another role. Her presence as a gym owner in Boston, and, later, in New York, established a direct link between America and the European gymnastics movement for women, a movement in which she and her husband, the free-thinking exercise radical, J. A. Beaujeu, were important figures.

Modern historians have generally dated the first wave of interest in women's exercise to the birth of the gender-specific calisthenics movement of the early 1830s. However, the Beaujeu's and several other exercise pundits recommended during the 1820s that women participate in exercises remarkably similar in nature and degree of physical difficulty to those prescribed for men. Furthermore, the arguments made to bolster women's participation in this earlier exercise movement tended to transcend ideas of female submissiveness. Advocates of women's gymnastics, unlike their counterparts in the milder calisthenics camp, viewed women's physical potential from a much more egalitarian perspective.

### The European Gymnastics Movement

German physical educator Johann Friedrich GutsMuths (1759-1839) emerged in the late eighteenth century as Europe's dominant theoretician on purposive exercise.[1] GutsMuths served for more than fifty years as the physical training instructor at the Schnepfenthal Philanthropic School, located near Gotha. Founded by Christian Gotthilf Salzmann (1744-1811), the school at Schnepfenthal required its male students to participate in both manual labor and gymnastics. By 1794, the gymnastics program there included such diverse activities as rope climbing, throwing the discus, climbing poles, jumping over a rope, and "lifting a weight hung on a rod and moved toward or from the hands according to the strength of the individual."[2]

In 1793, GutsMuths published his theories on purposive training in an enormously influential, two volume work entitled *Gymnastik fur die Jugen: Enthaltend eine PraktischeAnwisung zu Leibesubungen. Ein Beytraq zur Nothigsten Verbesserung der Korperlichen Erziehung*.[3] An English version, entitled, *Gymnastics for Youth or a Practical Guide to Healthful and Amusing Exercises for the Use of Schools. An Essay Toward the Necessary Improvement of Education; Chiefly as it relates to the Body*, appeared in London in 1800. Two years later, the first American edition appeared in Philadelphia.[4]

Based on his work at Schnepfenthal, GutsMuths' book primarily concerned itself with the fitness and exercise needs of boys. However, he also called attention to what he perceived as a decline in the health and vigor of women. "The hardy, active wife of the ancient German, from whom we are descended," he wrote, "was frequently delivered in the open field, in the midst of her toil. She bathed her loved offspring in the nearest brook, and wrapped him in cool leaves."[5] Rather than be concerned for the health and happiness of the women themselves, however, GutsMuths saw the problem in Lamarckian terms. His concern was that the "excessive delicacy of the female sex cannot fail of being too easily transmitted to the infant male." Quoting Rousseau, he claimed that "'When the women become robust, the men will become still more so.'"[6]

GutsMuths' successor and countryman, Friedrich Ludwig Jahn (1778-1852) believed that gymnastics could be a unifying force for German youth who had been denied their Teutonic heritage by the Napoleonic upheaval.[7] At the Graue Kloster school, where he began teaching in about 1809, Jahn began to play games with some of his students outside the gates of the city of Halle, and at the Hasenhide, an unwooded, slightly hilly stretch of empty land along the Spree River. Within a year, a rudimentary, outdoor gymnasium stood on the Hasenhide and eighty men and boys regularly gathered to exercise. Three years later, attendance had risen to five hundred.[8] By 1817, more than a thousand men regularly gathered at the Hasenhide to train.[9]

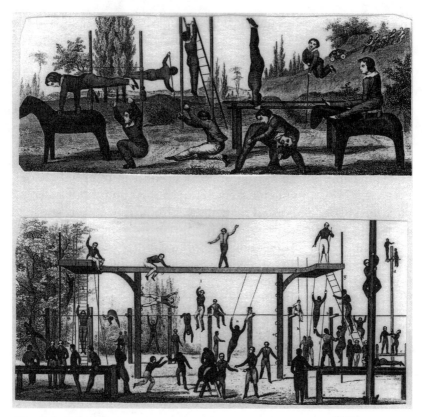

Figure 6: German-style gymnastics as practiced by schoolboys and grown men. Early nineteenth-century engraving from the Todd-McLean Physical Culture Collection, The University of Texas at Austin.

Jahn possessed a fierce commitment to German patriotism, an interest which dovetailed with his interest in physical training. Unlike GutsMuths, who viewed exercise from the perspective of the individual, Jahn saw training in nationalistic terms. Rather than referring to his system by the Greek word "gymnastics," Jahn called his exercises *Turnen* and his gymnasts *Turners,* to signify that his methods were distinctly German.[10] He published *Deutsches Volksthum,* his paean to German nationalism, in 1810, and released *Die Deutsche Turnkunst,* a long, rambling guidebook to German gymnastics and national unity, in 1816.[11] These books, and their incendiary ideas, struck a resonant chord in many German men who attended Jahn's increasingly elaborate training sessions at the Hasenhide, and many adopted his radical politics.

Jahn's charisma, his unique relationship with his students, and the rapid growth of other nationalistic Turner societies came to be seen as a threat by Prince Mitternich of Austria and by the Holy Alliance, who were struggling to maintain control of Germany. As Jahn's student followers engaged in increasingly open expressions of political defiance, authorities banned the student gymnastic groups and placed Jahn in prison.[12] Many of Jahn's students fled Germany—taking their gymnastic training with them—rather than face imprisonment. Carl Völker went first to Switzerland and then to London, where he opened a public gymnasium in the Spring of 1825.[13] Political refugees Charles Follen, Carl Beck, and Franz Lieber also left their homeland. Later, all three men played important roles in the introduction of German-style gymnastics to America.

Germany was not the only European country influenced by the late eighteenth-century interest in physical training. In 1798, Franz Nachtegall opened a gymnasium in Copenhagen which historians believe was probably the first private gymnasium devoted exclusively to physical training since the time of the ancient Greeks.[14] There, in the Fall of 1799, a young Swedish linguistics student named Pehr Henrik Ling came under Nachtegall's influence and learned German-style gymnastics. When Ling returned to his homeland, he took a job as fencing instructor at the University of Lund and began teaching the gymnastics techniques he had learned in Denmark.[15] Not content to simply copy the Germans, Ling studied physiology and anatomy and gradually developed his own system of "scientifically based" exercises; his system became known as Swedish Gymnastics and spread throughout the schools of Sweden.[16] Ling was highly regarded in Europe, particularly for his efforts in the area of remedial gymnastics. His exercise prescriptions were much more elaborate than those of his eighteenth century predecessors, and he made sure to assert the scientific foundations of his physiological prescriptions.[17] The therapeutic aspect of his interest in exercise proved an inspiration to dozens of later exercise entrepreneurs, who found that a living could be made by using what came to be known as the Movement Cure to treat poor posture, medical problems caused by tight lacing, and spinal curvature.[18]

Ling's work in the area of remedial gymnastics had an impact on the lives of many women. So, also, did his insistence that physical training be incorporated into the Swedish public schools. Ling suggested that school children could perform free-hand exercises while standing

beside their desks when no gymnastic equipment was available, or when the weather prevented outside play. Ling's system of school exercises consisted primarily of simple limb extensions, yet it was widely copied by other exercise advocates, including Catharine Beecher, Dio Lewis, Russell Trall, and many others.

### Phokion Heinrich Clias and
### The British Gymnastics Revolution for Women

Although some Britons were no doubt familiar with the German and Swedish experiments in physical training, the English enthusiasm for gymnastics can be traced to the arrival in London of Captain Phokion Heinrich Clias in 1822.[19] Clias (1782-1854) was living in Bern and training Swiss military troops when he published his first gymnastics book, *Anfangsgrunde der Gymnastik oder Turnkunst,* in 1816.[20] In 1819, following a successful stay in Paris, Clias produced a French edition of his ideas on exercise, *Principes de gymnastique,* reportedly the first gymnastics book published in France.[21] In approximately 1820, Clias met the British ambassador to Switzerland who asked him to work with the ambassador's slightly hydrocephalic son. Though the boy had visited a number of regular doctors, the regimen Clias suggested seemed to help the youth more than their traditional medical prescriptions, and the grateful ambassador invited Clias to move to England.[22] Appointed to a captaincy in the British Army, Clias became Superintendent of Physical Training for the Royal Military and Naval Academies in England, and he opened a private gymnasium in London.[23]

Shortly after his arrival, Clias brought out an English version of his text entitled, *An Elementary Course of Gymnastic Exercises; Intended to Improve The Physical Powers of Man.*[24] Clias's *Elementary Course* would, by modern standards, be considered a combination of gymnastics, remedial exercises and calisthenics movements.[25] It was also one of the first books to argue that the described exercise system was "practicable to the youth of both sexes." Clias believed that movements should be kept simple, "yet sufficient to develope their physical faculties, without occasioning any additional expense to parents, and even without depriving the children of one moment of time destined to their intellectual studies."[26]

In four lengthy chapters, Clias described simple arm and leg extensions as well as more vigorous exercises such as running, skating, jumping, swimming, parallel bar work, vaulting, wrestling, skipping

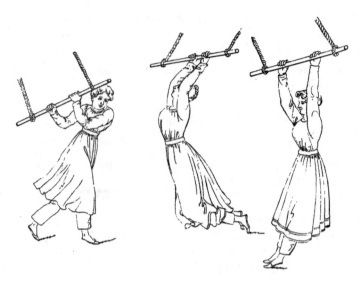

Figure 7: Exercises on the Flying Course from Clias's *Kalesthenie oder Uebungen zur Schoenheit und Kraft fuer Maedchen* (1829).

with a hoop, and the use of a specialized apparatus called the Flying Course. The Flying Course, or Giant Steps, as he also called it, consisted of two ropes securely tied to a trapeze-like handlebar.[27] The ropes then attached to a swivel in the ceiling or to a tall pole — so that the person using the apparatus could freely travel in a circle. Those using the Flying Course grasped the handles as they ran, dipped, or took giant steps to strengthen the legs. It was an exercise method that became especially popular with teachers of women students because the handles allowed the runners to catch themselves if they lost their balance.

To promote the book, and his own business interests, Clias gave public lectures and taught several courses of physical training to anyone who could afford to pay.[28] In a country imbued with neo-Classical idealism, Clias's unusually muscular physique apparently contributed to his ability to sell gymnastics to the British public. "The forms of Captain Clias are by far the most perfect of any man who has ever been exhibited in England," wrote one reviewer. "In him we discovered all those markings which we see in the *antique,* and which do not appear on the living models, from their body not being sufficiently developed by a regular system of Scientific Exercises, such as Captain Clias's."[29]

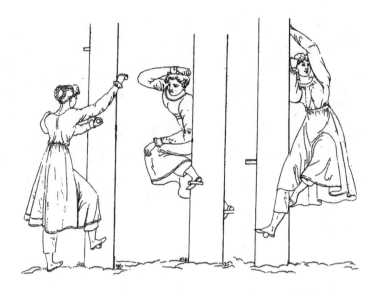

Figure 8: Clias called this apparatus the Column of Pegs and believed that it balanced the body as well as strengthened it. Illustration from Clias's *Kalesthenie oder Uebungen zur Schoenheit und Kraft fuer Maedchen* (1829).

During his years in London, Clias touched off an enormous interest in physical training for both sexes. One historian described Clias's impact thusly, "everywhere he seems to have given satisfaction. He was asked to apply his knowledge of medical gymnastics to cases of spinal curvature and others of similar nature; noblemen sent him their sons to train; and even the ladies requested, and received a course of lessons designed to meet their special needs."[30] In 1823, Clias reportedly had no less than fourteen hundred pupils, approximately four hundred of whom were women.[31] In 1826, *The American Journal of Education* reported that Clias had "superintended the training of over two thousand pupils."[32] The *London Medical and Surgical Journal* reported: "The regular and systematic method, thus taught in England, by Captain Clias, is not only well calculated to give the body its full degree of strength and activity, but, the mode of teaching, precludes every possibility of the occurrence of any accident."[33]

Despite the claims of safety, Clias's time in England was cut short when a student accidentally kicked him in the stomach with an iron-toed shoe and punctured his abdominal wall. Following a lengthy recuperation, Clias returned to Switzerland, where he wrote his first

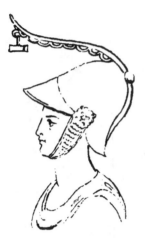

Figure 9: Weighted helmet to be worn for strengthening the neck and shoulders. From *Clias's Kalesthenie oder Uebungen zur Schoenheit und Kraft fuer Maedchen,* (1829).

book on women's exercise. Based on his experiences in England, where he worked with women as private clients and in the girls' schools at Chelsea and Greenwich, Clias wrote *Kalesthenie oder Uebungen zur Schoenheit und Kraft fuer Maedchen* and published it in 1829.

This seventy-four page book almost exclusively consisted of exercise descriptions. Clias did not enter into a long, philosophical argument on the appropriateness of his system for women, as he continued to believe that his exercises were genderless and would benefit both sexes. Instead, he devoted his time to describing exercises using wands, rings, the Flying Course, and a ladderlike pole on which women climbed in a circular motion to ensure total body development. Clias also described a large number of free-hand, extension exercises, toe touches, situps, and rope skipping. He even included a description of a weighted helmet designed to strengthen the neck and shoulders.[34]

Clias, like Ling, was especially concerned with the increasing prevalence of spinal deformities and ill health he perceived in young women, and he apparently devoted a considerable portion of his time in London to their treatment. He described several case histories of these treatments in his writings. Other hygienic authors reprinted these to demonstrate to their own followers the course of therapeutic exercise.[35] Clias's case studies give modern readers a rare insight into the use of exercise by women in the early nineteenth century. In 1827, for instance, an anonymous London physician included Clias's Case Three in his own text on health.

The patient in Case Three was a sixteen year old girl whom Clias identified as "Miss A. B." According to Clias, she had been under the care of another physician for some time when he was asked to take on her case and prescribe a course of exercise. Miss A. B. suffered from a battery of ailments. She had a distortion of the spine from the right to the left side; was extremely weak, particularly in the arms and the chest; had no appetite; slept only intermittently; and appeared "extremely pale and thin." She also seemed on the edge of developing tuberculosis, as she had what Clias described as an obstinate cough; her voice was nearly inaudible. Part of her problem, Clias believed, resulted from the pressure of her stays. In an attempt to straighten her spine, she had apparently worn exceptionally tight lacings for some time. Not only did the stays fail to help her scoliosis, they left her with a constant pain in her left side, where, Clias reported, "what are called the false ribs on the left side were bent one over the other, and forced inwards." So weak and debilitated was Miss A. B. that she could not hold her head erect. He wrote, "It was almost with repugnance that I engaged to employ my system of exercise in the case of a person who appeared to be nearly in a dying condition. . . ."[36] Clias's exercise prescription began on the twenty-second of October:

> Table of Gymnastic Exercise resorted to in this case, by which the reader will perceive the slow but gradual manner in which patients, in such cases, proceed from slight exercises to those which require greater strength and exertion.
> 1. To make prolonged inspirations sitting. 2. Prolonged inspirations, the patient standing, the arms fixed. 3. The same exercise, the arms hanging down. 4. The same, the arms extended horizontally. 5. The same, the arms fixed to a horizontal pole. 6. Deep inspiration, and counting a number without drawing the breath. 7. Movement of the feet on the ground, the patient sitting. 8. Deep inspiration, the patient lying on the left side, and leaning on the elbow. 9. In the same position to raise and lower the body. 10. Walking slowly and making deep inspirations. 11. Walking a little faster and counting several steps without drawing breath. 12. Bending without rising, the weak hands fixed above. 13. Beating time, with both hands fixed to the horizontal pole. 14. 15. Beating time, bearing a weight in the weak hand. 16. 17. Lifting up a small box from the ground with both hands, and then with the weak hand. 18. 19. 20. To declaim without moving and to sing without drawing breath. 21. 22. 23. 24. Movements of balance simple, in front and on one side. 25. 26. 27. 28. Develop other motions of the arms and to imitate the motion of sawing. 29. 30. These exercises with the weak hand only. 31. 32. To

draw upon a spring with the weak hand only, and then with the arms
and body fixed. 33. Seated on the ground, to rise with the assistance
of the arms, the feet fixed. 34. Lying down horizontally, to raise the
body without the assistance of the arms. Other exertions of a similar
kind, which it is not necessary to describe, follow these.[37]

Clias reported that by the twenty-seventh of November her cough
was gone, and he began to use massage on the weakened areas of her
body. By the twelfth of January she had an appearance of health, could
walk several miles with ease and "all the animal functions were perfectly restored."[38]

Clias remained in Switzerland through the 1830s and moved to
Paris in 1841 to assist with the training of the French army. He later
served as Superintendent of Gymnastic Instruction in the elementary
schools of Paris, and in 1843, brought out an expanded, French-lan-
guage edition of his women's book: *Callisthénie, ou Somascétique
Naturelle, Appropriée A L'Education Phyisique Des Jeunes Filles*, which
he dedicated to the Countess of Clermont.[39]

This French edition of Clias's thoughts on women and exercise was
much more detailed and sophisticated than his previous book. One
hundred and sixty-eight pages of text contained discussions of age-
specific exercises for toddlers, young girls, and, finally, women.
Copying texts published by other authors in the intervening years,
Clias divided the exercise section of the 1843 edition into chapters on
lower extremity training, upper extremity training and what he called
"complicated exercises," in which the arms and legs moved simultaneously. Young girls were shown exercising with their well-muscled
fathers, doing balancing exercises, and performing strengthening exercises such as situps and modified push-ups.

For older girls and adult women, simple limb extensions constituted the first phase of advanced work, followed by a series of exercises
using a bamboo cane, and, finally, the trapeze-like Flying Course. Clias
also included a section on swimming, or "natation," discussed the
physiological benefits of using a jump rope, and added a special chapter on curing spinal deformities.

Clias was frequently criticized for expecting too much of his
female students. As calisthenics replaced gymnastics in the 1830s as the
preferred exercise methodology for women, more than one expert condemned Clias for prescribing male exercises to female pupils.[40] In
reality, Clias's exercise system for women was neither strictly gymnastics nor strictly calisthenics, but a hybrid of the two forms. His simple

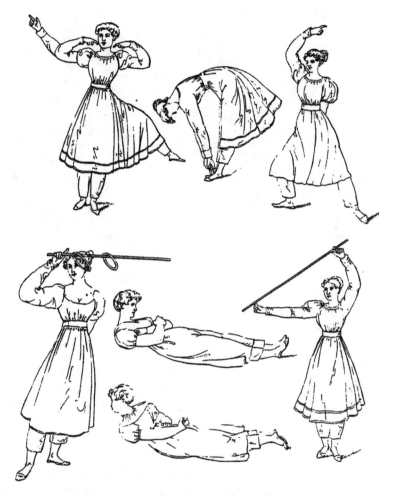

Figure 10: Exercise illustrations from *Clias's Kalesthenie oder Uebungen zur Schoenheit und Kraft fuer Maedchen* (1829).

limb extensions and wand exercises are classic calisthenics movements, but other exercises—such as the difficult Column of Pegs, the situps, push-ups, and even the Flying Course—suggest a more vigorous, gymnastic orientation. In choosing the word "calisthenics" for the title of his women's books, Clias undoubtedly reacted more to social pressure than he did to physical education dogma.

Although Clias was in London for less than four years, he apparently made a great impression on the British public. *The Dictionary of Medical Science* endorsed Clias's methods, writing: "The Gymnastics of

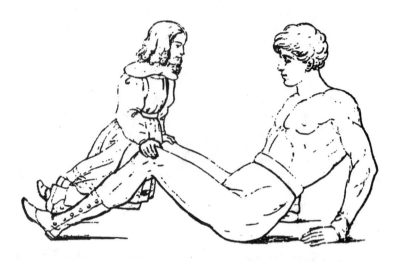

Figure 11: To strengthen the arms and expand the chest, Clias recommended that girls perform modified push-ups with their hands on their father's knees. Illustration from: Clias's, *Callisthénie, ou Somascétique Naturelle, Appropriée A L'Education Phyisique Des Jeunes Filles* (1843).

Captain Clias unite every advantage; and if considered minutely, will be seen to possess everything that is essentially useful in correcting numerous deformities, and in eradicating obstinate diseases."[41] Through his physical appearance, publications, ability as a master teacher, and work with the schools, Clias contributed to a growing climate of enthusiasm for gymnastics for both men and women in Great Britain. Though a nearly life-ending accident forced him to abandon the cause for a time, interest in gymnastics did not die with his departure. In fact, interest escalated as several new gymnastics experts stepped into the void left by Clias's forced retirement, bringing with them new approaches, and new ideas, to the question of women's exercise.

### Beaujeu's Radical System of Women's Gymnastics

Captain Clias had several competitors in mid-1820s Britain as enthusiasm for the new gymnastics fad escalated. German refugee Carl Völker, for example, who was sponsored by the philosopher Jeremy Bentham, opened a gymnasium in London near Regents Park in the spring of 1825; his gymnasium attracted many of London's upper-class

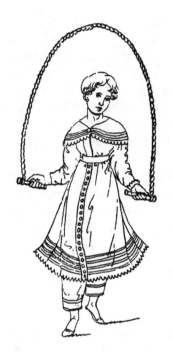

Figure 12: Clias's inclusion of rope skipping as a useful form of exercise was a
rarity in the early nineteenth century.
Illustration from: *Callisthénie, ou
Somascétique Naturelle, Appropriée A
L'Education Phyisique Des Jeunes Filles,*
(1843).

citizens.[42] As interest in gymnastics escalated, Völker organized several
classes for women which, according to a contemporary account, were
attended by "ladies of rank."[43] A "National Men's Gymnasium" was
established under his direction the next year, as was a gymnastics society, which had seven hundred members by year's end.[44] A visiting
American, John Neal, noted that gymnastics was "overspreading the
whole country far and wide—for women as well as for men, and for
little children as well."[45] Other evidence that a true gymnastics boom
existed in Britain during the middle years of the 1820s can be found in
J. A. Beaujeu's comment that, "the advantage of the system of gymnastic exercises is now-a-days so well known, and considered so
indispensable to the education of youth, that there is scarcely a school
in England in which they are not introduced."[46]

J. A. Beaujeu and his wife, Madame Beaujeu, are the most interesting—and the least well-known—figures of the 1820s women's
gymnastics movement. Beaujeu had originally planned to open a gymnasium in Edinburgh, but, finding the scientific community in Dublin
more open to his ideas about physical training, settled there instead, in
approximately 1824.[47] Located at 39 Dawson Street, Beaujeu's gymnasium offered classes for women on Tuesdays, Thursdays and Saturdays

from 11:30 to 1:30. He also supervised the physical training at the Royal Hibernian Military School, a co-ed institution for the children of soldiers, where he introduced four hundred boys and two hundred girls to gymnastics.[48] How many private clients attended his thrice weekly classes is unknown. However, based on his experiences with women in these two institutions, Beaujeu published, in 1828, *A Treatise on Gymnastic Exercises, Or Calisthenics For the Use of Young Ladies.* The purpose of this treatise was to help those unable to attend his classes to perform the same sorts of exercises at home.[49]

Beaujeu claimed to be the first person to have adapted the art of gymnastics to the capacities of the female sex, a claim which, if Clias did not immediately begin offering classes to women upon arriving in London, may be true.[50] In any case, Beaujeu was clearly influenced by Clias, whom he mentions frequently. Beaujeu dedicated his book to the Governors of the Royal Hibernian Academy and claimed in a self-aggrandizing dedication that his teaching methods had been endorsed by the College of Surgeons and Physicians, by several scientific bodies, and by numerous lords and gentlemen of Dublin.[51]

Beaujeu's book presented a startlingly vigorous exercise regimen designed to enhance strength and beauty for women. The illustrated, 120 page guidebook not only contained a lengthy section of difficult gymnastics movements, it discussed woman's physical potential in a significantly different tone than did other women's exercise texts of this era. Beaujeu believed that his contemporaries placed too much emphasis on intellectual learning and refinement for women at the expense of their health and vigor. "Is not our education depraved," he asked, "when it aims at a luxury and neglects our greatest and most essential want?" Women don't need lessons in refinement, he argued, "Let us tear the rising generation from our voluptuous habits, from the effeminacy of our degenerate manners, that we may, thereby, produce 'souls of fire, in iron hearts. . . .'"[52] Beaujeu's stated aim was to inspire other females to participate in "the immense advantages resulting from gymnastic exercises, for the promotion of health, and for the acquirement of all physical accomplishments."[53]

In the introduction, Beaujeu demonstrated a rare command of both the history and the present state of gymnastics. He gave credit to Jahn, Clias, GutsMuths, Salzmann, and Colonel Amoros of France; he discussed the various forms of medical gymnastics; he paid homage to the Apollo Belvedere and the Greek ideal; and he then launched into an elaborate rationale for recommending gymnastics for women.[54] He argued that gymnastics gave "strength, activity, and at the same time gracefulness to young ladies," traits that would help anyone get through life more easily.[55] Conscious of the concerns of parents who feared his exercise system might be too strenuous, Beaujeu reassured his readers that he had chosen his exercises for their ability to promote health and amuse the practitioner. These exercises, he wrote, are "incapable of wounding the most delicate feelings of modesty."[56] Beaujeu discounted the value of dance, arguing that it employed only a limited number of muscles and that its repetitiveness "renders it dull and monotonous." Purposive exercise was better, he argued, because it was, "founded on system, directed to a useful end, varied from ordinary pursuits, and conferring agility on the limbs, grace on the general movements, and strength on the animal economy at large . . . ."[57]

Absent from Beaujeu's instructions and introductory material are the usual antebellum admonitions regarding woman's inherent weakness, woman's need to improve her health in order to more ably fulfill her maternal functions, or the dangers of overdoing. In relatively straightforward language, Beaujeu opened his instructional section with a discussion on how to alternate upper and lower body exercises to maximize the benefits of training by not fatiguing one part of the body ahead of the other. Beaujeu further argued that the bodies of women should be gradually adapted to increasingly complicated exercises to "increase the firmness of the muscular fibre; for, if the bones of the human body acquire strength by exercise and motion, the muscular powers are still more benefitted."[58]

What seems entirely uncharacteristic, based on our traditional notions of nineteenth-century female exercise, is that Beaujeu then went into an extended discussion of how to deal with dislocations, joint problems, sprains, strains, overheating, and profuse perspiration. He advised his women gymnasts to perform each movement with a "determined firmness and presence of mind. Hesitation in the performance of any one," he wrote, "is always liable to expose the performer to danger, which determination and courage will in every instance totally prevent."[59] Determination, courage and firmness of mind were not female attributes most early nineteenth-century exercise advocates viewed as essential. But, then, neither did most antebellum exercise advocates worry that their system was vigorous enough to make a young woman pull a muscle, dislocate a joint, or break a sweat.

Beaujeu was also innovative in his organization of the book. Throughout his exercise descriptions, he listed the muscles involved in

the movement and provided a physiological rationale for the performance of each exercise. Executing a series of circles with the extended
foot, he explained to his readers, worked the *psoas magnus* and *iliacus
internus,* and was "calculated to give a graceful power of balancing the
body, on which good walking and dancing principally depend."[60] As to
the exercises themselves, he divided his system into three distinct
phases, each more difficult than the next. Those who had not been regularly exercising were instructed to start with the twenty preparatory
exercises. Beginning with the "primitive" or first position, the twenty
exercises comprising Beaujeu's first course of training gradually
increased in difficulty as the body accommodated to the demands of
regular physical training. From simple calf raises, Beaujeu's beginning
gymnast moved on to arm extensions, leg circles, punching movements, and, finally, to several types of marches.

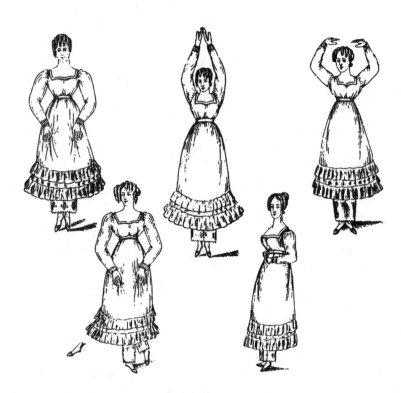

Figure 13: Preparatory Exercises from J. A. Beaujeu's *A Treatise on Gymnastic
Exercises,* (1828).

Having explained these rudimentary movements, Beaujeu next took his readers through ten difficult, "compound exercises, in which all the muscles of the trunk and the limbs, in fact all parts of the body, are called into action at the same time."[61] These compound exercises required several pieces of gymnastic apparatus: vertical parallel bars, horizontal bars, and a chair or box. They also required levels of strength and fitness which would be unusual even in an athletic, twentieth-century female. For instance, the third exercise in the new series is a palms-facing-away pull-up, or chin:[62]

> The pupil will take her position under the bar, raised a foot or more above her head. Having placed her hands thereon, will raise the body gradually by strength of the arms from the ground, the palms of the hands turned from the body, and the toes pointed to the ground, that the knees may be properly extended. The body to be raised until the chest be on a level with the bar, and the exercise to be repeated several times without putting the foot to the ground, and descending gradually by the exertion of the arms alone.[63]

Chinning movements such as this require a high level of upper body strength.[64] Furthermore, by placing the palms away from the body, Beaujeu actually made the exercise more difficult for women, since this position decreases the biceps' ability to help in carrying the load. Beaujeu didn't stop with chins, however. The seventh compound exercise is the dip between parallel bars.[65] The dip is another difficult exercises for women because of the relatively small size of the muscles in the female arm and shoulder. Based on this author's professional experiences in weight training, Beaujeu's inclusion of the dip indicates that his women gymnasts must have trained regularly, seriously, and with strength as a physiological goal. Simple calisthenics movements would not be enough to allow an average woman to perform either chins or dips.

Beaujeu placed even greater demands on his students' physical and emotional capacities, however, as the tenth compound exercise required girls to hang by the elbows on a horizontal bar while swinging back and forth.[66] Although this exercise did not require an unusually high degree of strength, it definitely required constitutional fortitude to deal with the pain such a position undoubtedly created in the arms and shoulders of these young women. Beaujeu admitted that the appearance of this exercise may "tend to alarm some timid persons," but he argued, nonetheless, that its utility to those suffering from "narrow and confined chests cannot be questioned."[67]

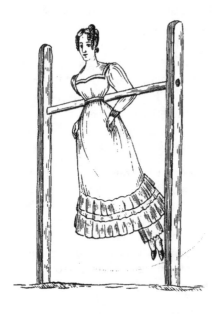

Figure 15: "Hanging on the Elbows backwards, and balancing," from J. A. Beaujeu's *A Treatise on Gymnastic Exercises,* (1828).

The final section of Beaujeu's text is a graduated series of Flying Course or "triangle" exercises. Beaujeu showed two arrangements for this piece of apparatus. He used it, as Clias did, by attaching it to a swivel and hook in the ceiling, and also by erecting a tall pole and attaching to the top of the pole several triangles so that four to five women could exercise at the same time. On the single triangle, Beaujeu demonstrated several difficult balancing exercises as well as more chins. On the Flying Course, in reality a hygienic Maypole, Beaujeu instructed his gymnasts to step forward with increasing speed until they were running around the pole. When their speed was sufficient, he explained, they should take giant steps so that their feet only "skim the earth." "There is no exercise . . ." Beaujeu maintained in a footnote, "more likely to contribute to health and strength than this."[68] Part of Beaujeu's preference for the Flying Course was that he felt it helped prepare young women to meet life's emergencies. He worried that so few women could run either swiftly or for an extended period of time, and he believed that by training on the Flying Course a woman could become much more prepared to deal with whatever physical demands her life presented. Beaujeu discounted his era's belief that women should be always delicate, and he noted that there were simply too many times in a woman's life when a modicum of speed and strength would be useful. We cannot overlook the fact, he argued, that dreadful

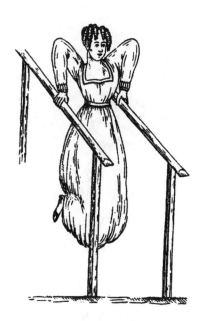

Figure 14: "To raise the Body by the Strength of the Arms on the Horizontal Bar." and "To descend and ascend between two Bars, the Knees bent." from J. A. Beaujeu's *A Treatise on Gymnastic Exercises,* (1828).

maladies occur which might have been averted "had we arrived some seconds sooner."[69]

In addition to the unusually high strength levels his exercises required and produced, and to his apparently egalitarian attitude toward women, Beaujeu's small textbook is noteworthy in another way. He appears to be the first author to recommend a distinct gymnastic costume for women. Beaujeu argued that to properly perform his exercises, women gymnasts should wear, "a pair of muslin or cotton trowsers, a little close above the ancle [sic]; they should take care to tighten their garters but slightly, in order that the bending of the foot or knee may not be impeded, and that in running, &c. these parts may acquire, without impediment, all the strength and elasticity of which they are susceptible."[70] Wearing the proper shoes was also important, Beaujeu argued, "Shoes with high uppers and quarters, having a double sole and no heel, are the best." Shoes of this type, he argued, help "form the limbs, and to give support to the parts during exercise."[71]

Historian Patricia Warner suggested, in her analysis of sport fashions, that some European girls began wearing ankle length trousers or pantaloons under their sheer, muslin, Empire-style gowns to preserve modesty as early as 1803. She also cited one expert who believed pantaloon costumes were used as exercise wear in British girls' schools as early as 1807.[72] Beaujeu cannot, therefore, be credited for inventing

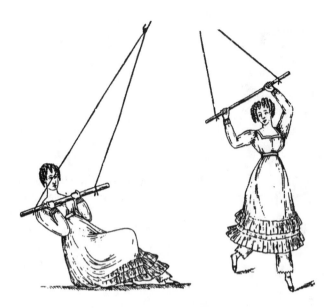

Figure 16: Flying Course and Triangle Exercises from J. A. Beaujeu's *A Treatise on Gymnastic Exercises,* (1828).

gymnastic dress for women, but he does appear to have been the first to address the question of appropriate training attire in print. Several other exercise books from the 1820s, examined in Chapter Four, contain illustrations of women in shortened gowns, with pantaloons underneath. However, none of these books discussed the question of appropriate dress for exercise and it is unclear whether their illustrations are of a legitimate gymnastic costume, or whether they are merely illustrations of a fashionable woman's walking costume.[73]

## Madame Beaujeu's American Gymnasium

It would be easy to dismiss Beaujeu's book as a European anomaly that had nothing to do with American women. However, Madame Beaujeu proved to be an important link in the introduction of women's gymnastics and calisthenics to America. Madame Beaujeu, whose birth name remains a mystery, learned gymnastics from her husband and assisted with the teaching at their private women's gym in Dublin, which they reportedly modeled after the "English Female Gymnasium."[74] In 1841, however, she appeared in Boston, where, as Mrs. Hawley, she opened an apparently successful school for the teaching of calisthenics and gymnastic exercises first at 339 Washington

Street and later, apparently, on the corner of Tremont and Bromfield Streets. Horace Mann described her Boston gym as "excellent" in the *Common School Journal* while women's health reformer, Mary Gove, enthusiastically reported the next year that, "this admirable establishment is well patronized, having at this time one hundred and seventy pupils from the most intelligent families in the city."[75] A report in the well-respected *Boston Medical and Surgical Journal* also praised Mrs. Hawley and her methods. "Very recently," the article began, "Mrs. Hawley, formerly Madame Beaujeu, of England, has commenced a series of calisthenic exercises for young misses in this city, which are recognized by very distinguished physicians of Philadelphia, New York and Boston as worthy of the patronage of parents." Anyone, the article promised, who took the time to visit Mrs. Hawley's gymnasium, "will be satisfied of the utility of her system."[76]

According to Gove, Mrs. Hawley operated her gymnasium for four years in Boston and then moved to New York City in either late 1845 or early 1846 where she opened another women's gymnasium.[77] *Doggett's New York City Directory* lists her gym at 136 Eighth Street and her residence at 396 Broadway for the years 1845-1846 and 1846-1847. She does not appear in the 1847-1848 *Directory* and there is no mention of a Mr. Hawley in either year.[78] How Madame Beaujeu became Mrs. Hawley and arrived in America must remain a mystery for future historians to solve. Efforts to determine how long Beaujeu's Dublin school remained open and when and how he died have also proved fruitless.

## Support for Women's Gymnastics

Beaujeu's book, and his difficult gymnastic system raise a number of interesting questions for scholars of women's exercise. First of all, did his vigorous gymnastic system actually help women live more healthy, physically active lives? Apparently, it did, for Royal Hibernian Military School physician, James William Macauley claimed in a letter dated 27 October 1827, that the introduction of gymnastics by Beaujeu had made a dramatic difference in the number of young women he saw in the school's infirmary. Prior to Beaujeu's arrival, Macauley reported, he saw a majority of the two hundred females of the school at one time or another during the course of a year. He attributed this high level of ill health to their lack of exercise and he argued that they became "much improved in carriage, health and appearance. . .[and] I have no doubt the above change is, in a great measure, owing to its influence."[79] Beyond this data, however, we can only speculate. So far, no personal accounts by women who participated in other early gymnastics programs have come to light.

Secondly, was Beaujeu's book simply an anomaly, or were there other exercise advocates who possessed similarly progressive attitudes toward women's physical capabilities in this era? The available evidence suggests that Beaujeu was *not* alone in his egalitarian approach to exercise. German ex-patriate Franz Lieber, who arrived in London in the late 1820s and then made his way to Boston to supervise Boston's public gymnasium, certainly sided with Beaujeu in an 1828 American magazine article on gymnastics. What is called calisthenics, Lieber argued, "appears to us founded on incorrect notions."[80] Educator William Bentley Fowle, as we shall see in Chapter Three, also operated from an equally modern perspective when he attempted, at the Boston Monitorial School for Girls, to establish a gymnastics program for his female students similar to Beaujeu's.

More substantial evidence that strength and gymnastics enjoyed a brief vogue in the 1820s can be found in an anonymously published 1828 Parisian imprint, *Calisthénie ou Gymnastique des Jeunes Filles, Traité Élémentaire Des Différens Exercises, Propres A Fortifier Le Corp, A Entretnir La Sante, Et A Preparer Un Bon Tempérament*.[81] This 163 page textbook had gone through ten editions by 1830, and was, according to historian Fred Eugene Leonard, based almost entirely on Clias's gymnastic exercises for young men. When the Philadelphia-based *Journal of Health* reviewed this text in 1830, it heartily sanctioned the book's theme of vigorous exercise, reminding its readers that although women were admittedly smaller and weaker in some ways than men, "we ought not to grant them [women] the privilege which some of their own number, and certain mawkish, male sentimentalists would claim for them, of being such frail and tender beings, as to be little better than interesting invalids."[82]

In this French text, the degree of strength required to perform some of the exercises is, again, exceedingly high. Opposite the title page we find a fold-out engraving of the Flying Course in use. In it the women's postures and garments indicate that they are running around this exercise May-pole rather than sedately walking. In the book, the author suggested as "indispensable apparatus" the parallel bars, a horizontal bar or chinning bar and a high-jumping device.[83] As to the exercises themselves, the author included, among others, full, deep-knee bends to strengthen the buttocks and legs; jumping from the ground and raising the knees as high as possible; the long jump, which

is illustrated as a jump across a ditch; the high jump at measured increments; parallel bar dips to open the chest and strengthen the arms; the
extremely difficult one-legged squat; and climbing a slanted ladder
while using only the hands and arms. Although the exercises are not
identical to Beaujeu's and differ, for instance, in their seeming preference for outdoor training, the physiological requirements and
philosophical underpinnings of these two books are amazingly similar.
These exercises require women to truly exert themselves. For Clias,
Beaujeu and the anonymous French author, strength is the desired
physiological goal, not merely grace and good carriage.

## American Magazines Spread the Word

A second question which needs to be asked, of course, is whether
the ideas contained in books such as these found an audience in
America. Apparently, they did, for the prestigious *Journal of Health*
printed a condensation of the French book, which not only lavishly
praised the book's message but went on to recommend the benefits of
parallel bar training for women. "After the pupil has learned to support
and balance herself on the bars," the *Journal's* article reported, "she may
give herself a forward progressive movement by advancing first one
hand and then the other." Having mastered this movement, the review
continued, she should proceed to "the movement by jumps—so that
the pupil, by resting firmly on her hands, shall give herself a quick
upward movement, letting both bars go at the same time, and lighting
a little in advance, both hands again quickly grasping the bars."[84]

*The Journal of Health,* "conducted by an association of physicians,"
played a major role in placing the exercise/health connection before the
American public. Dr. John Bell served as editor of the *Journal* which
appeared for the first time on 9 September 1829 in Philadelphia.[85]
According to phrenologist George Combe, who visited the United
States in the 1830s, the magazine had more than four thousand subscribers when its publishing company filed for bankruptcy in 1831 and
forced the magazine's demise.[86]

The *Journal of Health* came out strongly in favor of physical education for women in its very first issue. Parents, Bell argued, should avoid
"over anxiety for delicacy of complexion, in a daughter, or the appre-
hension that her limbs may become coarse and ungraceful, and her
habits vulgar," unnecessary fears which he believed barred too many
young women from the fresh air and exercise necessary to lifelong
health. "The bodily exercises of the two sexes ought, in fact, to be the

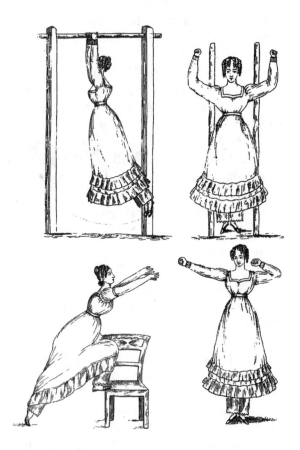

Figure 17: Illustration of various compound exercises from J. A. Beaujeu's *A Treatise on Gymnastic Exercises* (1828).

same," he continued forthrightly. "Both should be permitted, without control, to partake of the same rational means of insuring a continued flow of health and animal spirits . . . Girls should not," he emphatically stated, "therefore be confined to a sedentary life."[87]

*The Journal of Health* was not alone in promoting the idea of vigorous exercise for American women. Physician, lecturer, and gymnastics proponent, John G. Coffin, who inspired William Fowle, took over as editor of the *Boston Medical Intelligencer* in early 1826, and quickly added a subtitle to the magazine's masthead announcing that the magazine would be "devoted to the cause of Physical Education and the means of preventing and . . . curing diseases."[88] "Women in general," Coffin wrote, "from their relations and duties,

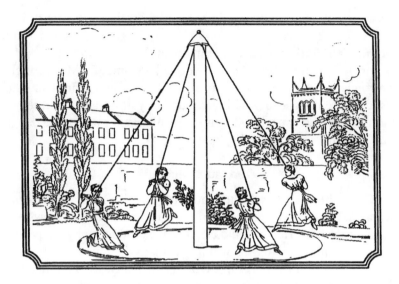

Figure 18: Illustration of the Giant Step or Flying Course from *Calisthénie ou Gymnastique des Jeunes Filles*, (1830).

need the preserving and invigorating movements of the gymnasium, more than men, and when they shall have realized their vivifying effects, will be as much attached to them."[89]

*The American Journal of Education* also pressed the question of women's education and women's exercise when it began publishing in January of 1826.[90] References to physical education and gymnastics appeared regularly in the *Journal,* whose stance on the question of female exercise was that "a slight infusion of the Spartan contempt of hardship," would go a long way toward improving the lives of American women.[91] Almost all the European books related to physical education and gymnastics were reviewed by the *Journal,* and true to their commitment to female education, the editors uniformly stressed the attention devoted to female exercise in these early texts. A review of Londe's *Medical Gymnastics,* for instance, appeared in April of 1826 and reminded readers that "corporeal exercise is necessary to both sexes," and urged women to select a variety of active and passive exercises for the development and preservation of their health and beauty.[92]

Evidence that the vigorous model of womanhood favored by Clias and Beaujeu found acceptance outside the medical and educational communities can be found in John Stuart Skinner's Baltimore-based

*American Farmer,* a magazine aimed at rural families. In an article entitled "Of the Exercises Most Conducive to Health in Girls and Young
Women," the author argued that many of the same sorts of exercises
performed by men should also be done by women.[93] More conclu-
sively, a later article claimed, "no absurdity is greater than that which
associates female beauty with great delicacy of body and debility of
constitution;" an appealing argument to any farmer with more daughters than sons and work to be done. [94]

### Too Much Muscle?

Clias, Beaujeu, and the anonymous author of *Calisthénie,*
demanded more than lip-service to strength and fitness. Their systems,
if followed as described, would clearly have produced physically competent young women who would, in many instances, actually be
superior to untrained males in strength and agility.[95] To flip her body
through the air and catch herself on a pair of parallel bars as the
*Journal of Health* recommended, a woman had to be strong, daring and
courageous. Furthermore, anyone following such a gymnastics regimen would have significantly increased in muscularity. Evidence that
some 1820s women trained sufficiently to produce true physiological
changes can be found in the disparaging comments of competing exercise promoter Bureaud Riofrey, who charged that the young women
who practiced gymnastics under Clias's supervision built too much
muscle. Their arms became "knotty and rough," Riofrey observed, and
their mothers forced them to stop before they looked like "pugilists."[96]

These training manuals and magazine endorsements suggest that
there were conflicting attitudes toward women, and their physical
capabilities, both in Europe and the United States in the 1820s and
early 1830s. While Clias, Beaujeu, his anonymous French cohort,
Lieber, Coffin, Dr. Bell and the association of American physicians who
published the *Journal of Health,* seem to be arguing, and demonstrating, that women's physical potential is virtually limitless, another group
of exercise experts positioned themselves to lead women's exercise in
more conservative, less physically demanding directions. In 1831,
William Grigg symbolically signaled the end of the 1820s women's
gymnastic movement when he sadly told a crowded lecture hall in
Boston

> It is thought by some, to be indelicate in a young female to romp and
> pursue the exercises of a boy. Indelicate! true it may be indelicate to
> use such means as are adopted in some foreign institutions. But there

are hundreds of exercises which may be employed, with which the most fastidious could find no fault. Indelicate! any exercise may be thought so by some, for the ultra fashionable think it indelicate to be healthy.[97]

As Grigg makes clear, the problem was not the idea of exercise for women but those exercises "adopted in some foreign institutions." During the next two decades, a widespread philosophical retrenchment on the nature of women's physical capacities dominated the women's exercise movement in America. In place of gymnastics, experts touted the benefits of calisthenics, remedial exercises and manual labor. However, not all Americans applauded the conservative approach to women's exercise. One American educator, in fact, went to great lengths to prove that gymnastics could be a suitable exercise regimen for American women.

[1]GutsMuths contributions are discussed in: Richard Mandell, *Sport: A Cultural History* (New York: Columbia University Press, 1984), 157-161; Robert K. Barney, "German Turners in America: Their Role in Nineteenth Century Exercise Expression and Physical Education Legislation," in Earle F. Ziegler, ed. *A History of Physical Education and Sport in the United States and Canada* (Champaign, IL: Stites Publishing, 1975), 111-120; Fred Eugene Leonard, "The First Introduction of Jahn Gymnastics into America, (1825-1830)," Parts I, II, III, IV, V & VI *Mind and Body* 12(September, October, November, & December 1905) and 12(January & February 1906): 193-198, 217-223, 248-254, 281-287, 313-319 and 345-351; and in Fred Eugene Leonard, "Johann Christopf Friedrich GutsMuths: Teacher of Gymnastics at Schnepfenthal, 1786-1835," *Mind and Body* 17 (January 1911): 321-326. Other sources include: Bernhard Reimer, "The Grandfather of German Gymnastics," *Mind and Body* 1(May 1894): 1-3; Ellen Gerber, *Innovators, and Institutions in Physical Education* (Philadelphia: Lea and Febiger) 115-121; and A. L. Cross, "Guts Muths: His Life and Ideas, in Relation to the Physical Training Movement," Unpublished paper, Luther Gulick Collection, Babson Library, Springfield College, Springfield, MS.

[2]Leonard, *Guide,* 75.

[3]J. C. F. GutsMuths, *Gymnastik fur die Jugen. Enthaltend eine PraktischeAnwisung zu Leibesubungen. Ein Beytraq zur Nothigsten Verbesserung der Korperlichen Erziehung.* (Schnepfenthal: Buchhandlung der Erziehunganstalt, 1793).

Volume One of *Gymnastics for Youth* raised philosophical questions surrounding man's need for exercise. Chapter titles included: "We are weak because it does not occur to us that we could be strong if we would;" as well as "Consequences of the common method of education, and especially the neglect of bodily training;" "All the means hitherto employed against lack of hardihood are insufficient;" and "Gymnastics proposed, and objections answered." The second, and longer volume gave specific exercise information on organizing an open air gymnasium, running, leaping, wrestling, climbing, balancing, lifting, carrying, pulling, dancing, walking, military exercises, bathing, swimming, manual labor, declamation, and fasting.

[4]C. G. Salzmann [J. C. F. GutsMuths], *Gymnastics for Youth: Or a Practical Guide to Delightful and Amusing Exercises For the Use of Schools, An Essay Toward the Necessary Improvement of Education, Chiefly as It Relates to the Body* (London: printed for J. Johnston, 1800); and, C. G. Salzmann, [J. C. F. GutsMuths], *Gymnastics for Youth: Or a Practical Guide to Delightful and Amusing Exercises For the Use of Schools, An Essay Toward the Necessary Improvement of Education, Chiefly as It Relates to the Body* (Philadelphia: William Duane, 1802).

Regarding the question of authorship, a bibliographical reference at Springfield College made by Luther Halsey Gulick in 1900 reads: "The author of this book is Johann Christoph Friedrich GutsMuths, who was a teacher of gymnastics under Salzmann at Schnepfenthal. American translators, knowing of Salzmann, never having heard of GutsMuths, and recognizing the high character of the book, concluded it was by Salzmann, and that GutsMuths (good courage) was a nom de plume. The translation is very free.

"The same book was published in French, in 1803, under the names of M. A. Amar Durivier and L. F. Jauffret. In this case, it was clearly a theft. However, the book appears to have aroused much interest." Historian Fred Eugene Leonard also attributes the book to GutsMuths, not Salzmann. Leonard, *Guide*, 76.

[5]Salzmann [GutsMuths], *Gymnastics for Youth*, 2.

[6]Ibid., 15.

[7]Fred Eugene Leonard, "Friedrich Ludwig Jahn, and the Development of Popular Gymnastics (Vereinsturnen) in Germany" Parts I & II. *American Physical Education Review* 12 (July & August 1905): 133-139 & 170-175.

[8]Hans Ballin, "Biographical Sketch of Friedrich Ludwig Jahn," *Mind and Body* 1(October 1894): 1-7. A fascinating, contemporary account of Jahn's life in Germany and the introduction of German gymnastics to the United States can be found in a lengthy book review, written by German ex-patriate and Jahn student, Franz Lieber. This review of Carl Beck's 1828 translation of Jahn's *Treatise on Gymnastics* appeared in the *American Quarterly Review* 3(March 1828): 126-150.

Jahn's biography is also included in: Henry Metzner, *A Brief History of the North American Gymnastic Union*, trans. Theodore Stempfel, (Indianapolis: National Executive Committee of the North American Gymnastics Union, 1911).

[9]Fred Eugene Leonard, *Pioneers, of Modern Physical Training* (New York: Association Press, 1915) 37.

[10]See Vera Olivova, "From the Arts of Chivalry to Gymnastics," *Canadian Journal of History of Sport* 12 (December 1981): 53-54, for a discussion of the ideological differences between GutsMuths and Jahn.

[11]F. L. Jahn, *Deutsches Volksthum* (Lübeck, Germany: 1810); and Friedrich Ludwig Jahn und Ernst Eiselen, *Die Deutsche Turnkunst zur Einrichtung der Turnplätze Dargestellt von Friedrich Ludwig Jahn und Ernst Eiselen* (Berlin: Kosten der Herausgeber, 1816). This work, with an introduction by Hugo Rühl, was reprinted in *Reclams Universal Bibliotek* (Leipzig: Phillipp Reclam jun., 1905).

[12]Leonard, *Pioneers*, 38. Upon his release from prison, in 1825, Jahn was forbidden to live in or near Berlin or any other city which contained a university or similar school for boys. He spent his later years in relative obscurity at Freyburg-on-the-Unstrut and apparently made no further attempts to organize gymnasts. Though Jahn was forcibly removed from the Turner movement he created, the movement did not die, nor was he forgotten. New life stirred in the Turner movement in the 1840s when, once again, Germans felt themselves losing control of their identity. By 1860, when the first convention and Turnfest was held at Coburg, more than a thousand adult Turners showed up representing 139 cities and villages. A second convention, at Berlin, held on the fiftieth anniversary of the founding of Hasenhide, included 2812 adult Turners, 1659 of them from outside the city.

As Germans began leaving their homeland in the late 1840s in record numbers, Turner societies spread into other parts of Europe and America. By 1861, there were approximately nine thousand registered members of the national American organization *Socialist Turnaround* and more than 150 different, individual Turner societies existed in the United States. In 1865, this group changed its name to the *Nordamerikanisher Turnerbund* and, by 1886, it included 231 societies and some 23,823 members. Throughout the nineteenth century, Jahn remained a true hero to Germans around the world. The fiftieth anniversary of his death and the one hundredth anniversary of his birth were celebrated in Germany as national holidays. For the full story of Jahn's later years and his continued influence, see Leonard, *Guide*, 96-108.

[13]Völker opened his outdoor gymnasium near Regents Park in London. Völker later ran an indoor gymnasium at Mr. Fontaine's riding school at Finbury Square. See: "Professor Voelker's Gymnasium, London," *American Journal of Education* 1 (July 1826): 430-432 and Leonard, *Guide*, 248.

[14]Leonard, *Pioneers*, 24-25. Nachtegall's gym was an outdoor facility, consisting of various ropes, "horses" and other gymnastic apparati in an open field. He began with only five pupils, had twenty-five at the end of his first year and by 1803-1804 had one hundred fifty members, both adults and children. So successful was Nachtegall that the king appointed him a "professor" of gymnastics at the university and put him in charge of training the

Danish military. In 1814, Danish law decreed that all schools must provide grounds and apparatus for gymnastics. Nachtegall's biography is also included in Gerber, *Innovators*, 177-81. By 1803, there were reportedly fourteen gymnasiums in Denmark. "Progress of Physical Education," *American Journal of Education* 1(January 1826): 21.

[15]D. W. Cheever, in "The Gymnasium," *Atlantic Monthly* 3 (May 1859): 537, claimed that Ling was inspired to pursue the study of exercise because of his experiences as a fencer.

[16]For an interesting description of Ling's methods written by one of his students, see: Harald Billberg, "Swedish Gymnastics," *Murray's Magazine* 9 (1863): 825-829.

[17]Besides Andry's *Orthopaedia*, Ling could have read Friedrich Hoffman, *"On Motion, the Best Medicine for the Body* (Halle, Germany: 1701); Friedrich Hoffman, *The Incomparable Advantages of Motion and of Bodily Exercises, and How They are to be Employed for the Preservation of Health* (Halle: 1819); Francis Fuller, *Medicina Gymnastica Or a Treatise Concerning the Power of Exercise with Respect to the Animal Economy and the Great Necessity of it in the Cure of Several Distempers* (London: printed by John Matthews, 1705); Simon André Tissot, MD, *An Essay on Diseases Incident to Literary and Sedentary Persons. With Proper Rules for Preventing their Fatal Consequences and Instructions for Their Cure* (Dublin: printed for James Williams, 1772); or Clement Joseph Tissot, *Gymnastique medicinale et chirurgicale, ou essai sur l'utilite du mouvement, on des differens exercises du corps, et du repos dans la cure de maladies* (Paris: Bastien, Libraire, 1780).

[18]In 1830, for instance, penmanship expert Dr. Shaw recommended attaching a weight and pulley to the front of the head to strengthen the neck and improve posture. "Cartesian System of Penmanship," *American Journal of Education* [New Series] 1 (August 1830): 378. See: Fred Eugene Leonard, "Per Henrik Ling and His Successors at the Stockholm Normal School of Gymnastics," Parts I & II. *Mind and Body* 12 (May and June 1905):74-79 & 102-105, for more complete information on Ling's therapeutic system.

[19]Peter McIntosh, *Physical Education in England Since 1800* (London: G. Bell & Sons, 1952), 78-79. See also: Fred Eugene Leonard, "Chapters From the Early History of Physical Training in America" *Mind & Body* 13 (December, 1906): 292; Deobold B. Van Dalen, Elmer Mitchell, and Bruce Bennett, *A World History of Physical Education* (Englewood Cliffs, NJ: Prentice Hall, 1963), 276-277, 285, & 290-292; and Fred Eugene Leonard, "The Beginnings of Modern Physical Training in Europe," *Mind and Body* 11 (November 1904): 239-241.

[20]P. H. Clias, *Anfangsgrunde der Gymnastik oder Turnkunst [Initial Reasons of Gymnastics or the Art of Gymnastics]* (Bern: 1816).

[21]P. H. Clias, *Principes de gymnastique* (Paris: 1819).

[22]These details of Clias's life are from the preface by U. Mockel in: P. H. Clias, *Kalisthenie oder Uebungen zur Schoenheit und Kraft fuer Maedchen [Calisthenics or Exercises for Beauty and Power]* (Bern: 1829).

[23][Franz Lieber] "A Review: Art. VI.—A Treatise on Gymnastics: Taken Chiefly from the German of F. L. Jahn. 8vo. Northampton, Massachusetts: 1828," *American Quarterly Review* 3 (March 1828): 139, reports that Clias was introduced to the British military leaders by the Duke of York and Duke of Wellington.

[24]Peter Henry Clias, *Elementary Course of Gymnastic Exercises; Intended to Improve The Physical Powers of Man* (London: Sherwood Jones and Co., 1823). All further references in this text are to the 1825 fourth edition. Clias adopted the more Anglo-Saxon "Peter," rather than "Phokion," for these English editions.

[25]Clias, *Gymnastic Exercises* (1823 and 1825), title pages. A review of the 1825 edition may be found in *The Journal of Health* 4 (27 October 1830): 51-53.

[26]Clias, *Elementary Course*, v.

[27]The Flying Course may have been developed by Don Francisco Amoros Et Ondeano, a Spaniard, who opened a gymnasium in Paris in 1817. He began working with the French military shortly thereafter and opened an enormous open-air gymnasium for military and civilian pupils in 1820. Van Dalen, Mitchell and Bennett, *A World History*, 278. More complete biographical information on Amoros may be found in Leonard, "The Beginnings," 237-239. Signor Voarino, in *A Second Course of Calisthenic Exercises; With a Course of Private Gymnastics for Gentlemen Accompanied with a Few Observations on The Utility of Exercise* (London: James Ridgeway, 1828) 93, gives credit for the invention of the "triangle" to Clias.

[28]Van Dalen, Mitchell and Bennett, *A World History*, 290-292. and Leonard, "Chapters," 292.

[29]Clias, *Elementary Course, The Literary Gazette* quotation appeared on 15 February 1823 and is included on page xix of the fourth edition.

[30]Leonard, "The Beginnings," 240.

[31]P. H. Clias, *Kalesthenie oder Uebungen zur Schoenheit und Kraft fuer Maedchen* (Bern, Switzerland: 1829) 9-10.

[32]"Progress of Physical Education," *The American Journal of Education* 1 (January 1826): 21.

[33] Quoted in Clias, Elementary *Course*, xix.

[34]Later in the century, American gymastiarch Dio Lewis would claim the invention of the "gymnastic crown" for precisely the same physiological purposes.

[35]*Buchan's Domestic Medicine*, for instance, included a case history of a young man's cure through gymnastics according to: "Progress of Physical Education," *American Journal of Education* (January 1826): 22.

[36]A Physician, *Sure Methods of Improving Health, and Prolonging Life; or, A Treatise on the Art of Living Long and Comfortably by Regulating the Diet and Regimen.* (London: by the author, 1827): 196-197.

[37]Ibid., 197-199. No steps were skipped in reproducing this exercise prescription. Apparently, steps 18, 19, and 20, for instance, were all more or less the same movement.

[38]Ibid.

[39]*Callisthénie, ou Somascétique Naturelle, Appropriée A L'Education Phyisique Des Jeunes Filles* (Besançon: Charles Deis, 1843). See Van Dalen, Mitchell and Bennett, *A World History,* 278 for the details of Clias's later years.

[40]See, for instance, Bureaud Riofrey, *Physical Education Specially Adapted to Young Ladies, 2nd ed.* (London: Longman, Orne, Brown, Green & Longmans, 1838), 76.

[41]*Dictionary of Medical Science,* vol. 52 (n. d.) 28-29. Quoted in Clias, *Elementary Course,* xix.

[42]The gym was located at Number One, Union Place. "Voelker's Gymnasium," 430-432.

[43]Lieber, "Gymnastics," 140. Völker played a role in the transmission of German gymnastics to America. A dedicated member of the gymnasium he opened in Regents Park in London was American author John Neal, a house guest of Jeremy Bentham's. Neal, who had apparently turned to the gym to relieve stress and fatigue, became so enamored of the benefits of gymnastics that he wrote a series of letters which were printed in the *American Journal of Education,* 1 (1826): 375 and 699-700, and in 2 (1827): 55-56. Upon his return from England in 1827, Neal gave lectures on gymnastics and opened his own gymnasium in Brunswick, Maine, which he operated for more than thirty years while continuing to pursue a law practice and a literary career. Information on Neal may be found in Leonard, *Guide,* 249-250; and in his autobiography, *Wandering Recollections of a Somewhat Busy Life: An Autobiography* (Boston: Roberts Brothers, 1869).

[44]"London Gymnastic Institution," *American Journal of Education* 1 (October 1826): 79-80. See also: "Prospectus of the London Gymnastic Society," *American Journal of Education* 1 (August 1826): 502-506.

[45]"Gymnastic Schools in England," *American Journal of Education* 2 (January 1827): 55. See also: [John Neal] "Gymnasium," *American Journal of Education* 1 (June 1826): 61.

[46]J. A. Beaujeu, *A Treatise on Gymnastic Exercises, Or Calisthenics For the Use of Young Ladies. Introduced at the Royal Hibernian Military School, Also at The Seminary for the Education of Young Ladies Under the Direction of Miss Hincks in 1824* (Dublin: R. Milliken and Son, 1828), 20.

[47]The author was unable to find any biographical information on Beaujeu in any standard work on the history of physical education. That Beaujeu's efforts were directed at women, and were primarily undertaken in Dublin, not London, may have kept his contributions out of mainstream historical

scholarship. That he recommended a vigorous, "unfeminine" approach to women's exercise no doubt added to his unacceptability to early physical educators. No information could be found on the role of Miss Hincks. Beaujeu, *Treatise on Gymnastics,* 24.

[48]Ibid., ix.

[49]"All the progressive exercises described in this work, are susceptible of being everywhere introduced; they may be performed in the smallest apartment and require no preparation, nor are they attended with expense." Ibid., 23.

[50]It is not known whether Clias began offering classes to women in London immediately after his arrival. If Beaujeu began his classes in 1824, it is possible that he predated Clias in his involvement with women.

[51]Beaujeu, *Treatise on Gymnastics,* vi-vii.

[52]Ibid., 7.

[53]Ibid., 19.

[54]Ibid., 7-19.

[55]Ibid., 18 &24. .

[56]Ibid., 19.

[57]Ibid., 19-20.

[58]Ibid., 40.

[59]Ibid., 40-41.

[60]Ibid., 60.

[61]Ibid., 87.

[62]Ibid., 90.

[63]Ibid., 90.

[64] During my twelve years of teaching weight training at The University of Texas in Austin, for instance, I would estimate that less than five percent of the college-aged women in my classes were capable of performing overhand (palms forward) chins, even after a twelve week course of strength training.

[65]Ibid., 94-96. The major muscle groups involved in the dipping motion are the triceps of the back of the arm, the anterior deltoid on the front of the shoulder and the pectoral muscles of the chest.

[66]Ibid., 98.

[67]Ibid.

[68]Ibid., 108.

[69]Ibid., 114.

[70]Ibid., 42.

[71]Ibid., 42.

[72]Patricia C. Warner, "Clothing the American Woman for Sport and Physical Education, 1860 to 1940: Public and Private" (Ph.D. diss., The University of Minnesota, 1986), 46. Another good source for information on women's exercise clothing is: Anne Wood Murray, "The Bloomer Costume and Exercise Suits," *Waffen-und Kostümkunde* (München: Deutscher Kunstverlag, 1982), 110-14. French historian Pierre Dufay reports, "En 1807

nous arrive de Londres la mode des pantaloons por les petites filles. Les exercises du saut se pratiquent en Angelterre dans les écoles de jeunes filles: c'est pour cela qu'on leur a donné de pantaloons. From: Pierre Dufay, *Le Pantalon Feminin* (Paris, 1906).

[73]Valerie Steele, *Fashion and Eroticism: Ideals of Feminine Beauty from the Victorian Era to the Jazz Age* (New York: Oxford University Press, 1985), 4, 52, 54, and 114. Women of fashion in the period 1825-1835 frequently wore their skirts, especially their daytime "walking costumes," above the ankles.

[74]Beaujeu, *Treatise on Gymnastics*, n.p. The English Female Gymnasium was probably a reference to Völker's gymnasium. It is not known whether the Miss Hincks mentioned in the lengthy title for Beaujeu's book refers to Madame Beaujeu or to some other Dublin schoolmistress who also followed Beaujeu's ideas about exercise.

[75]Mary S. Gove, *Lectures to Women on Anatomy and Physiology With an Appendix on Water Cure* (New York: Harper & Brothers, 1846) 218. See: Horace Mann, "Gymnasia," *The Common School Journal* 7 (10 June 1845): 12. See also: [Horace Mann], "Physical Exercise: Dr. Thayer's Gymnastic Apparatus, Boylston Hall, Boston," *The Common School Journal* 7 (16 June 1845): 179.

Although Mary Gove suggested that Hawley's gymnasium opened in 1841, it does not appear in *Sketches and Business Directory of Boston and Its Vicinity* until 1843. There are two listings under the name Hawley in 1843. "Hawley, B.W., Gymnasium, Washington," and Hawley, Beaujeu, Calisthenics School, 339 Washington," *Sketches and Business Directory of Boston and Its Vicinty for 1843* No. 151: 3 (Boston: Damrell, Moore and Coolidge, 1843), 72. In 1844 the single citation reads, "Hawley, B. W., Gymnasium, Washington," *Sketches and Business Directory of Boston and Its Vicinty for 1844* No. 152: 4 (Boston: Damrell, Moore and Coolidge, 1843), 70. There are no listings for 1845 or later. Hawley's home is listed at Bromfield Street in 1843. An article in the *Boston Medical and Surgical Journal* quoted by Gove, gives the gymnasium's address as the corner of Bromfield and Tremont Streets. *Boston Medical and Surgical Journal*, 219. No record could be found of Mr. Hawley.

[76]Ibid., 219.

[77]Ibid.

[78]John Doggett, Jr., *Doggett's New York City Directory for 1845-1846* (New York: John Doggett, Jr., 1845), 167; and John Doggett, Jr., *Doggett's New York City Directory for 1846-1847* (New York: John Doggett, Jr., 1846), 181.

[79]Beaujeu, *Treatise on Gymnastic Exercises*, 33.

[80][Lieber] "Gymnastics," 142.

[81]*Calisthénie ou Gymnastique des Jeunes Filles, Traité Élémentaire Des Differéns Exercises, Propres A Fortifier Le Corp, A Entretnir La Sante,. Et A Preparer Un Bon Tempérament* (Paris: 1828). All citations are from a copy of the tenth edition, published in 1830.

[82]"Calisthenics," *The Journal of Health* 2 (23 February 1831): 190.

[83]*Calisthenie*, 80.

[84]"Calisthenics," 192.

[85]George Combe, *Notes on the United States of America During a Phrenological Visit in 1838-39-40*. vol. 2. (Edinburgh, Maclachlan, Stewart & Co. 1841), 106-107.

[86]Ibid., 56. Combe noted that Bell was also the author of two health-related books: *Health and Beauty and Baths*.

[87]"Physical Education of Girls," *The Journal of Health* 1 (9 September 1829): 15.

Through the several years of the *Journal's* publication, a number of articles addressed the question of women's exercise. Admittedly, not all these articles advocated gymnastics as the only means of exercise for women. "Preservation of Beauty," published in the November 1830 issue, for instance, insisted on personal cleanliness, temperance at the table and "gentle and daily *Exercise* in the open air." "Preservation of Beauty," *The Journal of Health* 2 (24 November 1830): 89-90. For other *Journal* articles on women's exercise see: "Appropriate Exercise," *The Journal of Health* 1 (23 September 1829): 22; "Gymnastic Exercises, "*The Journal of Health* 1 (13 January 1830): 132; "In-Door Exercises, "*The Journal of Health* 1 (27 January 1830): 151-152; "Variety in Exercise," *The Journal of Health* 1 (28 April 1830): 243-244; "Benefits of Exercise," *The Journal of Health* 2 (27 October 1830): 51-53; "False Attitudes," *The Journal of Health* 2 (30 November 1830): 91-92.

[88]*Boston Medical Intelligencer* 4 (1826-1827):1.

[89]Editorial note by John G. Coffin in: William B. Fowle, "The Animal Mechanism and Economy," *Boston Medical Intelligencer* 5 (24 October 1826): 196-197.

[90]"Prospectus," *The American Journal of Education* 1 (January 1826): 3.

[91]"Thoughts on the Education of Females," *The American Journal of Education* 1 (June 1826): 352. See also: "Suggestions to Parents: Physical Education," *The American Journal of Education* 2 (May 1827): 289-292.

[92]Review of: Charles Londe, *Medical Gymnastics; or Exercise Applied to the Organs of Man, according to the Laws of Physiology, of Hygiene, and Therapeutics* (Paris: 1821); *American Journal of Education* 1 (April 1826): 235-239.

[93]"Of the Exercises Most Conducive to Health in Girls and Young Women," *American Farmer* 9 (26 October 1827): 254. Quoted in Jack Berryman and Joann Brislin, "The Ladies' Department of *The American Farmer,* 1825-1830: A Locus for the Advocacy of Family Health and Exercise," *Associates National Agriculture Library Today* 2 (September 1977): 11.

[94]*American Farmer* 9 (9 November 1827): 270-271. Quoted in Berryman and Brislin, "Ladies' Department," 11.

[95]Relying again on the author's experiences in teaching weight training at the University of Texas in Austin, there are many non-athletic, college-aged men who would find it impossible to perform dips and chins.

[96]Riofrey, *Physical Education*, 76.

[97]"Dr. Grigg's Lecture," *The Ladies' Magazine* 4 (November 1831): 517.

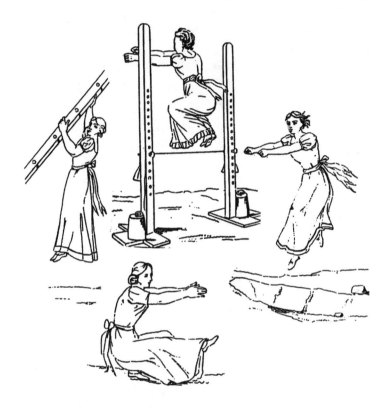

Figure 19: High jumping, long jumping, the one legged squat, and ladder climbing by the strength of the arms alone from *Calisthénie ou Gymnastique des Jeunes Filles*, (1830).

# Chapter 3
# William Fowle's Monitorial School for Girls:
# The First American Gymnastics Experiment

Despite the fact that the United States had declared its independence, early nineteenth-century Americans continued to look to Europe, particularly Great Britain, for ideas about health, fitness, and beauty.[1] Thus it was that at approximately the same time Clias, Völker, and Beaujeu introduced gymnastics to the British Isles, interest in purposive exercise also blossomed in the United States. The transatlantic seeding occurred in several ways.

Current European textbooks were highly prized possessions among America's intellectual elite who liked to feel connected to the educational reforms occurring in Europe. In Boston, for instance, William Bentley Fowle—a man who played a major role in the introduction of purposive exercise to American women—ran a bookstore in the early 1820s described as a "favorite resort for school teachers" that specialized in foreign texts.[2] Furthermore, book reviews of European exercise texts appeared with regularity in such reform-minded United States periodicals as *The Journal of Health* and *The American Journal of Education*, and bookstores other than Fowle's also sold European books.[3] News of the gymnastics revolution underway in Europe also reached America through the trips abroad that many American men made to complete their education. Medical students who could afford it, for example, tried to spend a year or so in Europe, usually in Edinburgh or Paris, to augment their training.[4] Some Americans even visited the German Philanthropic schools, or Amoros's gymnasium in Paris, or Clias's and Völker's gyms in London, and wrote home about what they saw in these new institutions.[5]

Sport historians have traditionally traced the beginning of school physical education in the United States to the introduction of gymnastics at the Round Hill School for Boys in Northampton, Massachusetts, in 1825.[6] Round Hill's claim to originality on this matter, however, appears to be based on rather shaky evidence. For one thing, it seems unlikely that not even one schoolmaster in the United States would have been motivated by the persuasive language of the 1802 American edition of GutsMuths's *Gymnastics for Youth* to experiment with GutsMuths's exercises. While no primary evidence has been found to corroborate this theory, nineteenth-century physical educator Edward

Mussey Hartwell does report in a historical review, published in 1885, that the Latin school at Salem, Massachusetts, had a "sort of gymnasium" as early as 1821. Apparently, Hartwell did not know the name of the person who built the gym and led the exercises.[7]

There is even greater reason to doubt Round Hill's pride of place when one looks at women's physical education in the early nineteenth century. As we saw in Chapter One, there can be little question that some of the female students of Sarah Pierce's Litchfield Academy practiced purposive exercise prior to 1820, even though historians may never know what the girls at Litchfield actually did in their private exercise sessions. We do know, however, that the students at William Bentley Fowle's Boston Monitorial School practiced vigorous gymnastics for a period of time and that Fowle apparently started gymnastics classes for his students before such formal classes began at Round Hill.[8]

In examining the early gymnastics movement in the United States, the present chapter focuses on the Round Hill-Boston Monitorial School controversy. As is the case in many other aspects of women's history, it appears that no previous historian has taken the time to investigate women's involvement in the 1820s American gymnastics movement. Although the Boston Monitorial School is cited by physical education historians for being the first school physical education program for women, new evidence suggests that the Boston Monitorial School should be considered the first bona fide physical education program for either sex. Future histories should credit William Bentley Fowle and his female students as pioneers in the introduction of gymnastics for school use in America.

### Fowle's Monitorial School Experiment

William Bentley Fowle opened the Boston Monitorial School at Washington Court on 14 October 1823 with eight students.[9] Begun as an experiment in Pestalozzian and Lancasterian educational theories, the school "was instituted not only to facilitate the acquisition of knowledge, but to render that acquisition a source of pleasure."[10] Three years later, when Fowle publicly reported the results of his experiment with gymnastics for women, seventy-five students attended the school, ranging in age from four to eighteen.[11]

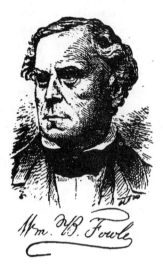

Figure 20: William Bentley Fowle (1795-1865) became headmaster of the Boston Monitorial School in 1823. In 1842, he began working with Horace Mann in the publication of the *Common School Journal* and served as its editor from 1848 to 1852. He published fifty books, sixty written lectures, and more than five hundred magazine and newspaper articles. Illustration from *National Cyclopaedia of American Biography.*

Fowle's only previous teaching experience was when he was hired by the group of citizens who began the Boston Monitorial School.[12] That job, as a teacher of "children of the poorest class in our city," apparently convinced Fowle of two things: (1) that the rigid discipline exerted by many schoolmasters in his era was an "evil tendency" and (2) that young women had as much right to a legitimate education as boys did.[13] Liberal and humane in his approach to schoolmastering, Fowle did not set himself noticeably apart from his students. Terror, Fowle argued, was not a proper tool for a good pedagogue.[14]

Nonetheless, Fowle apparently set high academic standards, and in his 80' x 30' school building provided his scholars with the latest textbooks and scientific apparatus.[15] Women at Fowle's school learned the same subjects as men did in their schools, and women scholars competed openly for advancement and monetary prizes. Unmoved by those who argued that he appealed "too powerfully to the principle of ambition" as an element of education, Fowle countered, "We encourage fair and honorable competition in every possible manner . . ."[16]

Late in the winter of 1825, physician John G. Coffin inspired Fowle to introduce gymnastics to his women students at the Boston Monitorial School. Coffin, who frequently used the pages of his *Boston Medical Intelligencer* to discuss his ideas on hygienic living, announced a three-lecture series on 22 February 1825:

> Dr. J. G. Coffin, of this city, is about to give three lectures on the following subjects: 1st. Physical Education in connection with

intellectual and moral culture as taught and practiced in the recent gymnastic seminaries of Germany, Denmark, Switzerland, France, &c. 2d and 3d. On the means of promoting health and preventing disease.[17]

Coffin was an avid proponent of gymnastics for both sexes and apparently argued in his lecture that the same sorts of exercises used to strengthen boys should also be used to improve the fitness and stamina of women.[18] In a letter to Coffin subsequently printed in the *Boston Medical Intelligencer* and, later, in the *Journal of Education*, Fowle reported that he had "noticed the feeble health of many of my students and encouraged them to take more exercise, but they wanted means and example, and little or nothing was effected."[19] Once he heard Coffin's lecture, Fowle wrote, he immediately implemented Coffin's suggestions regarding women and gymnastics. "The very day after your first lecture," he wrote to Coffin (making it late February or early March), "I procured two or three bars and as many pulleys and after I had explained the manner of using them, my pupils needed no further encouragement to action. The recess was no longer a stupid, inactive season; all were busy and animated."[20]

Coffin and Fowle both had to fight the public's idea that woman's physiology mandated a different degree and type of exercise from those used by men. Coffin contended that women actually needed gymnastics more than men did. Coffin wrote in 1826 that frequently he would be asked whether walking, riding, and domestic work were not better for women than the "queer motions and gesticulations of the gymnasium." "To answer briefly," he continued, "we say no, they are not!"[21] Fowle apparently faced similar opposition from concerned parents as he began to implement gymnastics at the Monitorial School. "My chief difficulty was in the proper exercise for *females*," he wrote to Coffin. "You know the prevailing notions of female delicacy and propriety are at variance with every attempt to render them less feeble and helpless,—and the bugbears of rudeness, romping &c. are sure to stare every such attempt in the face." In fact, Fowle continued, "It seemed as if the sex has been thought unworthy of any effort to improve their physical powers."[22]

Fowle, however, did not think women unworthy. Convinced by Coffin's lecture of the need for purposive exercise, Fowle persevered in his efforts and began to personally participate in the exercises with his students. His participation, he reported to Coffin, did not apparently lessen the students' respect for him or for his orders. In October 1826, he reported,

> I have finally succeeded in contriving apparatus and exercises enough to keep all employed in play [for] hours. Besides the ordinary exercises of raising the arms and feet and extending them in various directions, we have various methods of hanging and swinging by the arms, tilting, raising weights, jumping forward, marching, running, enduring, &c. &c.23

No longer, Fowle explained to Coffin, did he have any "anxiety about procuring suitable exercises, or in sufficient variety, for my pupils; and I believe the few parents whose more prim education led them to slander at my innovation, have surrendered their prejudices."24

Furthermore, Fowle happily reported to Coffin that the exercise regimen he implemented at the Boston Monitorial School caused what he considered to be positive changes in his students. "It may be recorded for the encouragement of others," he wrote, "that many weak and feeble children have at least doubled their strength and now disdain the little indulgences which were then thought necessary to them." He did not, however, lay claim to miracles. "I do not pretend that every dull child has been completely excited, nor that every wild one has been tamed, nor every vicious one reformed, but I do believe that no child has been made worse than she would have become without the exercises, while many, very many, have been essentially benefited."25

Philosophically, Fowle and his program aligned with the vigorous model of womanhood and exercise advocated by Wollstonecraft, Beaujeu, and Clias. Again, writing to Coffin, Fowle reported, "I would not conceal the fact that many hands have been blistered, and perhaps a little hardened by the exercises . . ." He continued, "I have yet to learn that the perfection of female beauty consists in a soft, small, and almost useless hand, any more than in the cramped, diminutive, deformed, and useless feet of the Chinese ladies."26 There was nothing wrong, Fowle argued, with walking and domestic work. He simply did not believe that such exercise alone was enough to produce the sorts of physiological changes women really needed. "I hope," he concluded, that "our young men, in selecting the mothers of their future offspring, will make it one condition of the covenant that they be healthy, strong, capable of enduring fatigue, encountering danger and helping themselves. . ."[27]

## A Question of Primacy

The Round Hill School for Boys opened its doors in two rented houses overlooking the Connecticut River Valley in the fall of 1823. Founded by George Bancroft and Joseph C. Cogswell on Pestalozzian educational theory, Round Hill aimed to educate the whole man—the intellectual and the physical.[28] Bancroft and Cogswell explained their commitment to physical training in the prospectus for their first class. "We would also encourage activity of body as the means of promoting firmness of constitution and vigor of mind," they wrote, "and shall appropriate regularly a portion of each day to healthful sports and gymnastics."[29]

According to historian Bruce Bennett, however, no real gymnastics program began at Round Hill during the first year or so of the school's existence. Not only were Bancroft, Cogswell, and their assistant teacher not qualified to teach gymnastics, Bennett argues, but the surviving student letters and diaries suggest that gymnastics were "quite subordinate to games and sports" in the first several years of Round Hill's life as a school.[30]

Historians who credit Round Hill as America's Plymouth Rock of gymnastics have generally cited Carl Beck's arrival at the school as the precipitating event of the movement.[31] Born in 1798, Beck had been one of the hundreds of boys who trained with Father Jahn at the Hasenhide outside Berlin. Like most Turners, Beck adopted Jahn's politics, as well as his love of exercise, and eventually fled to America to escape political persecution in his homeland.[32] Arriving in Philadelphia with fellow refugee Charles Follen in the fall of 1824, Beck met George Ticknor of Harvard University and, with Ticknor's aid, moved to Northampton to teach Latin and gymnastics at the Round Hill School.[33] Round Hill thus became the first school in the United States to hire a special teacher for physical education or gymnastics.[34]

Beck may have been the first hired physical educator in the United States, but did he actually begin teaching gymnastics prior to William Fowle? Described in student letters as a "splendidly formed and muscular man," Beck began at the Northampton school in the spring term of 1825.[35] Cogswell and Bancroft advertised their new gymnastics program in 1826 and claimed "that we were the first in the new continent to connect gymnastics with a purely literary establishment."[36] Beck

also claimed the preeminence of Round Hill in the preface to his translation of Jahn's *Deutsches Turnkunst*, published in 1828. "The school of
Messrs. Cogswell and Bancroft, in Northhampton, Mass., was the first
institution in this country that introduced gymnastic exercises as part
of the regular instruction, in the spring of 1825."[37] Based on the severity of New England's winters, however, it seems unlikely that Beck
could have begun actively teaching Jahn-style gymnastics before the
late spring or early summer of 1825. The gymnasium at Round Hill
was an outdoor, smaller version of the one at which Beck had trained
in Germany. Obviously, since it took time for the gymnastic apparati to
be built, the snow to melt, and the ground to thaw and dry, logic suggests that Fowle's *indoor* program, which he reportedly instituted the
day after Coffin's lecture, was the first real school gymnastics program
in the United States.[38] An 1826 article in the *Hampshire Gazette*
describing a typical day at Round Hill corroborates this theory. "The
hours from five till seven are designed for exercise and amusement. At
this time the classes in Gymynastics [sic] have their instruction, when
the weather permits."[39] In Massachusetts, before the advent of Daylight
Savings Time, it was still dark at seven until late in spring.

Several nineteenth-century authors, it should be noted, disputed
Round Hill's claims to innovation. Writing in *New England Magazine*
in 1890, Granville B. Putnam argued,

> The claim has been made that to Northhampton should be ascribed
> the honor of being the first to act in this matter, but I am inclined to
> confer the credit upon Boston, although admitting that but a very
> few months could have intervened between the adoption of gymnas-
> tic training by William B. Fowle in his 'Monitorial School for Young
> Ladies,' ... and the famous Round Hill School for boys ...[40]

Earlier, an 1861 biographical sketch of Fowle, which appeared in
Barnard's *American Journal of Education*, had claimed that Fowle introduced "regular and systematic physical exercise" to his students in
1824, noting that it was "the first instance of the kind, probably, in the
United States."[41]

More significantly, a recent find in the archives of the Boston
Public Library suggests that Fowle himself believed he had been the
first to implement gymnastics exercises in New England. The item is an
original 1826 subscription paper printed to raise money for the public
gymnasium in Boston. On the back are three inscriptions. The first
simply reads, "Original Subscription Paper for the first Gymnasium in

Boston—July 1826." On the opposite end and in a different hand is an inscription reading, "To the first Gymnastiarch in Boston, from a friend." Just below, in the same handwriting as the original (apparently Fowle's), is a second and longer handwritten message reading, "The above was written by Dr. Coffin who first called the public attention to Gymnastics by his Essays & Lectures. It is true that I was the first in New England who attempted to put in practice what many had studied theoretically . . . Boston, July 1826"[42] On the front side of this paper, and also written in what is believed to be Fowle's hand, we find that his name has been added to the list of organizers with the notation, "Wm. B. Fowle was afterwards added."[43]

### New England Flips Over Gymnastics 1825–1830

Throughout New England, interest in gymnastics and physical training escalated through the example and influence of men such as Coffin, Fowle, Ticknor, Beck, and Follen. After parting from Beck in Philadelphia, Follen learned English and joined Harvard's faculty in January 1826. Soon thereafter, he introduced the German system to Harvard's students and set up an outdoor gymnasium with the traditional German apparatus.[44] Almost immediately, Follen's efforts attracted attention, and the medical faculty issued a statement recommending the German system to Harvard's students. The elite student body, fascinated by Follen's purposive training system, passed its own resolution expressing readiness to follow his athletic advice.[45] Fired by the good reports of Follen's work at Harvard, a group of prominent Boston citizens proposed building a public gymnasium near the Boston Commons. A delegation of Harvard students encouraged the project, arguing that they had found their short experience with gymnastics to be "highly beneficial . . . the improvement in health has been perceptible . . . the cheerfulness which they produce, and the increased agility which results from them are remarkable."[46]

Two of Follen's first students, Cornelius C. Felton and Edmund Quincy, remembered those heady days with fondness nearly forty years later at the inauguration of another physical culture experiment—the first graduation exercises of Dio Lewis's Normal College in the fall of 1861. Felton, then president of Harvard, recalled the "extraordinary performances we went through . . . The class succeeded so well, that great crowds . . . were accustomed to drive out of Boston and station themselves around the college delta, which was covered with various machines—some of which looked marvelously like the gallows—with which we performed the gymnastic exercises of those times."[47] Quincy recalled that, although men were occasionally injured, he could not think of a single man who would not still attest "that he has derived advantage from the first principles of physical training which we received from the mouth and the example of Dr. Follen."[48] Daniel Webster was one of many prominent New Englanders who delighted in the gymnasium's opening. "I am highly pleased with the idea of a Gymnasium," he reported. "If it is desirable that there should be cultivated intellect, it is equally so, as far as this world is concerned, that there should be a sound body to hold it in."[49]

Charles Follen served as the gymnasium's first director, but in June 1827, he resigned and offered the position to Franz Lieber, another Jahn student and German expatriate. Lieber could not sustain the enthusiasm Follen initiated, however. Although four hundred gym members registered for 1827, only four remained by 1829 when Lieber closed the gym. This decline in gym memberships can partly be explained by Lieber's decision to open a swimming school to which many of the gymnasts turned in their search for novelty.[50] John Quincy Adams, the sixty-one-year-old president, no doubt helped the decline when he dove from the springboard at Lieber's new pool and declared swimming "superior to gymnastic exercise after hard intellectual exertion."[51]

Although the tenure of gymnastics was brief, nearly all the major men's universities and secondary schools adopted some form of German-style gymnastics during the period 1825 to 1830. The University of Virginia, at Thomas Jefferson's request, added the German system to its curriculum in 1824.[52] The New York High School introduced gymnastics during its first year of operation in 1825.[53] Yale began gymnastics in 1826; Amherst started later in the same year; and Brown University, Williams College, and Bowdoin soon followed.[54] The Noyes School at Andover, New Hampshire, offered gymnastics in 1826[55]; the Walnut Grove School at Troy, New York, built a small outdoor gymnasium that same year; and the Mount Pleasant Classical Institution required gymnastics twice a day between 1827 and 1829. The Berkshire High School at Pittsfield, Massachusetts, offered "gymnastics, riding, botanical and mineralogical excursions" in 1828. Utica High School opened in 1827 with an attached gymnasium; while the young Cornelius Felton, after teaching mathematics at Round Hill for a year, opened the Livingston County High School near Genessee, New York, advertising that part of each day would be dedicated to "health, physical vigor and gymnastics."[56] Someboys's schools even used the name "Gymnasium" in their title. Following extensive European travels in which they visited experimental schools and gymnasiums, Sereno and Henry Dwight, sons of Yale president Timothy Dwight, opened the New Haven Gymnasium on 1 May 1828, just a mile from Yale University.[57] In their prospectus, the Dwight brothers explained that "a part of each day is to be regularly devoted to Gymnastic exercises . . . . [which] are the best means of preserving health and invigorating the constitution."[58] L. V. Hubbard's school in Brookline, Massachusetts, was also known as the Brookline Gymnasium.[59]

Although men constituted a majority of the New Englanders involved in gymnastics, there were at least two schools besides Fowle's that advertised gymnastics for women prior to 1830. The coeducational Buffalo High School, modeled after New York High School, advertised in its prospectus that gymnastics would be taught to both the male and female students enrolled in 1828.[60] In Bridgeport, Connecticut, a similar school opened with gymnastics departments for both boys and girls.[61] Sadly, no documentation seems to have survived that could illuminate the nature of the gymnastics programs at these schools.

Organized gymnastics programs for men also developed in cities other than Boston during those years. Public and private gymnasiums opened throughout New England as the number of prominent individuals advocating gymnastics and other forms of purposive exercise continued to increase. In his letters home from England, John Neal had urged Americans to build gyms, even reporting in one letter that he had written to President Thomas Jefferson on the subject, offering to send a trained gymnastics teacher to the States, "recommended by Völker himself."[62] In 1827, when Neal returned to Portland, Maine, he opened a gym there that quickly had fifteen to twenty full classes of gymnasts. Subsequently, he opened gyms at Brunswick and Saco, Maine.[63] A gymnasium also operated in Philadelphia during those early years. Mr. Roper's Gymnasium received high praise in an 1830 issue of the *Journal of Health* followed by the reassurance that the dyspeptic will find there "every variety of contrivance" needed to regain health. The *Journal's* editor wrote, "Mr. Roper avails of, and copies from Salzmann, Jahn, Clias, and other approved gymnics, but although his is the only establishment of the kind in the city, he does not pretend, like other characters of much less merit and usefulness, to have a new and patent method, peculiar to himself, of giving strength and curing diseases."[64] Business was apparently good for Roper. In 1831, he opened a school for calisthenics at his gymnasium and employed his wife to oversee classes for women.[65]

## A Change in Sentiment:
### The Decline of Gymnastics for Women

Though Fowle, Coffin, and many of their peers believed women to be capable of more than light exercise, domestic work, and dancing, there remained a strong bias against the sorts of vigorous exercise Fowle advocated. While it is not clear just when Fowle eventually gave in to the expressed concerns of some of his students' parents and discontinued his vigorous program, it does not appear that his gymnastics experiment lasted more than a couple of years.[66] Fowle's capitulation to more conventional attitudes regarding woman's appropriate behavior and physical capabilities was symptomatic of a widespread reassessment of appropriate women's exercise. By the early 1830s, the tide carrying the vigorous exercises recommended by Beaujeu, Clias, and Fowle had ebbed for women. It was replaced by a building wave of enthusiasm for the lighter, and supposedly more feminine, exercise system known as calisthenics. Fowle's hope that "the day is not far distant when gymnasiums for women will be as common as churches in Boston" was not to be realized in his lifetime.[67] Nonetheless, Fowle maintained a lifelong commitment to health and exercise.[68] We can hope that he found some solace in the fact that his experiments at the Boston Monitorial School encouraged a few women to discover the benefits of strength, vigor, and endurance, and in the further fact that there were at least a few other people willing to promote gymnastics for women within New England at that time.[69] Perhaps Fowle would have been pleased to know that about 175 years later he is at last receiving credit for his trailblazing efforts on behalf of women and purposive exercise and that, while still not as common as churches, there is at last no shortage of women's gymnasiums in Boston.

[1]See Granville B. Putnam, "The Introduction of Gymnastics in New England," *New England Magazine* 3 (September 1890): 111-13, for a discussion of the transference of ideas about gymnastics from Europe to America. See also Nancy Struna, "Puritans and Sport, The Irretrievable Tide of Change, *Journal of Sport History* 4 (Spring 1977): 15-30; and William B. Walker, "The Health Reform Movement in the United States: 1830–1870" (Ph.D. diss., Johns Hopkins University, 1955).

[2]Fowle took over Caleb Bingham's bookstore at 44 Cornhill in April 1817. "William Bentley Fowle," *The American Journal of Education* 10 (June 1861): 603; and *National Cyclopedia of American Biography: Being the History of the United States as Illustrated in the Lives of the Founders, Builders, and Defenders of the Republic, and of the Men and Women who are Doing the Work and Moulding the Thought of the Present Time,* vol. 10 (New York: James T. White, 1909), 124.

[3]For examples of articles in American magazines about European gymnastic developments, see [John Neal], "London Gymnastic Institution," *American Journal of Education 1* (October 1826): 79-80; "Prospectus of the London Gymnastic Society," *American Journal of Education* 1 (August 1826): 502-503; John Neal, "Gymnastic Schools in England," *American Journal of Education* 2 (January 1827): 55-56; "Col. Amoros' Gymnastic School, Paris," *American Journal of Education* 1 (November 1826): 689-90; etc.

[4]Although American medical training in the latter half of the eighteenth century was unregulated and generally based on the apprenticeship or pre-ceptorial system, its knowledge base reflected that of Europe, particularly Scotland and Britain. For information on American medical education, see William D. Postell, "Medical Education and Medical Schools in Colonial America," *History of American Medicine: A Symposium* (New York: MD Publications, 1958): 48-54; William Frederick Norwood, "Medicine in the Era of the American Revolution," *History of American Medicine: A Symposium* (New York: MD Publications, 1958): 55-71; and William G. Rothstein, *American Physicians in the Nineteenth Century: From Sects to Science* (Baltimore: John Hopkins University Press, 1972), 26-38.

[5]Putnam, "The Introduction of Gymnastics in New England," 111-13.

[6]Betty Spears and Richard Swanson, *History of Sport and Physical Activity in the United States* (Dubuque, IA: William C. Brown, 1978), 80-81; Fred Eugene Leonard, *A Guide to the History of Physical Education,* 2nd ed. R. Tait McKenzie, ed. (Philadelphia: Lea and Febiger, 1927), 234-35; Deobold Van Dalen, Elmer Mitchell, and Bruce Bennett, *A World History of Physical Education* (Englewood Cliffs, NJ: Prentice Hall, 1963), 369; Emmett A. Rice, *A Brief History of Physical Education* (New York: A. S. Barnes and Co., 1927), 153.

[7]E. M. Hartwell, *Physical Training in American Colleges and Universities: A Report to the Bureau of Education* (n. p., 1885), 22.

[8]There are conflicting reports as to the proper name of Fowle's school. *The American Journal of Education* refers to it as the Boston Monitorial School in its several-part report on Fowle's educational experiment. See William Bentley Fowle, "Boston Monitorial School: Report to the Trustees, 23 December 1825," *American Journal of Education* 1 (January 1826): 29-42; and William Bentley Fowle, "Boston Monitorial School: Report to the Trustees, 23 December 1825," *American Journal of Education* 1 (February 1826): 72-80, 160-66. In a sketch of Fowle's life, however, it is referred to as

the Female Monitorial School. "Fowle," *Journal of Education,* 603. The *National Cyclopedia of American Biography,* 124. No catalog of the school could be found.

[9]Fowle, "Boston Monitorial School (February 1926): 165.

[10]Fowle, "Boston Monitorial School (December 1825): 29.

For insight into Pestalozzi's contributions to physical education, see Hans Ballin, "Johann Heinrich Pestalozzi," *Mind and Body* 2 (February 1896): 221-27. For information on Pestalozzian theory in America, especially its influence on Horace Mann, see Merle Curti, *Social Ideas of American Educators* (Totowa, NJ: Littlefield, Adams & Co., 1966), 29-30, 65-66, 123-24.

[11]Fowle, "Boston Monitorial School," 1 (February 1826): 164. In later years the school had more than one hundred students. Leonard, "First Introduction of Jahn Gymnastics," 314; and "Fowle," *Journal of Education,* 603.

[12]Details of the beginnings of the Monitorial School may be found in Fowle, "Boston Monitorial School," (February 1826): 164-65.

[13]Ibid., 74.

[14]Fowle, "Boston Monitorial School," 1 (January 1826): 40-41.

[15]Ibid., 165.

[16]Ibid., 76.

[17]"Notice," *Medical Intelligencer* 2 (22 February 1825): 168. The 1825 lectures were actually Coffin's second series of lectures on exercise. On 19 January 1820, Coffin advertised in the *Columbian Centinel,* a Boston newspaper that he would "begin a short series of lectures on Physical Education." Quoted in Walker, "The Health Reform Movement in the United States," 103.

[18]*Boston Medical Intelligencer* 5 (24 October 1826): 197. Information on Coffin's contributions may also be found in Edward Mussey Hartwell, *School Document No. 22: Report of the Director of Physical Training, December 1891* (Boston: Rockwell and Churchill, 1891): 12-13.

[19]Fowle, "Gymnastic* Exercise for Females," *American Journal of Education* 1 (November 1826): 698; Willam B. Fowle, "The Animal Mechanism and Economy," Boston *Medical Intelligencer* 5 (24 October 1826): 196-97.

The asterisk (*) related to a note by *Journal* editor J. G. Coffin that reads, "Would it not be well to avoid a term, the etymology of which renders it now so inapplicable, and to designate this department of the physical education, of females at least—by the phrase *hygeian exercise? Names,* it is true, are not commonly of very great importance. But the *fact* is that the term gymnastic is connected with an idea of coarseness, which in the early stage of the progress of this branch of education, might create a prejudice against it."

[20]Ibid.

[21]J. G. Coffin, "Intelligence, " *American Journal of Education* 1 (November 1826): 699.

[22]Fowle, "Gymnastic* Exercise for Females," 698.

[23]Ibid.

[24]Ibid.

[25]Ibid.

[26]Ibid.

[27]Ibid., 699.

[28]Joseph C. Cogswell and George Bancroft, *Prospectus for a School to be Established at Round Hill, Northampton, Massachusetts* (Cambridge: by the authors, 1823): 3. By 1827, Round Hill's high watermark, 135 boys attended the school (representing eighteen different states), and it employed ten faculty members.

Other sources of information on Round Hill School include John S. Bassett, "The Round Hill School," *American Antiquarian Society Proceedings, Part One* 27 (April 1917): 18-62; George E. Ellis, "Recollections of Round Hill School," *Educational Review* 1 (April 1891): 337-44; "Round Hill School," *American Journal of Education* 1 (July 1826): 437-39; George Shattuck, "Centenary of Round Hill School," *Proceedings of the Massachusetts Historical Society* 57 (December 1923): 205-209; Leonard, *Guide*, 233-35; and Ellen Gerber, *Innovators and Institutions in Physical Education* (Philadelphia: Lea and Febiger, 1971), 245-51. Fred Eugene Leonard also authored a six-part series entitled "The First Introduction of the Jahn Gymnastics into America, 1825–1830," *Mind and Body* 12 (September, October, November, December, January, February, 1905 and 1906).

[29]Cogswell and Bancroft, *Prospectus*, 17. Student letters indicate that approximately three hours each day were set aside for activity. Shattuck, "Centenary," 207.

[30]Bruce L. Bennett, "The Making of Round Hill School," *Quest* 4 (1963–1965): 58-59.

[31]See, for instance, Leonard, A Guide, 234-35; Spears and Swanson, *History of Sport and Physical Activity*, 80-81; Van Dalen, Mitchell, and Bennett, *World History*, 369; Rice, *Brief History of Physical Education*, 153.

[32]Leonard, *Guide*, 227-32. Biographies of Beck and fellow refugee Charles Follen may also be found in Fred Eugene Leonard, "The First Introduction of the Jahn Gymnastics into America, 1825–1830," *Mind and Body* 12 (September 1905): 193-98. See also Henry Metzner, *A Brief History of the North American Gymnastic Union: In Commemoration of the One Hundredth Anniversary of the Opening of the First Gymnastic Field in Germany by Friedrich Ludwig Jahn* (Indianapolis: National Executive Committee of the North American Gymnastic Union, 1911).

[33]Ticknor, who had studied at Gottingen, Germany, following his undergraduate work at Harvard, was well aware of the German gymnastics movement and its political overtones. Nonetheless, he apparently felt an immediate kinship with these refugees who had left their homeland to escape political oppression and decided to help them. He later helped Follen get a job at Harvard. George Ticknor, *Life, Letters, and Journals of George*

*Ticknor,* vol. 1 (Boston: Harper & Wells, 1876) 351. Ticknor lived in Germany from 1815–1817.

[34]Bennett, "Making of Round Hill," 54-55.

[35]Ibid., 59.

[36]Quoted in Gerber, *Innovators,* 247.

[37]Beck, Charles, *A Treating [sic] on Gymnastics Taken Chiefly from the German of F. L. Jahn* (Northampton, Simeon Butler, 1828), 3. Based on his work at Round Hill, and his American audience, Beck significantly altered the work of Jahn, omitting several chapters and including a chapter on dumbbells, an implement Americans were apparently quite familiar with by this time. According to an advertisement in *The American Journal of Education,* he sold the book by subscription for $1.75. "Treatise on Gymnastics," *The American Journal of Education* 2 (October 1827): 629-30.

[38]Fowle, "Gymnastic* Exercise for Females," 698.

[39]*Hampshire Gazette,* quoted in "Round Hill School," 439.

[40]Putnam, "The Introduction of Gymnastics," 111.

[41]"William Bentley Fowle," 608.

[42]"Gymnasium," broadside dated 26 June 1826, William B. Fowle File, Rare Books and Manuscripts, Boston Public Library, Boston MA.

[43]Ibid.

[44]E. L. Follen, *The Life of Charles Follen* (Boston: Thomas H. Webb and Co., 1844), 104-105.

[45]Leonard, *Guide,* 240.

[46]"Letter of the Deputation of the University to the Chairman of the Committee on the subject of establishing a Gymnasium in Boston," *American Journal of Education* 1 (July 1826): 444-45.

[47]"Commencement Exercises at the Normal Institute for Physical Education," *Lewis's New Gymnastics for Ladies, Gentlemen and Children and Boston Journal of Physical Culture* 1 (October 1861): 178.

[48]Ibid., 179.

[49]Paton Stewart, Jr., *Warren's Recommendation of Gymnastics* (Boston: n.p., 1856), 4. Quoted in John R. Betts, "Mind and Body in Early American Thought," *Journal of American History* 54 (1968): 794.

[50]Leiber's swimming school was quite successful and continued in operation for many years under the name Braman's Baths. "The First Boston Gymnasium," *Mind and Body* 6 (January 1900): 252-52.

[51]Betts, "Mind and Body," 794-95.

[52]Ibid., 793.

[53]"Course of Education in the New York High School," *The American Journal of Education* 1 (January 1826): 28.

[54]Leonard, "First Introduction, Part VI," 12 (February, 1906): 345-47. Dudley Allen Sargent claimed in a 1903 speech to the students of Springfield College in Massachusetts that schools in Maryland, South Carolina, and Mississippi also introduced gymnastics into their curricula. D. A. Sargent,

"The Achievements of the Century in Gymnastics and Athletics: Together With Notes and Questions," ts, Rare Books Room, Babson Library, Springfield College, Springfield MA.

[55] *American Journal of Education* 1 (June 1826): 378-79.

[56] Leonard, "First Introduction, Part V" 12 (January 1906): 315-16. See also Ralph Billett, "Evidence of Play and Exercise in Early Pestalozzian and Lancasterian Elementary Schools in the United States, 1809–1845," *Research Quarterly* 23 (1952): 127-35. Felton later became president of Harvard University and was a patron of Dio Lewis' Boston school.

[57] "Prospectus for the New Haven Gymnasium; A School for the Education of Boys, to be established at New Haven, Conn.; by Sereno E. Dwight and Henry E. Dwight," *American Journal of Education* 3 (February 1828): 115-16.

[58] Ibid., 115.

[59] L. V. Hubbard, "Brookline Gymnasium," *American Journal of Education* 3 (April 1828): 231-33.

[60] "Buffalo High School," *American Annals of Education and Instruction* 3 (April 1828): 233-35.

[61] Billett, "Play and Exercise," 134.

[62] "Gymnasium" *The American Journal of Education* 1 (January 1826): 61; "Gymnastic Exercises in London," *The American Journal of Education* 1 (June 1826): 375.

[63] John Neal, *Wandering Recollections of a Somewhat Busy Life: An Autobiography* (Boston: Roberts Brothers, 1869), 333-35.

[64] "Flannels—Dyspepsy—Gymnasium," *The Journal of Health* 2 (8 December 1830): 111.

[65] "Calisthenics," *The Journal of Health* 2 (23 February 1831): 193. In the 1850s, a James Roper opened a gym in New Orleans. Whether he was the same man is not known. *Crescent City Business Directory. Commerce of the City of New Orleans for the Year Ending 1857–1858* (n.p., n.d.).

[66] Leonard, "First Introduction of Jahn Gymnastics," V: 315.

[67] Putnam, "Introduction," 111.

[68] See, for instance, W. B. F. [William B. Fowle], "Health of Teachers," *The Common School Journal* 10 (1 August 1848): 234-37; and W. B. F. [William B. Fowle], "Physical Exercise," *The Common School Journal* 10 (1 September 1848): 266-68.

[69] Fowle continued to influence physical education in New England. Besides serving as the treasurer and chief executive officer for the building of the German-style pubic gymnasium in Boston, he also helped introduce the "lyceum lecture" to Bostonians, a lecture format that proved popular with health and physiology experts for the next several decades. In 1842, he took over the editorship of the *Common School Journal* and began to work closely with Horace Mann, assisting him in holding Teacher's Institutes throughout Massachusetts and other parts of New England. "William Bentley Fowle," 603-609.

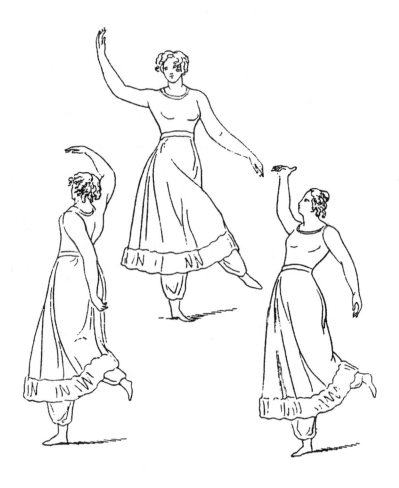

Figure 21: The perfect exercise for "ladies"—freehand calisthenics from G. P. Voarino's *A Second Course of Calisthenic Exercises* (1828).

# Chapter 4
# The Literature of Calisthenics

An arm swollen by physical exertion, a face suffused with the flush of violent effort, may be very becoming in a gentleman; but should we transfer them to a lady they would excite disgust rather than admiration.[1]

An 1827 reviewer of calisthenics books argued that two things were essential to the female character: decorum and grace. A woman's exercise "must strictly avoid collision with these," the reviewer warned, for gracefulness is nearly as important as a woman's health. Although granting that women needed some exercise, the author cautioned his readers that only those movements that fell within the boundaries of propriety and delicacy could safely be encouraged. "We . . . seldom make use of the triangle," he wrote, explaining that it created too much arm strength and caused the body to move "violently." "The greatest part of the exercises," the anonymous reviewer continued, "should consist of leg movements done while standing in one spot, a few balancing exercises, and those simple movements that help with graceful walking."[2] The pace should be slow and gradual, he explained, "because the female frame is more tender and delicate."[3]

Jean Jacques Rousseau would have smiled had he been able to read these sentiments in the *American Journal of Education*. In the late 1820s, this reviewer—and a significant number of other antebellum men and women—began to advocate the sort of distinct separation between men's and women's purposive exercise Rousseau had favored. Whether they resulted from German-style gymnastics, military drill, or the hard work of manual labor, the products of men's exercise were understood to be strength, vigor, and health. For women, Rousseau's spiritual descendants argued that the goals of exercise should be health and grace, a term nineteenth-century Americans used to describe physical attractiveness as well as easy movement.

Where Beaujeu and Fowle had argued for utilitarian robustness, the devotees of calisthenics favored a more ethereal model of beauty and fitness. Calisthenics proponents also generally adhered to the new, upper-class cult of femininity and embraced the idea that women should be slender, willowy, and pliant. Although calisthenics authors did not go so far as to argue that women should be frail, their strict adherence to the limited, decorous movements that came to be defined as calisthenics did not provide enough physical stimulation to produce significant changes in the fitness of women. Such exercises would produce none of the traditional aspects of fitness—strength, flexibility, and endurance. Sedate, constrained, and unexuberant, the calisthenics exercises of the antebellum era appear to modern readers to be almost a parody of exercise. The dance-like movements elicited no problems of decorum, however. No woman performing calisthenics needed to worry that her exercises appeared unfeminine, or that the routine would produce *too much* strength in her body.

Despite the many experts who continued to advocate more vigorous movements for women, calisthenics proliferated throughout England and America in the first two-thirds of the century and became the dominant form of school exercise. During these decades, the term *calisthenics* carried several meanings. Clias, for instance, used the word as the title for his women's exercise book, yet a significant part of his system consisted of vigorous gymnastics movements. Other early exercise books used the word as a catch-all phrase to describe any sort of exercise program aimed at women. After 1830, however, the term was most commonly used to refer to freehand, light, rhythmic drills performed almost exclusively by women and young girls. In some instances, handheld implements such as dumbbells and Indian clubs were used in calisthenics drills, but stationary apparati such as chinning bars and dipping stations were largely taboo. In this book, the criterion used to differentiate between calisthenics texts and gymnastics books was not whether the words *calisthenics* and *gymnastics* were used as they are in the late twentieth century but, rather, whether the book's primary philosophical focus favored light, nonstrenuous movements or the more demanding exertions of vigorous exercise. Even so, "calisthenics" meant different things to different people.

As was the case with the gymnastics movement, the first treatises describing calisthenics exercise for women appeared in Europe—primarily in England. In 1831, however, *A Course of Calisthenics for Young Ladies in Schools and Families* was published simultaneously in Hartford, Boston, New York, and Philadelphia, an event that rapidly accelerated the spread of this latest European exercise fad.

### Gymnastics for Men, Calisthenics for Women
### The Separation Begins

Professor Gustavus Hamilton is a forgotten figure in physical education history, yet his 1827 *Elements of Gymnastics for Boys and*

*Calisthenics for Young Ladies* may well have signaled the beginning of the antebellum era's formal separation of men's and women's purposive exercise. Heavily influenced by Rousseau's appeal for gender-based exercise, Hamilton, like Clias and Völker, opened a gymnasium in London in the mid-1820s. Unlike his competitors, however, Hamilton argued that women's exercise should consist only of simple, freehand calisthenics movements.[4]

Hamilton's rival in 1820s London was Signor G. P. Voarino, who released what appears to be the first English-language book dealing solely with exercise for women. *A Treatise on Calisthenic Exercises, Arranged for the Private Tuition of Young Ladies* was a short book, containing sixty-seven pages and nine illustrative plates.[5] Although he did not dedicate much space to his rationale, Voarino did take enough space to argue that his book contained "the most efficacious system hitherto invented" for women.[6] Like Clias, with whom he taught at several of the Royal Military schools, Voarino viewed exercise as a remedial therapeutic and as a means by which "the foundations of health and vigor" could be laid in young women.[7] Equally important, he believed, was his system's capacity to enhance the appearance of the women who performed his exercises. Performing calisthenics, he argued, would counteract "every tendency to deformity" and correct any flaws in a woman's figure.

The length and nature of Voarino's association with Clias is not known. Following Clias's return to Switzerland, however, Voarino attempted to create a niche for himself in London society by specializing in women's exercise. It does not appear that Voarino ran a gymnasium, *per se*, but he gave private lessons and worked with schools and claimed that his system was used in the most respectable women's seminaries in the greater London area.[8] He also suggested to those readers of his first book who wished to take classes in calisthenics that they contact his pupil, Miss Mason, who taught every Saturday morning.[9]

Although clearly influenced by Clias, Voarino did not embrace the more vigorous aspects of the Swiss gymnastiarch's philosophy regarding women's exercise.[10] Voarino warned that some exercises did not render women more physically appealing but, rather, were likely to produce injuries and create ungraceful attitudes.[11] Like Clias, he suggested using the triangle to enhance upper body strength, but in Voarino's exercises the feet of the women never left the floor, a fact that considerably decreased the strength-enhancing properties of triangle training.

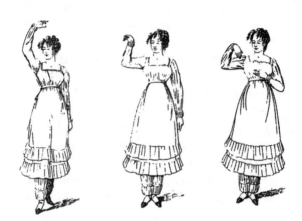

Figure 22: Elementary upper extremity exercises from Signor G. P. Voarino's
*A Treatise on Calisthenic Exercises* (1827).

Voarino opened *A Treatise on Calisthenic Exercises* with thirteen arm and shoulder exercises that primarily consisted of extension movements and arm circles without apparatus. The most vigorous of this first series is the last, shown in Figure 23, in which a small hop in place is performed as the women swing their arms overhead and change foot positions.[12]

Following these thirteen upper extremity exercises, Voarino described eleven "elementary"—and relatively nonstrenuous—exer-

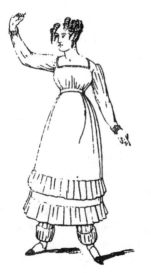

Figure 23: To perform Voarino's most difficult elementary exercise, a woman placed her heels in line, then took a small step forward on the right leg raising the right arm above the head. Returning the right arm to her side, a small skip was then taken to change feet, the left leg then being forward as the left arm is raised above the head. Illustration from: G. P. Voarino's *A Treatise on Calesthenic Exercises* (1827).

cises for the lower body. Voarino advised women to march in place, raising their knees as high as possible "without changing the position of the body."[13] The other exercises in this series consisted of leg extensions to the front, rear, and the side, as well as several "zigzag" exercises in which one leg crossed in front of the other as the exerciser either marched in place or took small skips from side to side.[14] The most strenuous exercise of this series is a deep-knee bend performed while standing on tiptoe.[15]

Keeping with the nomenclature of his era, Voarino then described "complicated exercises" that involved the simultaneous movement of the arms and legs. Thirteen of Voarino's more advanced exercises were, again, to be done in place, such as Exercise One:

> She must bring the right arm stretched forward on a line with the shoulders, bending the right knee in raising the heel; the same movement is to be made backward, bringing the heel to the ground, the right hand to be placed on the chest, and the left arm is to perform the same exercise as the right; then the right and left alternately, and afterwards both at once.[16]

Following this initial series of complicated exercises, Voarino described an additional thirteen complicated exercises in which small steps punctuated the arm movements.[17]

Voarino recommended only one piece of apparatus other than the triangle in his first book: a wooden cane. For this wooden implement, Voarino described twenty-one exercises that varied only slightly from his freehand movements. Although the women are holding an implement in their hands, there is no sense in Voarino's language or in the illustrations that cane exercises were particularly strenuous. Like Nicholas Andry in the eighteenth century, Voarino recommended the cane exercises to increase flexibility in the shoulders, chest, and neck, and to impart to them, according to Voarino, "a graceful firmness and elasticity."[18]

The only section of Voarino's work that might be described as at all vigorous is his final chapter describing eight triangle exercises.[19] Holding on to the trapeze-like handle, Voarino's pupils squat partly down, for instance, or lean forward, or run in circles, or perform modified chins in which their feet never leave the ground.[20] Voarino later claimed that this series of exercises produced suppleness and sufficient vigor for whatever physical demands may be placed on the female body.

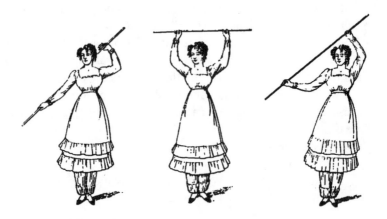

Figure 24: Exercises using wooden canes from: Signor G. P. Voarino's *A Treatise on Calisthenic Exercises* (1827).

Encouraged by the success of his first book, the following year Voarino published *A Second Course of Calisthenic Exercises; With A Course of Private Gymnastics for Gentlemen.*[21] In the book's dedication to the Duchess of Clarence, Voarino explained that his calisthenics system paid the strictest attention to decorum, "to remove the objections of the most delicate or fastidious." Those who followed his method, he explained, again, will find "that elasticity and grace which give an indescribable charm to the female form and carriage."[22]

Although Voarino included a brief chapter discussing the relative merits of exercise for women, there was little new material in his sec-

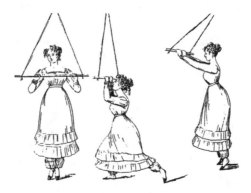

Figure 25: Triangle exercises from Signor G. P. Voarino's, *A Treatise on Calisthenic Exercises* (1827).

ond book. The only real innovation was Voarino's introduction of a series of exercises to be done with a large hoop. Used as the bamboo wands had been—to increase flexibility in the shoulders—Voarino specified that hoops should be equal in diameter to the length of a woman's arm. To protect the hands from calluses, he suggested padding the one-inch-thick wooden circles with cotton and wrapping them with a ribbon.[23]

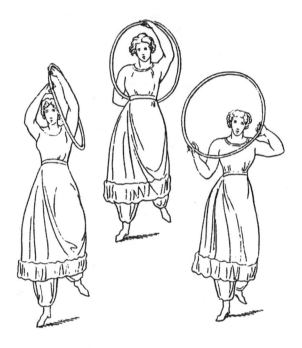

Figure 26: Hoop exercises from Signor G. P. Voarino's *A Second Course of Calisthenic Exercises* (1828).

Voarino argued that exercise strengthened women by improving their circulation and thereby freeing their bodies of impurities.[24] Even if his exercises were performed rapidly and for a large number of repetitions, however, it is unlikely that they created significant cardio-vascular improvements by modern standards because the exercises were relatively stationary and required little exertion. While they undoubtedly aided in shoulder and arm flexibility, his exercises appear to have done little to increase flexibility in other parts of the body. Furthermore, despite the claims of an 1831 American reviewer that Voarino's exercises "are very well calculated to give strength, not only to the arms and shoulders, but also the back," there is little evidence from his books to suggest that any significant strength improvements could occur by performing the exercises as described in his text.[25]

Although Voarino's work represented a serious retrenchment in the physical education community's stance on woman's potential, his views were not nearly as conservative as those of exercise doyen Donald Walker, who, in the 1830s, led women's exercise to even less physically demanding levels. Enraptured by the new upper-class cult of femininity, Walker's vision of woman's physical needs and her physical potential cast a pall over the expansion of women's physical education for many years to come.

## Donald Walker's *Exercises For Ladies*

Donald Walker rose to prominence as an expert on physical training with the publication of an extremely successful book, *British Manly Exercises*.[26] Although *Tom Brown's School Days*, published later in the century, was more influential in the field of competitive sports, *Walker's Manly Exercises* was undoubtedly the most influential book on purposive exercise published in England during the nineteenth century.[27] Written for the upper classes, Walker's book served as well as a guide to appropriate, gentlemanly behavior as to appropriate exercise. When Walker published a companion volume in 1835, *Exercises for Ladies*, it received close attention from the upper classes. It also served as a guidebook to those women aspiring *to* the upper classes.[28] Page after page of endorsements appear in the second edition of *Exercises for Ladies*, all uniformly praising Walker for defining a system that would enable a woman to become an "ornament to her sex, an honour to her race, and a fine specimen of British woman."[29]

Besides its insistence on decorous, less strenuous movements, *Exercises for Ladies* strongly emphasized the aesthetic value of exercise. Although Walker briefly examined the issues of health and reproductive capacity, he placed far more emphasis in his text on physical appearance, arguing that "few young women are exempt from some degree of deformity."[30] Although the deformity in many cases was "*embonpoint*," or obesity, Walker also paid serious attention to spinal and postural malformations that resulted from what he described as "one-sidedness." Too many tasks, he argued, used only one arm or caused the body to bend to the side. Exercise that "requires an equal and similar use of the other side," he explained, could relieve such problems. He cautioned, however, that these corrective movements must not require more strength than women *already* possessed, must not cause any sort of inconvenience, and must preserve beauty and grace.[31] As prominent British physician George Birkbeck observed in a letter to Walker, it was not enough for exercises to create physical improvements in women. The movements themselves must also be "attractive," or else women would not want to perform them. [32]

*Exercises for Ladies* contained few athletic surprises, except for Walker's introduction of a new piece of apparatus—the Indian scepter, a smaller and more ornamental version of the larger Indian clubs already being used by the British military. Walker insisted that scepter exercises were the "most useful and beautiful" exercises ever introduced into physical education and that they had "vast advantages over the dumbbells."[33] Walker further claimed that his text marked the first time this apparatus had been described in any book, although it is not clear whether Walker means Indian clubs or only the smaller Indian scepters.[34]

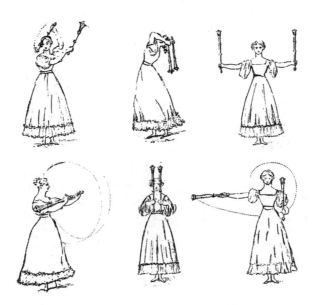

Figure: 27: A sampler of Indian sceptre exercises from the second edition of Donald Walker's *Exercises for Ladies* (1835).

Used to train the upper body, Walker's Indian scepters measured approximately twenty-four inches in length, had a smaller handle for ease in holding, and had lead inserted in the knob on the larger end to make them precise in weight. For women, Walker argued that scepters should weigh either one, one and a half, or two pounds.[35] With the implements, women performed many of the same sorts of limb extensions and chest expansions Voarino recommended, as well as swinging movements requiring slightly greater vigor. Many of the published endorsements Walker included in his book praise the "beautiful," "amusing," and "novel" Indian exercises.[36]

In addition to the Indian scepter exercises, Walker's 288-page text included simple limb extensions and "Spanish Exercises" using a three- to four-foot inflexible rod or cane. He also included a section on dumbbell training, noting that dumbbells had been used in Great Britain for some time, even in "school-exercise for the instruction of ladies."[37] He suggested that girls between the ages of six and ten should use dumbbells weighing three to four pounds, while older female students needed dumbbells weighing four to six pounds.[38]

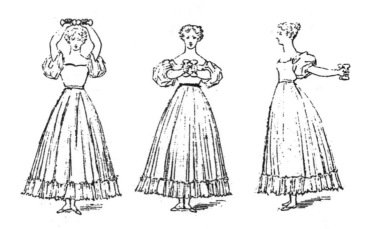

Figure 28: Dumbell exercises from the second edition of Donald Walker's *Exercises for Ladies* (1835).

For the lower body, Walker understandably preferred his namesake. "Of all exercises, walking is the most simple and easy," he wrote, nonetheless suggesting that there must be decorous limits to the method of walking employed for exercise. A lady should never take a step longer than the length of her foot, he contended, and the pace should at all times be natural—even tranquil—with no appearance of hurrying. "Nothing can be more ridiculous," he asserted, "than a little woman, who takes innumerable minute steps with great rapidity, to get on with greater speed, except it be a tall woman, who throws out long legs as though she would dispute the road with the horses."[39] Walker did not consider either running or leaping "congenial" activities for women, cautioning his readers against the propensity of these activities to shock the reproductive organs and appear unattractive.[40]

There were two other forms of exercise that Walker felt merited adoption for women: dancing and what he called the "Gymnastique de Tronchin," or light housework. Dance, he told readers, was "the most suitable to females," as it contributed greatly to the improvement of the figure and, when habitually practiced, increased the strength, suppleness, and agility of the body. Walker also saw medicinal reasons for young women to dance. "It is particularly suited to females in whom ennui and inaction have produced habitual indisposition," he wrote.[41] Walker warned, however, that too much dance would unbalance the body and create so much muscle in the lower limbs that they would become out of proportion to the upper body. To maintain symmetry, Walker argued, women should practice his Indian scepter exercises.[42]

"The Gymnastique De Tronchin," according to Walker, was especially useful for women of the "middling condition," who would find in "useful occupations" both the amelioration of their physical problems and a cure for their mental agitations, troubled sensibilities, and nervous irregularities.[43] Tronchin, architect of this new scheme to call housework exercise, was a "philosophical physician" who had persuaded women on the Continent that luxury and sedentary living were the principal causes of women's nervousness and disease.[44] Though the foregoing statement sounds positive, Walker quickly qualified his remark by warning that there were definite limits to the degree of work that could be considered ameliorative. Domestic work must be restrained, he explained, just as a woman's walking gait should be. Her household activities must never require violent or difficult movements. Walker maintained that it was "a matter of disgust to see women, in our large towns, bending like the savages in America under the weight of burthens, or gaining a livelihood by the most toilsome labours . . ."[45] He wished to limit his "ladies" to the relatively sedentary tasks of needlework, cooking, millinery, dressmaking, haberdashery, hairdressing, and child care.[46] Cleaning, laundry, and wood chopping—household labors that might have provided some useful exercise—were apparently to be left to the servants, who, though also female, did not require exercise advice from Walker.

*Exercises for Ladies* reinforced the growing social bifurcation of women's activities. By suggesting that certain tasks were beneath "ladies," Walker strongly reinforced the cult of true womanhood's belief that hard work should be delegated to women and men of the lower classes. For the record, however, the activities in Walker's "Gymnastique de Tronchin" were even less energetic than the notions regarding domestic exercise then prevalent in America. For one thing, Walker's domestic suggestions all related to indoor activities, most of which could be done while seated. Furthermore, Walker's "Gymnastique de Tronchin" cannot be truly classified as "exercise" if we continue to work with a definition that includes as one of its conditions that exercise movements should increase respiration. Needlework and hat making may be necessary activities, but they are not purposive exercise. However, Walker's reputation as an expert on physical training made his book extremely influential. If contemporary reports can be believed, many people on both sides of the Atlantic took his restrained approach to women's exercise all too seriously.

### Bureaud Riofrey: Utilitarian Fitness

One person who objected to Walker's approach was French physician Bureaud Riofrey. In *Physical Education Especially Adapted to Young Ladies*, published in an English language edition in 1838, Riofrey argued that women's exercise "should not be reduced to mere mechanical movements of going backward and forward with a wand, or Indian scepter."[47] Walker's system, Riofrey maintained, simply consisted of "raising and bending the arms like puppets."[48] However, Riofrey cautioned, the vigorous gymnastics favored by Clias and Beaujeu were also unsuitable for women. It was inappropriate to train "like the Greeks," Riofrey wrote, when men and women no longer lived like the Greeks.[49] As he put it, "The gymnastics we recommend cannot be compared to those practiced in Lacedemonia, where young girls wrestled in public, and swam across the Eurotas; neither are they similar to those of Clias."[50] Riofrey claimed that his system was a compromise between these extremes and that it would create utilitarian fitness in women. His exercises would not produce too much muscle, he contended, yet they were sufficient to make women more attractive, less fearful, and more physically competent.[51] "A young lady may, during ten years, learn to move the Indian scepter, and would feel timid and awkward going up a ladder," he explained. Physical education's goal, he argued, should be to prepare women, as well as men, for the demands and emergencies of day-to-day living.[52]

Although the philosophical base of Riofrey's system sounds more liberating than Walker's, his actual system departed very little from those of his more conservative predecessors. The exercise section of his massive, 574-page book (which discussed physiology, childbearing, and many other aspects of women's health) opened with simple limb extensions, then featured three wand exercises, and, finally, recommended Walker's Indian scepter over the dumbbell for upper body training. Riofrey suggested that after women mastered these gentle exercises, they should move to what he called "portico exercises," or gymnastic exercises of "a more quiet nature" than those practiced by boys.[53] In this series, Riofrey explained the use of the triangle, warning readers that the "wonderful feats" recommended by Clias should not be attempted. On the other hand, Riofrey believed girls should learn to climb both wooden and rope ladders in case they ever needed to board a ship or escape from a burning building. He also urged women to learn to mount a horse, pass from one boat to another, maintain equilibrium in a small boat, dive, and swim.[54]

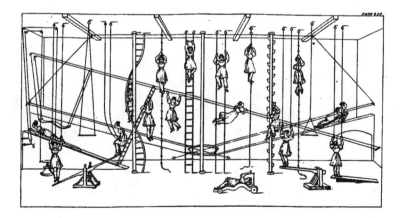

Figure 29: Riofrey titled this illustration "Gymnasium for the Normal and Anormal State." Note the above-the-knee gymnastic costumes and the many unusual apparati. Illustration from Bureaud Riofrey's *Physical Education: Specially Adapted to Young Ladies* (1838).

An illustration opposite the title page of Riofrey's book is somewhat misleading. It depicts several difficult gymnastic-type exercises that he did not describe in the text. Women, wearing gymnastic costumes of pantaloons and above-the-knee skirts, are shown climbing slanted ladders using only the strength of their arms, climbing the column of pegs advocated by Clias, climbing a knotted rope, and raising their bodies toward the ceiling by climbing two parallel ropes.[55] Also depicted were women using a seesaw, standing on a springboard, and using several curving, therapeutic devices designed to help pull the back into proper alignment.

Although he cautioned against the passions of the waltz and the too-quick pace of the *galope,* Riofrey concurred with Walker and the growing antebellum sentiment that dancing could be sufficient exercise for women and would create harmonious bodily development. He warned readers, however, that too much dancing could create dire problems. He painted a grim picture of the physical condition of opera dancers who concealed "misery" beneath their fancy dresses and gave way to fatigue as soon as they left the stage. "Nearly all have bad health," he wrote, "and those wonderful feats that surprise the public, are rather the effect of nervous excitation, maintained by public applause, than by real strength."[56]

Riofrey also stressed the important contributions that exercise could make to a woman's childbearing capacities through its improvement of her overall health. He agreed with Rousseau and maintained that another equally powerful rationale for including a regular system of purposive exercise in a woman's life was that such a course of training would improve a woman's appearance and increase her marketability as a wife. Arguing against the finishing schools of his era, which encouraged women to specialize in the upper-class accomplishments of fancy needlework and music as a means to attract the attention of a potential husband, Riofrey contended that a young woman's time could be better spent by attending to physical exercise. "It is forgotten," he wrote, "that there is often more attraction in beauty of figure, and brilliancy of health than in any other accomplishment."[57] Health and beauty were "inseparable," he continued, and no woman could expect to achieve them who had not been involved with physical education in her childhood.[58] Like Rousseau, Riofrey argued that women were inherently weak, delicate, and more likely to become ill than were men. He argued, however, that woman's congenital weaknesses could be significantly moderated by proper training. For

Riofrey, such training meant dance, first and foremost, followed by calisthenics and a few light gymnastic exercises to prepare women for
times of emergency.

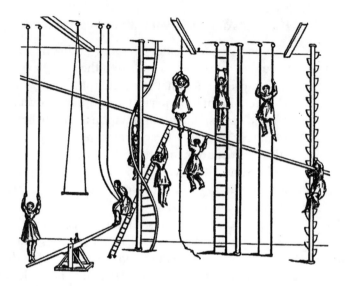

Figure 30: Illustration of a women's gymnasium from Daniel Jacques's *Hints
Toward Physical Perfection: Or the Philosophy of Human Beauty* (1859).

It is difficult, of course, to quantitatively measure Riofrey's influence. Based on the endorsements included in the second edition,
Riofrey's book and its utilitarian approach to women's fitness received
considerable approval from European journalists. It further appears
that he had excellent professional connections in Europe where he
served as editor of the *Continental and British Medical Review*. He also
belonged to the Faculty of Medicine in Paris, the Westminster Society
in London, and the Anatomical Society of Edinburgh.[59] In America,
Riofrey's ideas served as the foundation of the women's exercise section of Daniel H. Jacques, *Hints Toward Physical Perfection: Or the
Philosophy of Human Beauty*, released by Fowler and Wells in 1859.[60]
Jacques especially liked Riofrey's suggestions regarding the climbing
exercises and included a drawing entitled "The Girls' Gymnasium,"
which is nearly an exact copy of the illustration appearing in Riofrey's

second edition.[61] Riofrey's ideas reached an even wider American audience when Jacques's book appeared as a serial in Fowler and Wells's *The Water Cure Journal and Herald of Reforms* beginning in April 1857.[62]

### The First American Women's Exercise Text

In 1831, *A Course of Calisthenics for Young Ladies in Schools and Families* explained that calisthenics had "stood the test of experiment" in Europe, and then prophesied that it would not be long "before the practice of Calisthenics shall be perfectly familiar to every female school in the United States."[63] This anonymously published book is important not only for its ability to accurately predict the future but because it was the first textbook for physical education written by and for women. Furthermore, it provides modern scholars with some of the best evidence available on what constituted calisthenics in antebellum America.

The anonymity of the book's prescient author, however, has puzzled historians for more than a century. Written as a series of letters "by a mother," the initial "M" is given as the only evidence of authorship. Historian Fred Eugene Leonard reported in 1906 that he could find "no internal evidence of the real authorship," but said that he believed the book to be Catharine Beecher's work.[64] History textbooks such as Spears's and Swanson's *History of Sport and Physical Activity in the United States,* and Van Dalen's, Mitchell's, and Bennett's *A World History of Physical Education* have likewise attributed the book to Beecher and have credited her, in large part because of her supposed authorship of this work, with the birth of the American calisthenics movement.[65]

Although the fact that it was published in Hartford, in 1831, suggests a link to Catharine Beecher, she made no mention of the work in any of her later writings, including her *Educational Reminiscences and Suggestions,* in which she wrote at some length about her efforts on behalf of calisthenics.[66] According to Beecher's biographer, Katherine Sklar, the childless Beecher was busy in 1831 promoting a new book on moral philosophy and preparing to move to Ohio with her father.[67]

So who was the author if it was not Beecher? Sarah Hale, who reviewed the calisthenics text in the February 1832 issue of *The Ladies' Magazine,* reported that it was "prepared by a Mother, who was led to the subject of Physical Education by circumstances connected with her own family." Hale glowingly recommended the book to her readers, noting that the author had rejected all the "objectionable" parts of calisthenics such as "romping," and rendered the text perfectly "safe and appropriate to young girls."[68] A tantalizing clue can be found in the introduction to Bureaud Riofrey's book on physical education for women. In that introduction, Riofrey gives credit to the various experts who contributed to the formulation of his theories. According to Riofrey, his ideas came from Locke, Rousseau, Salzmann, Gall, and a "Mrs. Leigh" from America.[69] While I have been unable to trace Mrs. Leigh beyond this reference, it is possible, though certainly not proven, that since Riofrey's book appeared four years later than *A Course of Calisthenics*, and since no other book on calisthenics was apparently published in America during this half decade, Riofrey's "Mrs. Leigh" was the author of the 1831 treatise. To continue such speculation a step further, it is also possible that Mrs. Leigh was the anonymous Englishwoman who introduced calisthenics to Catharine Beecher and her students in 1827.[70]

Regardless of authorship, the 1831 treatise is important. "M" noted in her introductory remarks that she relied on earlier English and French texts in putting together her course of exercises and that she chose from these texts those movements she deemed useful and suitable for young ladies. "M" reassured her readers that "no circumstances could render it necessary, to adopt those very vigorous exercises, which have been invented for boys."[71]

The book consisted of nine "letters" and sixty-two engravings demonstrating proper exercise techniques. In Letter One, the author explained that her aim was to publish a handbook of calisthenics exercises that could be used by both mothers and school mistresses.[72] In her second letter, the author addressed a problem that haunted women's exercise throughout the nineteenth century: the impact of the increasing demands of intellectual education on the health of American women. "It is astonishing how many perish by what has been called 'the disease of education,'" she wrote.[73] In language atypical of Beecher's normal stance on woman's situation, "M" argued that the requirements of an upper-class woman's education were more demanding than were the educational expectations imposed on men. She alleged that by the age of eighteen, women were expected to be "finished," meaning that they had mastered Greek and Latin, were skilled in the sciences, spoke a modern foreign language, had mastered drawing, had become adept at dancing and music, and had learned the skills of housewifery. "The other sex," she wrote, "will go on with these same studies till one or two and twenty . . . What is the inference?" she asked rhetorically. "That their natural abilities are superior? But who will allow this to be the fact?"[74]

In Letter Three, the author outlined the causes of ill health among young women, citing as contributing causes the long hours girls spent at school on backless seats, limited play and outdoor exercise, and poor sleeping arrangements that contributed to postural problems. In addition, "M" warned against tight lacing and the powerful influence of fashion, arguing that they curbed the naturally playful instincts of the young and set a standard of beauty based on frailty, poor posture, and insipidness.[75] Inculcating young women with the belief "that it is unladylike to be active and healthy," was, she argued, perhaps the greatest crime perpetrated against a young woman's health. "In fitting girls to appear well in this society whose watchword is 'gentility,'" she declared, "they often become dull and stupid; mere automata . . . spiritless specimens of prim perfection . . . ."[76] Her program of calisthenics, "M" wrote in Letter Four, would ameliorate women's physical and attitudinal problems because:

> 1. They bring every part of the system into action. 2. Expand the chest. 3. Bring down the shoulders. 4. Make the form erect. 5. Give grace to motion. 6. Increase muscular strength. 7. Give a light elastic step in walking. 8. Restore the distorted or weakened members of the system. 9. Prevent tight lacing. 10. Promote cheerfulness. 11. Render the mind more active. 12. They are conducive to general health.[77]

As to the exercises themselves, "M" relied on several new pieces of equipment for women. To the wands and triangles used by earlier advocates, "M" added the oscillator, the patent spring, weight-lifting exercises, and an unusual tongueless bell with a wooden handle that weighed approximately a pound. "M" explained that the bells should be struck together, so they would create pleasant tones as accompaniment to the calisthenics movements. "M" recommended that her triangle be attached to a ring in the ceiling, and her illustrations showed women using the triangle to swing by their hands, slide forward and lower their body close to the floor, and run in circles until centrifugal force allowed them to swing freely.[78] To expand the chest and create flexibility in the shoulders, she suggested taking a four-foot-long bamboo wand and, with a widely spaced grip, lowering it behind the body while the arms remained straight. She also described overhead cane lifts, freehand arm extensions, and arm circles like those seen in other exercise texts.[79]

"M" next included a series of weight-lifting movements she described as "Exercises to bring down the Shoulders." The weight-lifting movements were necessitated, the author explained, by the many "indolent" girls who threw a shawl carelessly around themselves and then shrugged their shoulders to keep it in place. This action, "M" explained, plus the hunching forward so common in studying caused the shoulders to "lose that graceful fall, that beautiful slope so universally admired in the female figure."[80] Although "M" maintained that dumbbells would also work for this series of exercises, she recommended using clock weights of four to five pounds, covered by a soft fabric to protect the hands.[81]

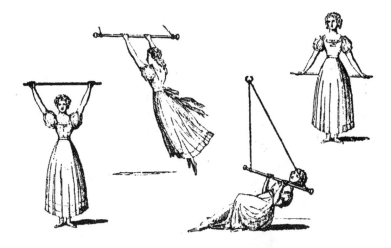

Figure 31: Triangle and wand exercises from the anonymously published, *A Course of Calisthenics for Young Ladies* (1831).

The author expressed disapproval, however, for those women's schools that were using weights as "heavy" as eight or nine pounds for similar exercises. This disagreement suggests that women's purposive exercise was more widely practiced in the United States in this era than modern historians have so far documented.[82]

"M" turned to other forms of resistance training to correct posture. She recommended walking with a "large octavo" on the head, joking that "some books will do better for the outside of the head than the inside."[83]

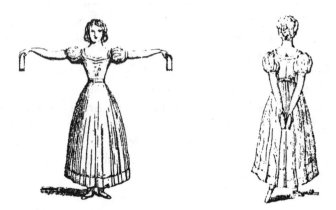

Figure 32: "The Weight Exercises," as depicted in *A Course in Calisthenics for Young Ladies* (1831).

For those women whose stooped and rounded shoulders could not be remedied through simpler exercises, "M" urged the use of the patent spring, a device she found superior to the more common exercise of suspending a weight behind the head by a strap.[84]

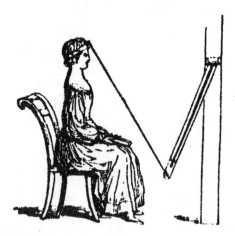

Figure 33: Instructions for the Patent Spring from *A Course in Calisthenics for Young Ladies* (1831): "The girl ... sits in a chair, with the band around her head, and pulls up the string. You will say, perhaps, that it looks a little Irish to pull the head down to keep it up, for this is in fact the mode employed; the spring acts with a great deal of force to return to its place; in order to prevent this, the head must be held very straight, and the muscles of the neck and shoulders are thus brought into vigorous exertion."

The author's next series of exercises promised to unify strength with beauty through slow, graceful movements that look remarkably like dance steps. "M" first explained the "five basic positions," observing that these were to dancing and calisthenics what the eight notes were to music. Following these, she gave instructions for a variety of freehand exercises, a curtsey, and a series of dance-like movements such as the Spanish Step, for which "M" advised using the tongueless bells as rhythmic accompaniment.[85]

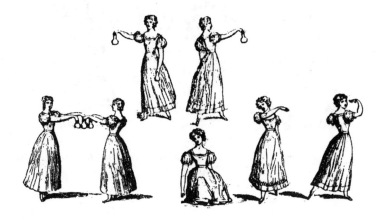

Figure 34: Calisthenic and tongueless bell exercises from *A Course in Calisthenics for Young Ladies* (1831). The Spanish Step is shown at the far right.

Perhaps the most philosophically interesting reading in *A Course of Calisthenics* occurs in the sixth letter, which "M" devoted to the subject of jumping. Like Riofrey, "M" argued that women needed to be physically prepared to meet emergencies that might occur during their lifetime. Jumping exercises could be useful, she argued, in case "a house is in flames; a carriage is driven by an unskillful or a drunken coachman, or when riding upon an unmanageable horse." "M" recognized that some arbiters of female behavior frowned on jumping for women, but defended her position by arguing that she was not trying to create "a race of fearless Amazons," but to instill a sense of nobleness and superiority of mind in young women, attributes she considered the cornerstones of true courage. Many women exhibited daily the kind of courage she called "fortitude," she argued, but "the occasions for active courage seldom occur; when they do, it is disgraceful to exhibit a weak cowardice."[86] The "scientific" way to improve jumping, she explained, was to mark a line about five feet away from where the jumper stood and have that person jump toward the line.[87]

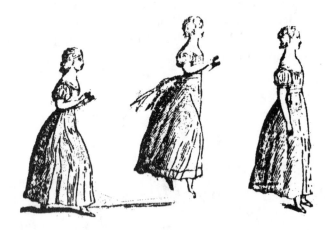

Figure 35: Jumping exercises from *A Course in Calisthenics for Young Ladies* (1831).

The most novel exercise in "M's" text appeared in Letter Eight, in which the workings of the oscillator or "Patent Dormant Balance" were described. "M" recommended this particular brand as the "best machine in use, for the cure of the lateral curvature of the spine."[88]

Invented by James K. Casey "and a lady," this early exercise machine consisted of a series of ropes and pulleys and a platform on which the exerciser stood. To work the machine, a woman reached as high overhead as possible and grasped the ropes attached to the weights. Then, by pulling on the ropes with first one arm and then the other, the platform was shifted from side to side, and "the weights are raised, and of course much muscular strength is exerted."[89] "M" argued that these pulling movements would balance the back and pull an offending spinal curvature into proper alignment.

In summation, "M" expanded upon her ideas of the appropriate relationship of the sexes and the role exercise played in that delicate balance. She argued strongly against her era's increasingly prevalent idea that femininity and weakness must be handmaidens of the same master. "It has been thought *vulgar*, to possess 'rude health,' " she

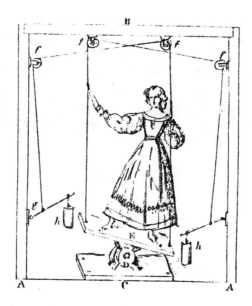

Figure 36: The Oscillator, or Patent Dormant Balance, from *A Course in Calisthenics for Young Ladies* (1831).

argued, claiming that to ignore women's physical education was to nurture "fragile, delicate creatures, who must wither, or be swept away by the first rude blast of real life to which they are exposed."[90] Although she essentially agreed with those physicians and authors, like Rousseau, who contended that the natural constitution of the female sex was delicate, and that God had made man stronger in order that he may, among other things, look after women, "M" insisted that it was improper and degrading for women to exacerbate this difference. "On the contrary," she argued, "it is our duty, religiously, sacredly to preserve our constitutions . . . we should increase our own firmness and vigor . . . *The varied and arduous duties which woman is called upon to perform, require vigorous health.*"[91]

Furthermore, "M" observed, women have been misled into worshiping "erroneous ideas of what constituted female elegance and beauty."[92] The "horror" of being dumpy and stout kept many women from eating normally, she argued, adding that the new model of beauty had become a shadowy, sylph-like being, "Of so thin and transparent a hue, you might have seen the moon shine through. . . The delicate, interesting beings," she continued, "withering like a rose bud ere it expands, have called forth not only sympathy, but admiration and affection."[93] Holding up the image of the ancient Greeks as an alternative ideal, "M" argued that the symmetrical bodies displayed in their statuary could only be accounted for by their commitment to physical training. What American women needed, she concluded, was a similar commitment to purposive exercise and a paid, trained calisthenics teacher in every women's school.[94]

## The Spread of Calisthenics

From these early texts, the calisthenics movement of the antebellum era blossomed. In America, the movement strove to achieve a philosophical middle ground between the insipid, elitist approach recommended by Walker and the vigorous strength and independence recommended by gymnastics devotees such as Beaujeu and Fowle. Propriety remained an issue for the next several decades, and the restrained movements of calisthenics did not threaten society's vision of appropriate feminine movement. Furthermore, calisthenics, as "M" noted, would not turn a girl into an "Amazon." There was no danger when performing these exercises that women would become so strong, healthy, and self-confident that they might like to explore the world outside their homes. It was, in other words, an exercise system ideally suited to its period in American history. For, during 1830 to 1860, as many feminist historians have suggested, the prevailing ideology that directed women's lives was the notion of separate spheres of influence. Men had the world of business and commerce; women had their home and family. Calisthenics allowed women to be just fit enough to fulfill that limited role. Strength may be an "ornament" to man, wrote one reviewer of calisthenics books, "but it is far from being so to the softer sex."[95]

During the next several decades, and largely because of "M's" groundbreaking efforts, increasing numbers of American educators experimented with the system in their schools. Leading this movement were two women—Mary Lyon at Mount Holyoke College and separate sphere enthusiast Catharine Beecher—who kept calisthenics in the forefront of exercise for women for the next thirty years.

[1]"Reviews," *American Journal of Education* 1 (August 1827): 489.

[2]Ibid., 490.

[3]Ibid., 488.

[4]Gustavus Hamilton, *The Elements of Gymnastics for Boys and Calisthenics for Young Ladies* (London: 1827).

[5]Signor G. P. Voarino, *A Treatise on Calisthenic Exercises Arranged for the Private Tuition of Ladies* (London: printed for N. Hailes, 1827).

[6]Ibid., 2-3.

[7]Ibid.

[8]Signor G. P. Voarino, *A Second Course of Calisthenic Exercises: With a Course of Private Gymnastics for Gentlemen: Accompanied with a Few Observations on the Utility of Exercise* (London: James Ridgeway, Boosey and Sons, Royal Exchange, and Rolandi Italian Library: 1828), 27, 80.

[9]Ibid., 68. In a footnote on page vi of P. H. Clias, *Kalesthenie oder Uebungen zur Schoenheit und Kraft fuer Maedchen* (Bern, Switzerland: 1829), 9-10. Clias quoted a Miss Marion Mason whom he described as *his* former pupil.

[10]Fred Eugene Leonard, "Chapters from the Early History of Physical Training in America, Part II: The Introduction of 'Calisthenics' for Girls and Women (Dating from around 1830)," *Mind and Body* 13 (December 1906): 292.

[11]Voarino, *A Treatise on Calisthenics*, 4.

[12]Ibid., 16.

[13]Ibid., 17.

[14]Ibid., 20-21.

[15]Ibid., 23.

[16]Ibid., 25.

[17]Ibid., 34-42.

[18]Signor Voarino, *A Second Course of Calisthenic Exercises*; 26. See Chapter One for information on Nicholas Andry.

[19]Ibid., 59. "The balance is a moveable instrument, supported by means of a hook, strongly fixed in the center of a room, from which two cords are suspended; and at the extremities of which is fixed a stick, made of a very dry piece of ash wood, four feet in length, and an inch and a half in diameter. The middle of the stick should be wrapped with any sort of soft substance, such as cotton, velvet, &c. to prevent it from hardening the hands. In order to prevent the cords from twisting, a swivel must be used, so that the balance may turn in any direction."

[20]Ibid., 59-64.

[21]Voarino, *A Second Course*, iv. Voarino dedicated it to the Duchess with her permission.

[22]Ibid., vi.

[23]Ibid., 27.

[24]Ibid., 13.

[25]"Calisthenic Exercises," *The Journal of Health* 2 (27 April 1831): 250.

[26]"Craven" [Donald Walker], *British Manly Exercises; In Which Rowing and Sailing Are Now First Discussed* (London, 1834). This book stayed in print throughout the nineteenth century. An eleventh edition, "Carefully Revised," entitled *Walker's Manly Exercises; Containing Rowing, Sailing, Riding, Driving, Racing, Hunting, Shooting, and Other Manly Sports* was published in 1888 by George Bell and Sons.

[27]Thomas Hughes, *Tom Brown's School Days* (London, 1857) was a novel extolling the virtues of athletic games in the British public schools. It inspired the athletic movement of the late nineteenth century in which amateur sporting competition became equated with manliness and teamwork, attributes considered essential to British gentlemen. For information on the importance of Hughes' work, see Bruce Haley, *The Healthy Body and Victorian Culture* (Cambridge: Harvard University Press, 1978), 145-55.

[28]Donald Walker, *Exercises for Ladies Calculated to Preserve & Improve Beauty and To Prevent and Correct Personal Defects, Inseparable from Constrained or Careless Habits Founded on Physiological Principles* (London: Thomas Hurst, St. Paul's Church Yard, 1835). A second edition was released in 1837. All quotations are from the 1837 edition.

[29]Quoted in Walker, *Exercises for Ladies,* 293; originally in the *New Monthly,* March 1836.

*The Lady's Magazine* for February 1836 reported that "a more important work to the fair sex than *Walker's Exercises for Ladies* has not for years issued from the press." Blackwood's *Lady's Magazine* for June 1836 called it a "first class work" and "invaluable." *The Gentlemen's Magazine* for August 1836 reported, "Were we to follow the guidance of our own feelings, we should transcribe a great part of this work, which has been introduced into our publisher's family *with great success.*" *The Educational Magazine* for February 1836 said, "There are few works addressed to ladies which will afford them more really useful information. Mr. Walker writes like a philosopher, a scholar, and generally a man of refined taste." Glowing reports also appeared in *The Metropolitan Magazine* for February 1836; *Tait's Magazine* for February 1836; and *The Monthly Review* for March 1836. Newspaper reviews are also quoted from the *London Times* (8 February 1836); *The Spectator* (9 January 1836); *Bell's Life in London* (9 January 1836); *Frazer's Literary Chronicle* (16 January 1836); *The Observer* (9 January 1836); *The Globe* (12 January 1836); and the *Weekly Belle Assembly* (6 February 1836). In addition, Walker included quotes from sixteen provincial papers. All quotes are included on pages 293-96 of the 1837 edition.

[30]Walker, *Exercises for Ladies,* xi.

[31]Ibid., xiii-xviii.

[32]Ibid., viii.

[33]Ibid., xx.

[34]Ibid.

[35]Ibid., xxiii.

[36]Dr. George Birkbeck especially liked Walker's use of the Indian scepter "which by its elegance, variety and moderation, will, I doubt not, when your work has been extensively circulated, become a general favorite. Indeed I am not acquainted with any modifications of action, which in conferring grace, facility and power, can be compared with the Indian Exercise." [Ibid., viii]. Dr. James Copeland wrote, " Of the safety and efficacy of the exercises you recommend, I have no doubt. The Indian Scepter Exercise is the most efficient and most graceful of any hitherto devised." [Ibid., ix].

[37]Ibid., 105. Walker cited Renaissance physician Hieronymous Mercurialis's *de Arte Gymnastica* as the inspiration for the British fad of dumbbell training.

[38]Ibid., 105-106.

[39]Ibid., 128.

[40]Ibid., 131-32.

[41]Ibid., 188-89.

[42]Ibid., 184-85.

[43]Ibid., 264-65.

[44]Ibid., 264.

[45]Ibid., 265-66.

[46]Ibid., 265.

[47]Bureaud Riofrey, M.D., *Physical Education Specially Adapted to Young Ladies*, 2nd ed. (London: Longman, Orme, Brown, Green, and Longmans, 1838), 247.

[48]Ibid., 256.

[49]Ibid., 252-53. The first edition appeared in French, in 1835.

[50]Ibid., 252-53. Riofrey discussed the pros and cons of Clias's gymnastics and Walker's system on pages 76-79.

[51]Ibid., 253.

[52]Ibid. 247-48.

[53]Ibid.

[54]Ibid., 252-55. Regarding swimming or "natation," Riofrey noted on pages 256-57 that Italian women swam in a special dress made for that one purpose. Women in Paris, he reported, frequented two large plunge baths where they learned to swim in loose dresses, whereas London was so far without a swimming facility.

[55]On page 254, however, Riofrey argued that rope climbing is unsuitable for women.

[56]Ibid., 265.

[57]Ibid., viii.

[58]Ibid., vi.

[59]Ibid., 575-79, title pages.

[60]D[aniel]. H. Jacques, *Hints Toward Physical Perfection: Or the Philosophy of Human Beauty; Showing how to Acquire and Retain Bodily Symmetry, Health*

*and Vigor, Secure Long Life, and Avoid the Infirmities and Deformities of Age* (New York: Fowler & Wells, 1861 [1859]), 163.

[61]Ibid., 163.

[62]D[aniel]. H. Jacques, "Hints Toward Physical Perfection; or, How to Acquire and Retain Beauty, Grace, and Strength, and Secure Long Life and Continued Usefulness," *The Water-Cure Journal and Herald of Reforms* 23 (April, June, 1857): 77-78, 123-26; and 24 (July, August, September, October, November, December 1857): 3-5, 29-30, 53-55, 77-79, 100-102, 116-17.

[63]*A Course of Calisthenics for Young Ladies in Schools and Families With Some Remarks on Physical Education* (Hartford, CT: H. and F. J. Huntington, 1831), 6.

[64]Fred Eugene Leonard, "Chapters from the Early History of Physical Training in America. Part II: The Introduction of 'Calisthenics' for Girls and Women (Dating From About 1830)," *Mind and Body* 13 (December 1906): 291. In this article, Leonard basically attributes the calisthenics movement to Catharine Beecher.

[65]Betty Spears and Richard Swanson, *History of Sport and Physical Activity in the United States* (Dubuque, IA: William C. Brown, 1978), 73; Deobold Van Dalen, Elmer Mitchell, and Bruce Bennett, *A World History of Physical Education* (Englewood Cliffs, NJ: Prentice Hall, 1963), 370. John Betts also attributed the book to Beecher in "Mind and Body in Early American Thought," *Journal of American History* 57 (1968): 799.

[66]Beecher, *Educational Reminiscences*, 65-67.

[67]Sklar makes no mention of this anonymous text in her biography of Beecher. Beecher published *The Elements of Mental and Moral Philosophy, Founded Upon Experience, Reason and the Bible* in Hartford in 1831. In a telephone interview, Sklar said she had turned up no references to the book in her research on Beecher's life.

[68]"A Course of Calisthenics for Young Ladies in Schools and Families; With Some Remarks on Physical Education," *The Ladies Magazine* 5 (February 1832): 91.

[69]Riofrey, *Physical Education*, xviii.

[70]See Chapter Six for Beecher's introduction to calisthenics.

[71]*A Course of Calisthenics*, 1.

[72]Ibid., 6.

[73]Ibid., 14

[74]Ibid.

[75]Ibid., 17-26.

[76]Ibid., 24.

[77]Ibid., 26-27.

[78]Ibid., 30-31.

[79]Ibid., 32-36.

[80]Ibid., 36.

[81]The heavy pendulums used in clocks would have been readily available in

most parts of America during this period, while dumbbells, though available, were less likely to be found outside of large cities.

[82]*A Course of Calisthenics*, 36-37.

[83]Ibid., 38.

[84]Ibid., 41-42.

[85]Ibid., 45-54.

[86]Ibid., 56.

[87]Ibid., 57.

[88]Ibid., 60-61.

[89]Ibid., 62.

[90]Ibid., 75.

[91]Ibid., 77.

[92]Ibid.

[93]Ibid.

[94]Ibid., 80.

[95]"Reviews," 488.

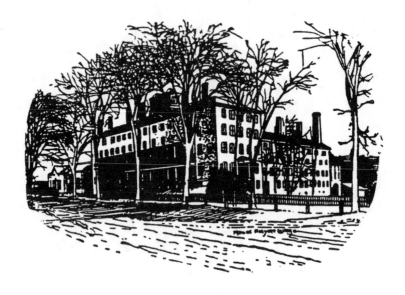

Figure 37: Mount Holyoke Female Seminary as it looked in the mid-nine-teenth century. Illustration from *National Cyclopaedia of American Biography*.

# Chapter 5
## "I Practice Calisthenics Every Day and Like It Quite Well": Mary Lyon, Mount Holyoke, and American Calisthenics

When Mary Gove introduced calisthenics to the female students at her school in Lynn, Massachusetts, around 1835, many of her students' parents became upset.[1] Yet two or three years later, Gove reported, when another woman opened a school in Lynn and advertised that calisthenics would be part of the curriculum, "it was considered a recommendation of her school." It is not difficult to understand, Gove pointed out, that "public sentiment is changing."[2]

That change in public sentiment can be traced to several influences. Although the texts of Hamilton, Voarino, Walker, Riofrey, and "M" played important roles, Mary Lyon, founder of Mount Holyoke Female Seminary, was chiefly responsible for the acceptance and dissemination of calisthenics throughout America in the 1830s and early 1840s.

Mary Lyon shared both "M's" vision of healthy, vibrant womanhood and the anonymous author's commitment to introduce calisthenics to the girls's schools of America. Early in her career, Lyon vowed to establish an endowed college of higher education in which young women could be trained for careers in teaching. As she became convinced of the benefits of exercise, Lyon's aspirations broadened to encompass not merely an endowed college for women, but a college in which intellectual education and physical education received equal attention. Lyon finally realized her dream in 1837, when Mount Holyoke Female Seminary opened its doors to students. Although she has received little credit for it from sport historians, Lyon's efforts at Mount Holyoke resulted in the codification of an American system of calisthenics and in the training of America's first female physical education teachers.[3]

### Influences on Mary Lyon's Vision of Appropriate Exercise

It is impossible to completely trace the beginnings of Mary Lyon's interest in purposive exercise. As a subscriber to the *American Journal of Education*, however, Lyon undoubtedly kept up with the latest educational innovations and probably read some of the magazine's reports of the 1820s gymnastics revolution underway in Europe. It is likely that she even purchased some of the books on exercise reviewed by the journal.[4]

The greatest influence on Mary Lyon's ideas about exercise, however, was her good friend and enduring colleague, Zilpah Grant, with whom Lyon taught intermittently during the period 1826 to 1830.[5] Although the details are sketchy, Zilpah Grant had apparently introduced some form of purposive exercise to her female students at Derry, New Hampshire, by 1826, a year before Catharine Beecher introduced "calisthenics" in her school. The fact that a tendon "in the heel was parted from its fastening" while Grant performed these exercises, raises the intriguing question of what Grant considered suitable exercise for women. According to L. T. Guilford's biography of Grant, her "suffering was great," and she needed crutches for two full years after the injury in May 1827.[6] Grant was not the only early American woman so injured. Emma Willard, at the Troy Female Seminary in Middlebury, Vermont, also suffered a similar injury in the 1820s while practicing "calisthenics." These two injuries help make sense of Catharine Beecher's comment, in her 1827 catalogue for the Hartford Female Seminary, that some New England schools "require of young ladies vigorous physical exercises suited only to the strength of young gentlemen."[7] Whether or not Grant or Willard modified their systems after their injuries is unknown. Despite her suffering, however, Grant's commitment to purposive training did not waver, and she continued to require exercise at her schools through the end of her academic career.[8]

In 1830, Mary Lyon settled into full-time employment with Zilpah Grant at the Ipswitch Female Seminary in Massachusetts. There, according to Guilford, "Education of the muscles and grace and ease of motion were systematically taught by a series of calisthenics arranged by Miss Grant. They were performed usually with singing, and the various figures and movements afforded a lively and beautiful recreation."[9] According to Mount Holyoke historian Persis Harlow McCurdy, "Miss Grant arranged a system of calisthenics for her school [at Ipswitch], and when Miss Lyon opened Mount Holyoke she took this with her as she did some other of Miss Grant's methods."[10] Lyon stayed at the Ipswitch school through 1834, and ran it on her own during another lengthy illness Grant suffered. During these years calisthenics of an undefined nature remained an integral part of the curriculum at Ipswitch Female Seminary.[11]

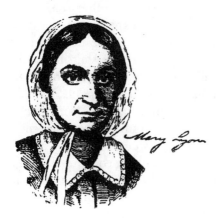

Figure 38: Mary Lyon in an engraving from the *National Cyclopaedia of American Biography.*

## Mary Lyon's Views on Exercise

Mary Lyon was already teaching calisthenics to her own students before her move to Ipswitch, however. A letter to Lyon from Abigail Tenney—who studied with Lyon in Buckland, Massachusetts, in 1828-1829 and later became a teacher in her own right—explained that half of Tenney's female students practiced calisthenics, a fact she hoped would please Miss Lyon.[12] Two other letters from former students also corroborate Lyon's advocacy of calisthenics. Harriett Fairchild reported to her mentor in 1832 that she offered calisthenics and composition at a select school in Derry, New Hampshire. That same year, Hannah White wrote to Lyon that she had tried to "mimic you a little here," and that she included chirography, drawing, reading, spelling, calisthenics, and composition in her curriculum.[13]

Calisthenics were important to Lyon because of her concern with the health of America's young women. "The value of health to young ladies is inestimable . . ." she wrote, "but not enough has been *done*, in our systems of education, to promote the health of young ladies."[14] Like many of her peers, Lyon was religiously conservative, even puritanical, in her ideas about appropriate behavior. She equated idleness with sin and believed that exercising helped bolster a person's moral stamina as well as physical fitness. "Those who enjoy bodily idleness, enjoy sin," she wrote on one occasion. "Exercise is part of the constitution of man . . . every organ is strengthened by it."[15] Lyon even told one young woman at Mount Holyoke who asked to be excused from calisthenics in order to have more time to read and pray that she could not grant her request, for exercise was also a religious duty.[16]

Shortly after opening Mount Holyoke in November 1837, Lyon composed a *Book of Duties* that outlined her expectations for both teachers and students. In addition to an hour of domestic work each day, Lyon expected Mount Holyoke girls to run up the stairs inside the new school building rather than walk, and to spend an hour outdoors before breakfast each day in which they walked at least a mile. To make sure they covered the desired distance, Lyon installed half-mile posts on the roads leading out of South Hadley.[17] In the winter, when snow made walking difficult, Lyon still required the students to spend at least forty-five minutes outdoors.[18] Although walking continued to be a focus of Lyon's exercise regimen, it appears that it did not continue to be a *daily* activity for all students. A walking record card has survived from the second term of 1847 on which Eliza Jenkins recorded her daily mileage over a thirteen-week period. She walked only four days a week, always on Mondays, Thursdays, Fridays, and Saturdays. In two weeks out of the thirteen, Eliza walked a full two miles on each of her outings, giving her a total of eight miles for the week. In other weeks, however, her total distance was as little as two miles.[19] A letter from Lydia French, a Mount Holyoke graduate in 1857, also suggested that the walking requirement was somewhat flexible. Lydia explained to her friend, Kate, that she had little free time at Mount Holyoke because of all the extracurricular activities, including the school's concern with physical education. "My time is as fully occupied as can be . . ." she wrote. "We are required to walk a mile every day . . . . If we do not spend an hour in walking, we are required to spend it in some sort of recreation."[20]

As for the school's manual labor requirement, Lyon explained in a letter to a friend in 1834 that she favored manual labor for her students but did not want it to become a significant focus of the school's curriculum or identity.[21] She viewed the domestic work as an adjunct to the regular curriculum and required it of all the students, although the girls were not paid for their work. Mount Holyoke's students shared in carrying wood and maintaining the fires throughout the school and did much of the school's washing, cooking, cleaning, ironing, and sweeping. One member of the original 1837 class remembered her manual labor experiences warmly. "There was real genuine working exercise in those days," she wrote. "The pupils really swept and dusted long halls and stairways . . . made bread, did the laundering and a thousand and one things that make up housekeeping." Before open house, she explained, the girls worked especially hard. "How well I remember the first housecleaning preparatory to public examinations and an open house. The delicate hands that scrubbed doors and windows inch by inch, that not a stain or flaw would be discovered in the new temple, till hands and heads were weary, yet how they laughed and made fun of it all!"[22]

Not all the students viewed their domestic exercise so positively. A student in 1863 claimed that the only real benefit she received from her domestic labor was that the hour's break in her study routine mentally refreshed her. "Sleeping at night," she claimed, "is just as well."[23] Lyon, however, was satisfied with her decision to require manual labor. Domestic exercise, she wrote, was "peculiarly fitted to the constitution of females . . . Our young ladies study with great intensity, but they are just as vigorous the last of the term as ever." Indeed, Lyon reported, "the vivacity and apparent vigor of our young ladies near the close of the winter term . . . was noticed by gentlemen of discrimination."[24]

## Calisthenics at Mount Holyoke

During Mary Lyon's lifetime, the primary exercise focus at Mount Holyoke was on calisthenics. Lyon appears to have allowed little latitude; each student participated, every day, unless she was ill. Margaret Huntting wrote in 1846, "I practice calisthenics every day and like it quite well, we are all obliged to practice, as they think it conducive to health."[25] Lucy Goodale, a Mount Holyoke student in 1838, described how organized the calisthenics classes were: "The Young Ladies here are divided into three classes in calisthenics, one for each spaceway. They exercise every evening from half past eight to nine o'clock. This gives them new vigor for study in the remaining hour before retiring."[26] According to Poet Emily Dickinson's correspondence, calisthenics classes were reduced to fifteen minutes a day by the late 1840s, but still required of every student.[27] In the 1860s, when Lizzie Morley entered Mount Holyoke, calisthenic exercises were still performed on a daily basis in the hallways for a period of fifteen minutes.

Mary Lyon not only defined the system of rhythmic drills she wished her students to follow, she regularly observed the classes and frequently took part in the exercises in the opening years of the academy.[28] A student who attended Mount Holyoke the year it opened wrote:

> I feel an electric thrill as I see Miss Lyon on her inspecting tour fall in line with us, her bright eyes and rosy cheeks aglow with half-suppressed enthusiasm and with the little characteristic shrug. I hear

again her urgent encouraging voice, "Now young ladies, try that again! a little more force! ah, yes, I knew you could! Now that is better. Stand erect!" and with the sweet silent laugh, the lovely turbaned head disappeared to look in on another class, leaving with us a new access of vigorous endeavor.[29]

By 1845, calisthenics at Mount Holyoke had evolved into two distinct types of activities. There were the hallway exercises, done by all the female students, and special, exhibition calisthenics practiced by the senior class. Margaret Huntting wrote to her cousin in 1846, "O how I wish I could practice as the seniors do. O it is a beautiful sight to see them . . ."[30] In both cases, it appears that music played a role in the performance of the exercises. Generally, the girls sang to accompany their movements, and, in the late 1840s, these calisthenic songs were published in a small booklet, which was updated and reissued in 1856.[31] At some early point in the seminary's history, an unheated room over the school's woodhouse was designated as a sort of gymnasium. There is no indication that the girls at Mount Holyoke wore any sort of specialized dress for their workouts until the 1860s when the school program switched to Dio Lewis's New Gymnastics.[32]

As to the system employed in the early years of Mount Holyoke, it appears to have combined freehand exercises and some handheld apparatus work. A Mount Holyoke student from 1837 recalled that wands arrived in the middle of the term. "That opening year we often waited to have things made that we needed, and we had taken many lessons before the wands were in evidence—not fairy wands, but quite substantial affairs which we grasped at either end, and carried in various ways holding them over the head, in front and back, etc." With their wands, she reported, they marched "singly and double, with joined wands, meeting, parting, with always, left! right!"[33] Though few other clues remain from the first decade of the school's operation as to what constituted calisthenics at Mount Holyoke, we do know from the comment above and from Mary Lyon's reminder in the *Book of Duties* that she did not want these exercises to be as easy to perform as quadrilles or other line dances. "Care should be taken," Lyon warned her teachers, "that the exercise does not become like dancing in the impression it makes on observers."[34]

## Exhibition Calisthenics

By the middle of the 1840s, however, the exhibition calisthenics at Mount Holyoke must have looked remarkably similar to dance. Several student letters from the end of the 1840s report favorably on the calisthenics exhibitions held on holidays and at graduation by members of the senior class. Margaret Huntting, at Mount Holyoke in 1846, discussed the Thanksgiving Day exhibition in a letter to an unnamed cousin. Margaret asked her cousin to relay to her Uncle Gilbert that she was working on the step that "Mademoiselle Blengy took in crossing the stage, that possibly I may be able to show it to him again as that is the step used here in Calisthenics . . . I think it is beautiful."[35] In 1848, Mary Ware was forced to stay at Mount Holyoke during the Thanksgiving holiday. Ware reported to her friend, Anny Batchelder, that following the traditional Thanksgiving dinner, the remaining students and the more than seventy guests "repaired to the seminary hall which was beautifully ornamented with evergreens and paper flowers and the tables were tastefully spread and trimmed." There, according to Ware, the choir sang, and then "came the calisthenics class and it was the prettiest sight I ever saw of the kind—Sixteen young ladies with wreaths of green and white upon their heads entered the room and such pretty steps and figures as they took, and kept time by their own singing. I think you would like to have seen them."[36] The following year, on the heels of Lyon's unexpected death on 5 March 1849, only three guests joined the Mount Holyoke students for Thanksgiving dinner, but the calisthenics exhibition went off as usual.[37] Annie Walker described the festivities for her father: "We all took seats round the hall, and soon [the] sound of distant music fell upon the ear; a door open and twenty-four young ladies, with myrtle wreaths on their heads came out singing. 'We Come, We Come, a Happy Band.' They practiced calisthenics for our gratification about fifteen minutes," Walker reported, "and then departed in the same manner as they entered singing. 'Good Night Dear Friends' &c."[38]

It is not known who taught the earliest classes in calisthenics at Mount Holyoke, but in the middle of the 1840s, Mary Chapin, an 1843 Mount Holyoke graduate, assumed leadership of the classes. Chapin, though still young, became acting principal in 1850, following Lyon's death, and it was she who directed the calisthenics exhibitions described above. Chapin passed responsibility for the classes on to Mary Titcomb in the fall of 1850.[39]

## Mary Titcomb and Calisthenics in the 1850s

During Titcomb's tenure at Mount Holyoke, students kept calisthenics notebooks in which they copied the detailed instructions for their various drills. The three calisthenics notebooks examined by the author were virtually identical in content and revealed that by the 1850s, the calisthenics classes at Mount Holyoke were divided into three series of movements, none of which required any sort of gymnastics apparatus. The first series of exercises consisted of gentle warm-up movements and what may best be called "social exercises." Beginning in an erect position, feet placed heels together at a sixty-degree angle, the students raised their arms, touched their foreheads, and let their hands fall back to the sides. Then, both the right and left legs were extended and brought back into line before the "slow walking dip" was executed with a pointed toe. Taking eight paces, the students next executed the "Formal courtesy," and then as they increased their walking pace, they performed arm exercises by raising their hands overhead, turning the palms upward, making their elbows meet behind their back, and so on. Next came the "Double formal courtesy," then "Courteseying around the circle," and then "Shaking hands around circle." The girls next spent time working on their posture and social graces. They marched with a book on top of their heads. They practiced "presenting a chair," properly sitting down and rising from a chair, the "slight courtesy," the "Double slight courtesy, leaving and entering a room, and "Introducing." The final exercises of the first series included raising the hands and looking over the alternate shoulder and "Walking the step called Spanish step."[40]

The second series of exercises demanded slightly greater effort from the Mount Holyoke girls. In this series the pace quickened, the arm movements were more pronounced, and a series of leaps, springs, and hops were used to accelerate the pulse rate. Singing "Of Late so Brightly Glowing," the girls executed movements such as the Double Spring: "Heels together skip twice on the left and right foot alternately;" and the "Quadruple Spring," whose instructions read: "Hands in front and at the side. A slight courtesy and change the position of the feet: right foot to the right side. carry it to the left-side beyond the left foot, point right again to the right and bring it to the first position." As the exercises became more complicated, the instructions in the calisthenics manuals became more difficult to understand. For instance, "The High Step" reads:

Throw the right foot to the right-side returning it with a spring, throwing the left foot to the left side at the same time return the left to its place with a spring, throwing the right to the front at the same time, bring the right foot to its place with a spring. Throwing the left back at the same time, bring the left to its place throwing the weight to the right-side at the same time counting eight &c.

The "High Step Complicated," "School Step," and "School Step Complicated" completed the second series of calisthenics exercises.[41]

In the 1850 notebook attributed to Mary Titcomb, the third series of exercises consisted entirely of elaborate marches in which the object was to form interesting patterns on the floor. Section leaders led columns of followers in figure eights, spirals, crescents, crosses, stars, and other forms using the side step, school step, the Spanish step, and promenade step. New combinations of movements continued to evolve, apparently. The 1851 calisthenics notebook kept by Anna Benton King, for instance, gives details of more complicated, patterned marches that do not appear in Titcomb's 1850 notes. These new marches use two or more columns of girls working together to form patterns such as "The Wreath," in which two concentric circles of girls sang "My Heart is Entranced" while circling and weaving in and out using the Spanish step, side step, and numerous curtseys. "The Garland" and "Star Promenade" are similar group movements and appear to resemble the patterned movements of modern drill teams or marching bands.[42]

In the early 1850s, Mary Titcomb published these three series of exercises in a small, twenty-three-page, green booklet called *Calisthenic Exercises*.[43] Titcomb herself could not remember the exact date of the book's publication but did recall later in her life that "the little book was prepared while I was teacher there, as I had charge of the Calisthenics Classes most, if not all of the time. Doubtless I had suggestions and advice from others about the exercises," she wrote, "though I remember nothing definite . . . there *may* have been some brief written or printed directions (though I can recall none), for most of the exercises were *practically* in existence when I entered the Seminary." "My work," Titcomb continued, "was chiefly bringing them into a printed form—or rather a form suitable to be printed." According to Titcomb, there "were no other special exercises for physical training" during her time at Mount Holyoke Seminary.[44]

## Teacher Training

One aspect of Mount Holyoke's involvement with calisthenics that needs further examination is the role Lyon played in training young women to become teachers of calisthenics. In January 1846, for instance, Mary Lyon wrote to a Miss Backus about the possibility of coming to Mount Holyoke to train to be a teacher of gymnastics. "We can give you a place a short time as a member of our family," Lyon wrote. "The classes in calisthenics are so arranged that you can practice three times a day with classes in different parts of the course. I hope you will make your plan to stay as long as will be necessary in view of our teachers to become a superior teacher in this branch."[45] This letter is one of the earliest references found by this author regarding the training of female physical educators in the United States. How many other women pursued similar courses of training at Mount Holyoke is not known. However, since Mount Holyoke's primary educational focus was teacher preparation, and since all Mount Holyoke students learned and practiced calisthenics, it seems safe to assume that many of them carried this exercise system with them to their new teaching assignments. Certainly the letters from Mary Lyon's early students, cited above, suggest that they felt they had been prepared by Lyon to be physical as well as intellectual educators.

## The Decline of Calisthenics

By the early 1860s, as George Barker Windship and Dio Lewis led American women's exercise to more vigorous levels, some Mount Holyoke students began to regard the calisthenics drills as outmoded and insipid. Chafing under the restrictions of her new school, Lizzie Morley said the girls called the fifteen-minute sessions "Hop Meeting" and she wrote an elaborate satire entitled "Mode of Operations in Case Mount Holyoke Seminary Takes Fire," which took dead aim at Mount Holyoke's calisthenics requirement:

> In case the Seminary takes fire, the young ladies have permission to enter the North Wing Parlor and inform Miss Chapin of the fact. She will then send for the bell girl, and have a long bell rung. When all the young ladies will assemble in the Seminary hall, Miss Chapin will take her accustomed seat, and then bid the young ladies "good morning." And then say "As a fire has broken out it will be necessary to have some benevolent work done, any that are willing to aid in it may rise." . . . The scholars pails in hand will proceed to the river having formed themselves into a procession arranged alphabetically

taking the promenade step. After having filled their pails, they are to return to the Seminary taking the side step.

Morley's satire ended with the now-homeless Mount Holyoke girls assembling in the South Hadley graveyard, maintaining their ladylike decorum to the end.[46] Other Mount Holyoke students also found the exercises too restrained and confining. Writing to her friend Helen Savage, Love Brown complained, "Their [Mount Holyoke's] exercise is only a fatiguing process—the main object being to look well and show off."[47]

### Influences on American Calisthenics

The decorum and restraint that so troubled Morley and Brown in the 1860s were, of course, precisely what allowed calisthenics to become such a popular system of exercise in the period between 1830 and 1850. One person responsible for selling this concept of restrained exercise to the masses was not a physical educator *per se* but magazine publisher Sarah Josepha Hale, America's foremost arbiter of fashion and upper-class virtue.

In both her *Ladies Magazine* and in her later *Godey's Ladies Book,* Hale defended the idea of separate spheres of endeavor and influence but insisted that woman's homebound duties still required proper training in both intellectual and physical education.[48] Hale tackled the question of women's physical education in the first issue of her *Ladies Magazine,* writing "Strengthen their physical powers," and you may then "give energy to their intellects, brilliant tints of beauty to their persons, animation to their spirits, and grace to their manners."[49] Through the years, Hale reprinted for her women readers a number of physical education articles from other magazines and reprinted lectures that dealt with the question of physical education.[50] In 1832, when Johann Caspar Spurzheim, the eminent European phrenologist, delivered a series of lectures in Boston, Hale made sure to stress the phrenologist's "earnest emphasis" on women's need for exercise and to report that he considered calisthenics as the best system of exercise for women.[51] Hale also devoted considerable space to the ideas of Dr. William Grigg, who became so enraptured with Spurzheim's advocacy of calisthenics that he proposed beginning a fund drive to establish a "calisthenium" in Boston.[52] According to Hale, the calisthenium was long overdue, and she applauded the fact that "several influential gentlemen are making exertions to have it opened, under the patronage of one or more of our popular female schools."[53]

In January 1831, in a lengthy piece entitled "Physical Education of Woman," Hale made clear her personal convictions on the question of appropriate exercise. In it Hale argued that women must look at exercise and health as social and personal issues resulting from improper education. Hale contended that women needed to study physiology—a subject largely forbidden to them because of its "indelicate" nature—so that they understood their bodies and learned how to safeguard their health and that of their children. "Two things are needed in Boston, and perhaps everywhere else," Hale declared. "One is a woman, who . . . will learn to demonstrate the anatomy of the chest and abdomen, at least, to all females . . . The other needful thing is a system of calisthenic exercises in a proper place, with proper apparatus—and under a scientific and practical instructer [sic]."[54]

Hale's article was representative of an ideological change that occurred in the early 1830s regarding the subject of physical education. No longer content to simply teach exercise, the new "physical educators" preached, as Hale did in her article, that what Americans needed was a bifurcation of physical education into the study of human physiology and the practice of exercise. This divided approach became the most commonly accepted definition of "physical education" during the antebellum years, and it found its chief advocate for women in the person of Catharine Beecher.

Unfortunately for the course of women's exercise, however, the 1830s and 1840s enthusiasm for the new science of physiology—which is exactingly detailed in historian James Whorton's *Crusaders for Fitness*—led many people to believe that physiological knowledge alone was sufficient to maintain health.[55] Once a woman understood the placement of the organs in her abdominal cavity and how badly those organs could be damaged through tight corsets, bad eating habits, and inadequate elimination, the argument went, she could take the necessary steps to maintain her health by simply following the nonnatural maxims of moderation. Secondly, the new interest in physiology reinforced the idea that women were, indeed, different from men. As the rhetoric surrounding the ideology of separate spheres solidified into a national mantra, these newly understood physiological differences were used to impress upon women the idea that their exercise should be substantially less difficult than that attempted by men.

Catharine Esther Beecher seized on these ideas in the 1850s to open a new chapter in the story of American calisthenics. Although Beecher did not author the first woman's book on exercise, and although she was not the first woman teacher to introduce purposive training to her female students, she did play a very important role in the dissemination of calisthenics throughout the United States and in shoring up the social barriers that tried to contain women's exercise within the construct of separate spheres. Her success in these endeavors, however, can be partly attributed to the influence of Mary Lyon and her corps of students and teachers. Lyon's students, like Beecher's protégés, carried their calisthenics training with them to their new teaching assignments. Had Mount Holyoke's founder not died at such an early age, her legacy as a physical educator might not have been so easily obscured by Catharine Beecher's self-serving, inaccurate claim of having "invented" calisthenics.

[1]Mary S. Gove, *Lectures to Women on Anatomy and Physiology with an Appendix on Water Cure* (New York: Harper & Brothers, 1846), 218. Gove was the first person to use an anatomically correct mannequin in her physiology lectures to women.

[2]Ibid. In the 1840s, as Gove became involved with hydropathy, she continued to recommend calisthenics, walking, and domestic labor for women's exercise. See, for example, Mary Gove Nichols, *Experience in Water Cure: A Familiar Exposition of the Principles and Results of Water Treatment in the Cure of Acute and Chronic Diseases* (New York: Fowler & Wells, 1849), 73-74.

[3]The two best sources on Lyon's life and her struggle to build Mount Holyoke Female Seminary are Elizabeth Alden Green's *Mary Lyon and Mount Holyoke: Opening the Gates* (Hanover NH: 1979); and Edward Hitchcock's *The Power of Christian Benevolence Illustrated in the Life and Labor of Mary Lyon* (Northampton: Hopkins, Bridgman, and Company, 1852). The best source on her early years of teaching is L. T. Guilford, *The Use of a Life: Memorials of Mrs. Z. P. Grant Banister* (New York: American Tract Society, 1885). See also Gladys Haddad, "Social Roles and Advanced Education for Women in Nineteenth-Century America: A Study of Three Western Reserve Institutions," (Ph.D. diss., Case Western Reserve University, 1980).

[4] Green, *Mary Lyon*, 46. See also Guilford, *Use of a Life*, 66-68.

[5]During the 1820s, Lyon taught in a number of schools, as it was common for women teachers to hold summer sessions in one town, winter sessions in another.

[6]Guilford, *Use of a Life*, 82.

[7]Catharine Beecher, *Catalogue and Circular of the Hartford Female Seminary* (Hartford: by the author, 1827).

[8]Harriet Webster Marr, *The Old New England Academies* (New York: Comet Press Books, 1959), 163; and Green, *Mary Lyon*, 57.

[9]Ibid., 105.

[10]Persis Harlow McCurdy, "The History of Physical Training at Mount Holyoke College," *American Physical Education Review* 14 (1909): 139.

[11]Green, *Mary Lyon*, 65. See also [Sarah Hale], "Female Seminaries," *Ladies Magazine and Literary Gazette* 6 (March 1833): 142.

[12]Abigail Tenney Smith to Mary Lyon, 24 October 1831. Quoted in Green, *Mary Lyon*, 81.

[13]Hannah White to "My dear Miss Lyon," 6 November 1832. Mount Holyoke College Library/Archives, South Hadley MA. Harriett Fairchild to Mary Lyon, 22 June 1832. Quoted in Green, *Mary Lyon*, 81.

[14]Hitchcock, *The Power of Christian Benevolence*, 297.

[15]Quoted in Mildred S. Howard, "History of Physical Education at Mount Holyoke College, 1837–1955." Unpublished typescript, Box 1, Physical Education Department Records. Mount Holyoke College Library/Archives, South Hadley, MA.

[16]"Mary Lyon Memorabilia," 61, Mount Holyoke Library/Archives, Mount Holyoke College, South Hadley, MA.

[17]Howard, "History of Physical Education at Mount Holyoke College," 2.

[18]In 1862, the walking requirement increased to two miles per day.

[19]Eliza Jenkins's card entitled "Walking during the second term, South Hadley, January 22, 1847." Box J/3, Mount Holyoke College Library/Archives, South Hadley, MA.

[20]Lydia French to "My dear Kate," 10 October 1854. Photostat copy, Mount Holyoke College Library/Archives. Original letter on deposit with the Minnesota Historical Society, St. Paul, MN.

[21]Mary Lyon to Hannah White, 1 August 1834, quoted in Green, *Mary Lyon*, 115.

[22]Quoted in McCurdy, "Physical Training at Mount Holyoke College," 139.

[23]Ellen Parsons, "A Plea for a Gymnasium," An Oration Given at the 1863 Mount Holyoke College Seminary Graduation, ts., College History Collection, Mount Holyoke College Library/Archive, Holyoke, MA).

[24]Quoted in Mildred S. Howard, "A Century of Physical Education," *Mount Holyoke Alumnae Quarterly* 19 (February 1936): 213. Physical Education Departmental Records, Mount Holyoke College Archives, South Hadley, MA.

[25]Margaret Huntting to Laura Howell, 9 December 1846. Mount Holyoke College Library/Archives, South Hadley, MA.

[26]Lucy Goodale to her family, March 1838. Included on p. 3 of typed notes deposited by Mildred Howard in Mount Holyoke College History Collection, Mount Holyoke College Library/Archives, South Hadley MA.

[27]Quoted in Haddad, "Social Roles and Advanced Education," 68.

[28]McCurdy suggests that Lyon wrote out the original series of exercises and that these written instructions were then passed from teacher to teacher. "No one was especially trained to teach them," she noted, "but anyone who had

taken them was considered qualified to teach a class." McCurdy, "Physical Training at Mount Holyoke," 141.

[29]Ibid., 144.

[30]Margaret Huntting, to "My Dear Cousin," 9 December 1846. Mount Holyoke College Library/Archives, South Hadley, MA.

[31] *Songs for Calisthenics* (Springfield: Horace S. Taylor, 1849) and *Songs for Calisthenics* (Northampton: Hopkins, Bridgman & Co, 1857).

[32]In 1862, when Mount Holyoke introduced the Dio Lewis system of New Gymnastics, the school adopted the shortened skirts and pantaloons Lewis recommended for gymnastics attire.

[33]Quoted in McCurdy, "Physical Training at Mount Holyoke," 144.

[34]Mary Lyon, *Book of Duties*, Mary Lyon Papers, Mount Holyoke College/Archives, South Hadley, MA.

[35]Margaret Huntting, to "My Dear Cousin," 9 December 1846. Mount Holyoke College Library/Archives, South Hadley, MA.

[36]Mary Ware to Anny Batchelder, 1 December 1848. Mount Holyoke College Library/Archives, South Hadley, MA.

[37]Lyon died of erysipelas, a streptococcus infection of the skin and mucous membranes. Green, *Mary Lyon*, 310.

[38]Annie Walker to "My dear, dear Father," 25 December 1849. Mount Holyoke College Library/Archives, South Hadley, MA. Punctuation and capitalization have been added to this quote for clarity.

[39]Mary Titcomb graduated in 1850 and returned the following fall as a teacher. She taught at Mount Holyoke until March of 1852, returned following an illness in the fall of 1853, and taught through August 1856, when ill health again forced her to resign. She received the highest salary of any teacher in the school: $120. "Biographical notes on Mary Titcomb," compiled by Mrs. J. B. Clark, Physical Education Department Records, Mount Holyoke College Library/ Archives, Mount Holyoke College, South Hadley, MA.

[40]See calisthenics notebooks kept by Anna King Benton (1851), Mary McLean (1851), and one attributed to Mary Titcomb (1850). Physical Education Department Records, Mount Holyoke College Library/ Archives, Mount Holyoke College, South Hadley, MA.

[41][Mary Titcomb], "Calisthenics," handwritten manuscript (1850), 2-3. Physical Education Department Records, Mount Holyoke College Library/Archives, Mount Holyoke College, South Hadley, MA.

[42]Anna Benton King, "Calisthenics, Mount Hol. Fem. Sem. 1851," handwritten manuscript, 7-8. Physical Education Department Records, Mount Holyoke College Library/ Archives, Mount Holyoke College, South Hadley, MA.

[43][Mary Titcomb], *Calisthenic Exercises* (n.p., n.d.). The copy of this booklet in the rare book room of Springfield College has "Miss Titcomb, 1852" written on the cover. A second copy is on file at Mount Holyoke.

[44]Mary Titcomb to Miss Blakely, 14 January 1909. Mary Lyon papers, Mount Holyoke College Library/Archives, South Hadley, MA..

[45]Mary Lyon to "My dear Miss Backus," 30 January 1846. Mary Lyon papers, Mount Holyoke College Library/Archives, South Hadley MA.

[46]Lizzie Morley, "Mode of Operations in Case Mount Holyoke Seminary Takes Fire," 28 November 1862. Folder 5.10. Unpublished manuscript in Edward Williams Morley Collection, California Institute of Technology Archives, Pasadena, CA.

[47]Love Brown to Helen Savage, 11 August 1866. Student Files. Mount Holyoke College Library/Archives, South Hadley, MA.

[48]"Introduction," *The Ladies' Magazine* 1 (January 1828): 1. Hale argued that "no experiment will have an influence more important on the character and happiness of our society, than the granting to females the advantages of a systematic and thorough education."

[49]"Female Education," *The Ladies Magazine* 1 (January 1828): 25, 26.

[50]Hale regarded "The Physical Education of Girls," which appeared in volume one, number one of the *Journal of Health* as excellent, and reprinted it in the January 1830 issue of the *Ladies Book*. See "The Journal of Health," *The Ladies' Magazine* 3 (January 1830): 46-47. Hale also reprinted "Rules for a Young Lady," which recommended "domestic exercise," and the *Journal's* "A Physician's Advice on the Education of Girls," which suggested a combination of domestic exercise and outdoor walks. "Rules for a Young Lady," *The Ladies' Magazine* 3 (May 1830): 239-40.

[51][Sarah Hale], "A Chapter to be Read," *The Ladies Magazine and Literary Gazette* 5 (1832): 518.

[52]Ibid.

[53]Ibid. It does not appear that such a women's gymnasium actually opened in the 1830s.

[54]Ibid., 34. One example of the influence of Hale's thought can be found in the fact that this very passage was used by John Bolles in a lyceum lecture, "The Influence of Woman on Society" later that year. See *The Ladies' Magazine* 4 (June 1831): 261.

[55]James Whorton, *Crusaders for Fitness: The History of American Health Reformers* (Princeton: Princeton University Press, 1982), 38-131.

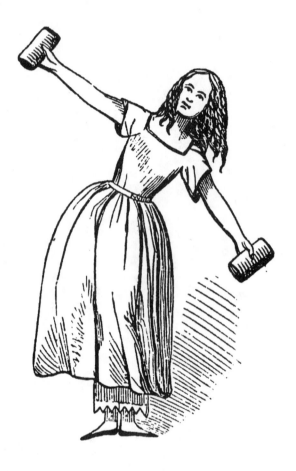

Figure 39: Young girl with "corn-bags" from Catharine Beecher's *Calisthenics Exercises for Home, Schools and Families* (1856).

# Chapter 6
## Becoming Catharine Beecher:
## Antebellum Proponent of Women's Exercise

During the three decades prior to the start of the Civil War, Catharine Esther Beecher possessed one of the most consistently persuasive voices in North America on matters of feminine exercise.[1] What set Beecher apart from other exercise authors of her era and contributed to her lasting reputation as a major figure in the history of women's exercise was not, however, originality. Beecher's reputation evolved largely as a consequence of her distinguished New England lineage and through the sophisticated promotional campaign she organized to sell her books on health and exercise in the mid-1850s.

While Beecher is widely regarded by historians as the most significant American popularizer of calisthenics for women, little attention has been paid by these same historians as to how, at age fifty-six, Beecher came to publish a work on calisthenics. Kathryn Sklar's excellent biography of Beecher filled in many gaps in our understanding of this complicated woman, but it paid almost no attention to Beecher's involvement with purposive exercise. James Whorton's casual handling of Beecher is typical of many sport histories: "Calisthenics and light gymnastics for women had been recommended by earlier reformers, most notably Catherine [sic] Beecher (and many of Beecher's exercises had been adopted and modified by Lewis)."[2] Even the two primary monographs in scholarly journals examining Beecher's physical culture ideas paid little attention to the true sources of her athletic inspiration.[3] This chapter, then, examines the influences that helped to produce Catharine Beecher's beliefs on exercise. It argues that Beecher should be regarded as a popularizer of physical training, not an innovator. Her involvement with purposive exercise can, in fact, be traced directly to four significant individuals in her life: Sarah Pierce of the Litchfield Female Academy; an anonymous Englishwoman who taught Beecher calisthenics; Dr. Elizabeth Blackwell, the first American woman to receive university training as a physician; and the movement cure specialist, Dr. George Taylor, who worked with Beecher just prior to the publication of her first exercise book.

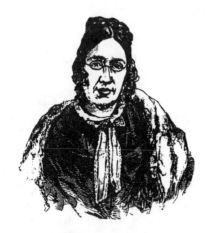

Figure 40: Catharine Beecher in
an engraving from Sarah Hale's
*Biography of Distinguished
Women.*

### Catharine Beecher and the Litchfield Female Academy

Born on Long Island in 1800, Catharine Beecher was the eldest
child of the influential, evangelical minister Lyman Beecher. She
reportedly began life with a "delicate and scrofulous constitution" that
kept her from walking until she was two years old. She soon passed this
early period of invalidism, however, and later claimed to have enjoyed
an active, healthy childhood. She reported, "As to exercise, the whole of
childhood and youth, up to eighteen, was one long play-spell out of
doors . . . The result was that I can not recall the memory of a single
day of sickness from infancy to the age of twenty."[4]

Part of the reason Catharine felt so well as a child might be
because, in 1810, she and her family moved from Long Island to
Litchfield, Connecticut, where she soon found herself enrolled at Sarah
Pierce's Litchfield Female Academy.[5] At the academy, ten-year-old
Catharine had her first introduction to purposive training.
Reminiscing about her early years at the school, Beecher recalled that
Pierce "had a quiet relish for humor and fun," which she tried to trans-
mit to her students.[6] "Her great hobby was *exercise for health*," Beecher
wrote, reporting that Pierce took a morning and evening walk each
day, "exhorting her pupils to the same." As a consequence, Beecher
elaborated, "every pleasant evening witnessed troops of young people
passing and repassing through the broad and shaded streets."[7] Beecher
remained a student at Pierce's school for six years, but whether she participated in exercises other than walking during these years is not
known. Her time at the Litchfield Academy left its mark, however.
Although she later disparaged the quality of the intellectual education

she received at the school, Beecher never forgot the personal example of Miss Pierce's dedication to exercise.[8] Pierce's insistence on regular, health-promoting exercise undoubtedly provided Beecher with a model for the incorporation of physical training into women's schools when she embarked upon her own career as an educator.

### Catharine Beecher's Quest for Health

Beecher's adult health problems began in 1822 when she received word that her fiancé, Alexander Metcalf Fisher, had died in a shipwreck.[9] After several months in which she was virtually incapacitated by her grief, Beecher decided that she must dedicate her life to public service. She felt her only professional option was to teach, so she apparently threw herself headlong into the organization of her first school, nearly exhausting her already limited physical reserves. What later became known as the Hartford Female Seminary opened in rented rooms over the White Horse Harness Shop on the town's main street in 1823. It was Beecher's hope, according to Sklar, to draw on the example of the Round Hill School for Boys and Emma Willard's Troy Female Seminary and create at her new home in Hartford, Connecticut, a boarding school where all aspects of a young woman's life could be regulated.

Although proud of her ambition and recent accomplishments, Catharine's brother, Edward, grew concerned with the way she disregarded her health during the early days of her professional career. He urged her to take time for herself and to use exercise as a form of medical therapy: "The mind cannot bear intense application to any one subject for a long time, without interruption," he cautioned Catharine, "nor will the body, without much care, bear it. I would advise you, therefore, to take *much exercise*."[10] Apparently, Catharine took her brother's concerns to heart. Reflecting on this period later in her life, Beecher recalled that after the school had opened, she tried to get eight hours of sleep a night, tried to wear healthful dress, and generally took one to two hours of exercise each day in the open air.[11]

For the first several years of her time in Hartford, Catharine's exercise of choice was horseback riding. She and her younger sister, Harriet, who taught with her at the school, rode each morning on two rented horses named Music and Dancing.[12] Later, Catharine purchased a beautiful, white horse whom she called Rollo. The Beecher sisters were generally not alone on these exercise rides; students and other teachers often accompanied the young headmistress and her sister.[13]

Abolitionist Angelina Grimke took part in one of the Beecher sisters's riding excursions in 1831 during a visit to Hartford, and reported that Catharine, in an attractive green riding dress, rode at the head of a cavalcade of students. "The contrast was handsome—she is an expert rider."[14]

It would be interesting to know whether Catharine practiced calisthenics on her own during her early adult years. Although calisthenics became part of her school's curriculum in 1827, at no point in any of Beecher's writings does she claim to have personally participated in the sessions. Despite an apparent intellectual understanding of the remedial value of exercise and the importance of moderation in matters of rest, food, and recreation, Beecher suffered a major nervous breakdown in 1829. For several months, she retired from all school work, and she reportedly could not read, write, or even listen to a conversation.[15] Beecher attributed her condition to overwork and her flaunting of the non-natural Laws of Health. Nearly twenty years later, she warned a group of teachers to "beware yourselves of the rocks on which I have fallen, and shipwrecked health irretrievably."[16]

Beecher returned to her work at the Hartford Seminary the next year, but her health never fully returned. She continued to suffer from what she described as a "singular susceptibility of the nervous system to any slight wound, bruise or sprain." Apparently, this problem manifested itself in an inflamed sciatic nerve that caused a semiparalysis in one leg.[17] As Kathryn Sklar observed, however, Beecher's primary ailment seemed to be the same sort of ephemeral nervous prostration suffered by so many other wealthy and upper middle-class women in this era. Sklar reasoned that Beecher's response to the internal tension she felt because of her assertive public role was periodic debility. According to Sklar, this allowed Beecher to be periodically dependent, without actually renouncing her desire for independence.[18]

In any case, whether Beecher's problems were physical, emotional, or a combination of the two, they were certainly real to her. Over the next several decades, sciatica, nervousness, and vision problems periodically sabotaged her efforts to promote the new women's professions of teaching and domestic economy. To cure these maladies, Beecher, like most reasonably affluent Americans of her day, sought medical assistance from both regular and irregular medical practitioners. In the mid-1840s, for instance, she visited a clairvoyant who sought help for her among the spirit world, and she worked with a hypnotist who conducted eight mesmerizing sessions within a period of ten days. Beecher also visited a number of allopathic medical practitioners who tried such remedies as prescribing a teaspoon of carbonate of iron three times a day, bleeding her, applying an irritating ointment to her spine, dosing her with camphor until temporary deafness set in, and recommending rhubarb three times daily as a purgative. On other occasions, Beecher endured other exotic remedies: Turkish hot air baths, galvanism, Russian baths, chemical baths, vapor baths, sulfur baths, and sun baths.[19]

The medical therapeutic Beecher found most beneficial, however, was the water cure, and she spent time in at least twelve different hydropathic institutions during the 1840s and early 1850s.[20] In these expensive, often luxurious, resort-spas, Beecher enjoyed cultured companionship, a retreat from her battles on behalf of education for women, and some medical solace.[21] She also participated at these spas in regular, purposive exercise.

Hydropathy was an enormously popular medical therapeutic for women in the middle years of the nineteenth century, and at least 213 different water cure centers opened in the years between 1840 and 1880 in the United States.[22] Water cure specialists attempted to cure disease by immersing their patients in water at a variety of temperatures, applying cold compresses, using steam baths, and internally administering large amounts of pure water.[23] Many water cure physicians specialized in the treatment of female reproductive complaints and a nineteenth-century nervous disorder called neurasthenia, which was most frequently associated with women.[24] In her 1855 physiology primer, *Letters to the People on Health and Happiness,* Beecher detailed a three-month hydropathic regimen she had once followed:

> At four in the morning packed in a wet sheet; kept in it from two to three hours; then up, and in a reeking perspiration immersed in the coldest plunge-bath. Then a walk as far as strength would allow, and drink five or six tumblers of the coldest water. At eleven A.M. stand under a douche of the coldest water falling eighteen feet for ten minutes. Then walk, and drink three or four tumblers of water. At three P.M. sit half an hour with the feet in the coldest water, then rub them till warm. Then cover the weak limb and a third of the body in wet bandages and retire to rest. This same wet bandage to be worn all day and kept constantly wet.[25]

Walking and other forms of exercise played important roles in most water cure establishments, and, consequently, many adult women had their first experiences with purposive training while they were in residence at such institutions. Nearly all water cure specialists agreed on the therapeutic benefits of regular exercise and prescribed it just as they did sitzbaths and mineral waters. Mrs. M. L. Shew, wife of the nation's leading water cure practitioner, Dr. Joel Shew, wrote in 1844 that exercise "is an important matter in the success of the Priessnitz method and in the water cure generally."[26] Beecher reported that "after every bath the patient is required to bring on a glow by exercise in the open air, and as baths are taken four and five times a day, this secures a considerable amount of pure air for the lungs as well as exercise for the lower limbs."[27] Walking was the preferred exercise modality for the seriously ill, Mrs. Shew observed, but as strength returned to a patient, jumping, hopping, skipping, and running should be included in the exercise program, even for women.[28] According to Beecher, several water cures adopted "a system of calisthenics that exercises all the other muscles of the body."[29]

Although the water treatments may not have healed by themselves, the spare, healthy diet, relaxed dress, and regular exercise that were so much a part of the water cure's hygienic regimen frequently worked wonders. Although Beecher's medical condition proved to be beyond the capacities of hydropathic practitioners, she did not abandon her quest for health; and, after a series of inconclusive and frequently unpleasant hydropathic treatments, she discovered a different and far more effective medical remedy.[30] As she told her readers in *Letters to the People on Health and Happiness,* "I was led to an institution where the main reliance was placed on *exercise,* in connection with a strict obedience to all the laws of health."[31]

### The Influence of Dr. Elizabeth Blackwell

Beecher arrived at this new therapeutic mecca through the influence of Dr. Elizabeth Blackwell, the first American woman to earn a university degree in medicine. Like many physicians of her era, Blackwell maintained an eclectic approach to medical theory, especially in the early years of her practice.[32] When her old friend from Cincinnati, Catharine Beecher, came to consult with her about her physical problems in the early 1850s, Blackwell suggested that Beecher try exercise. She loaned Beecher several European books on physical training and took the then middle-aged Beecher to the offices of Dr. George H. Taylor, the foremost proponent of the movement cure in America.[33]

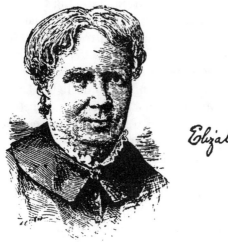

Figure 41: Elizabeth Blackwell in an engraving from the *National Cyclopaedia of American Biography.*

Born in England in 1821, Blackwell had first met the Beechers when she and her family moved to Cincinnati, in 1838.[34] The teenaged Blackwell became close friends with Catharine's younger sister, Harriet Beecher Stowe, and Elizabeth often took care of Harriet's children, so Harriet would be free to write.[35] Although Catharine was away from Cincinnati most of the years Blackwell lived there, she did come home from time to time, and served as both a friend and a role model for young Elizabeth.[36] In 1845, when Blackwell decided to become a physician, she found little support among her family or friends.[37] Even her good friend Harriet considered the idea "impracticable," though she did finally allow that "if carried out it might be highly useful."[38]

The story of Blackwell's fight to receive a medical diploma is now so well known that it need not be recounted here.[39] What is less well known regarding Blackwell's medical education, however, is that following her graduation from Geneva Medical College in 1849, and a subsequent residency at *La Maternite* hospital in Paris, she went to London to do a second residency at St. Bartholomew's Hospital. There, in addition to her hospital duties, the young physician also took classes from "Professor Georgii" in the latest European exercise fad—the Swedish Movement Cure.[40] Georgii was at Ling's Swedish Central Gymnastic Institute from 1829 to 1849 and served as head teacher there from 1840 until his departure. Although two other Swedes—

Govert Indebetou and C. Erenhoff—trained in Ling's methods had preceded Georgii to London, it was his arrival that truly launched the system in England. The program Georgii introduced to London—which Blackwell and then Beecher helped transfer to America—was Ling's Swedish system of free and remedial gymnastics. Beecher, in particular, became enraptured with the Ling mystique. In her *Letters to the People on Health and Happiness*, she described Ling as a "distinguished Swedish philanthropist" and went on at great length to point out the scientific basis of Ling's suggestions regarding exercise.[41]

The exercise sessions with Professor Georgii proved unexpectedly useful to Blackwell. When she returned to the United States in 1851 and attempted to open a medical practice at 44 University Place, New York City, Blackwell could find no patients willing to run the risk of being treated by a female physician. To establish her credibility and advertise her new medical practice, Blackwell decided to deliver a series of public lectures on the physical education of women.[42] On 1 March 1851, a brief notice appeared in the *New York Times* announcing the six-lecture series at a price of two dollars.[43] Blackwell later confessed, "These lectures . . . gave me my first start in practical medical life."[44] The next year, Blackwell published the lectures in book form as *The Laws of Life With Special Reference to the Physical Education of Girls.*[45]

Curiosity compels one to wonder about the content of the conversations between Blackwell and Beecher. It would be interesting to know, for instance, which French and English books on exercise Blackwell loaned Beecher. It would also be interesting to know what Beecher thought of Blackwell's approach to womanhood and exercise. Blackwell was far more egalitarian in her attitudes toward the sexes than was Beecher, and the young physician argued in her book on exercise that women needed physical strength as well as physical fitness. Unlike Beecher, who up to this point in time had maintained in her writings that women could find adequate exercise in housework and light gardening (if they did the work themselves rather than hiring servants), Blackwell maintained that women needed more and more vigorous forms of exercise. "The ordinary exercise of walking and domestic occupations," she wrote, "does not bring the majority of these muscles into active play." On the contrary, Blackwell explained, women need "special movements, which shall produce this wide activity, and thus strengthen every muscle and place it under the control of our will."[46] In America, Blackwell believed that those special movements could best be learned at Dr. George Taylor's Institute of the Swedish

Movement Cure, located at the corner of Sixth and Thirty-eighth
Streets in Manhattan.

### The Movement Cure

George Taylor had just graduated from medical school when
Beecher followed Blackwell's advice and visited his Institute in 1853.[47]

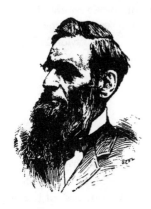

Figure 42: George H. Taylor in an engraving from the *National Cyclopaedia of
American Biography.*

Although new to the profession, Taylor was not afraid to blaze his
own trail as a physician. He may have employed hydropathy and other
eclectic medical remedies at times, but Taylor centered his practice
around exercise. He argued—well before any of the cardiovascular
studies of the twentieth century—that a direct relationship existed
between the body's ability to utilize oxygen and its general, overall
health. Unlike modern sports medicine specialists who tout the health-
prolonging benefits of slender, aerobically trained bodies, however,
Taylor fixed on the idea of chest size and muscularity as key components of health. He argued that increasing the size of the chest
increased the body's "oxidizing capacity" and thereby created health
improvements for his patients. Only truly vigorous exercises, Taylor
contended, could create the desired increase in chest size.[48]

Taylor was one of the first physicians/physical educators to use
physical measurements as an indication of the progress of his
patients.[49] At the end of her six-week movement cure, Beecher
reported with considerable pride that she had to enlarge her clothing
by three inches around the chest and by two inches around the waist.[50]

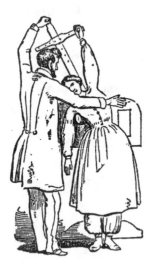

Figure 43: This illustration shows one of Taylor's favorite exercises for chest expansion. As the patient pushed the machine's handles overhead, the physician, or "operator" as Taylor called the person assisting the patient, would clap the patient on the side of the chest to vibrate the lungs and free up more air space. From: George Taylor, M.D., *An Illustrated Sketch of the Movement-Cure* (1866).

According to Taylor, a four-inch increase in chest expansion was not at all uncommon with his methods.[51] Taylor also measured the success of his system by its ability to increase muscle mass. He believed that his specific movements could direct the "vital powers" of the body into those areas requiring an increase in size or power.[52] In his *Illustrated Sketch of the Movement Cure,* Taylor listed many differences between his system and other competing exercise therapies, but the first difference listed was that "the movement cure increases muscle."[53]

At Taylor's Manhattan offices in the early 1850s, patients such as Beecher employed a variety of remedial exercises depending on their physical problems. Disordered digestion, biliousness, headaches, constipation, diarrhea, pulmonary disease, disorders of the uterus, nervousness, infantile paralysis, spinal curvatures, anemia and hysteria—all had an appropriate set of exercises assigned to them to offset their pernicious effect upon the body. Taylor, as Ling had done, differentiated between generalized exercise, which he called gymnastics, and the specific movements that made up his therapeutic medical arsenal. According to Taylor, anyone could lead an exercise class, but to properly prescribe the special movements that healed the body required scientific training, an understanding of physiology, and, "for their greatest success, certain mental and moral qualities in the practitioner calculated to gain and keep the confidence of the patient."[54] Taylor further divided his exercises into "single movements" deemed useful for correcting uneven bodily development, and "passive movements," such

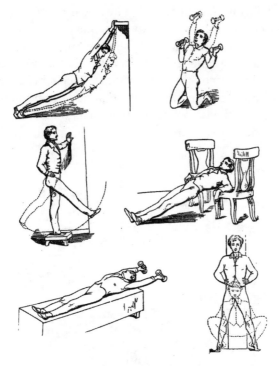

Figure 44: A sampler of movement cure exercises from George Taylor's instruction manual for home training—*Health by Exercise* (1879).

as massage, shaking, and kneading. His single movements—some of which Beecher adapted for her calisthenics text—were exercises done with dumbbells or weights, in which the general object was to work one muscle, or group of muscles, at a time.[55] These single movements consisted of limb extensions, dumbbell swings, deep-knee bends, and a wide variety of stretches. In other exercises favored by Taylor, a partner provided extra resistance and helped increase the range of motion in certain positions. Taylor also experimented with and invented various types of exercise machines.[56]

Beecher claimed in *Letters to the People on Health and Happiness* that she entered Taylor's institute in order to see whether his system "was scientific or empirical and whether it was taken from Ling as a whole or in part." She stayed under Taylor's care for eight weeks, however, and did exercise for six of those weeks. She pronounced the experience "entirely satisfactory . . . even where it was not scientific but empirical." According to Beecher, she took no medicines or water treatments at Taylor's institute, relying instead on a "strict obedience to the laws of health, and a system of vigorous exercises, commenced moderately, and increased daily till the nervous and muscular system were brought up to a tone and power which seemed wonderful, especially in a community of chronic invalids." Beecher claimed that her experience created "a general vigor . . . that had not been experienced for years . . . [and] the weak limb seemed to gain more than from any previous method of treatment."[57]

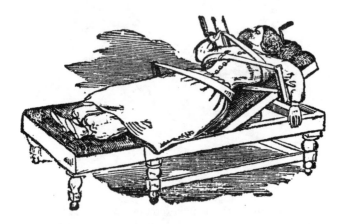

Figure 45: To cure spinal curvature, Taylor suggested the "Combination Couch" and strong rubber bands which attempted to pull the person's spine back in line in an early form of traction. From: *An Illustrated Sketch of the Movement Cure,* George Taylor (1866).

Beecher's newfound strength did not last long. Although she apparently believed that the movement cure would bring her to the "fair prospect of an entire cure," a clumsy railroad employee accidentally knocked her against a moving train that caught her clothing, pulled her down, and dragged her for a considerable distance. "The fright, the jar, and the strain on a weakened limb" were too much for Beecher. She had another of her nervous attacks and retired from active life for most of the next year. By 1855, when *Letters to the People on Health and Happiness* appeared, she still had not recovered sufficiently to try the movement cure.[58] Ironically, the one bright note in this incident—the $2,500 settlement Beecher received from the railway—also eluded her in the end; her bank failed shortly after she deposited the check.[59]

### A New Career:
### Promoting Women's Health and Exercise

Beecher's experiences with Blackwell and Taylor stimulated her to embark on a physical culture campaign in the mid-1850s. Prior to this time, Beecher had discussed matters relating to health and exercise in several of her books, but only in relatively general terms.[60] For instance, her 1829 essay, *Suggestions Respecting Improvements in Education*, and her 1841 book, *A Treatise on Domestic Economy for the Use of Young Ladies at Home and at School*, shared the same hygienic-educative theme: women needed intellectual *and* physical education to properly fit themselves for their lives as homemakers and mothers.[61] Beecher argued in these early works that good health and the physical exercise that enhanced that health were essential to a woman's ability to properly fulfill her socially-determined roles as homemaker and mother. Beecher believed that women had a moral obligation to their families and their country to treat health and exercise matters seriously.[62] "What is the profession of a woman?" she asked rhetorically in 1829. "Is it not to form immortal minds, and to watch, to nurse, and to rear the bodily system . . . upon the order and regulation of which, the health and well-being of the mind so greatly depends?"[63] By the mid-1850s, when Beecher published *Letters to the People on Health and Happiness*, she had come to believe that "woman is the Heaven-appointed guardian of health in the family, as the physician is in the community . . . ." Every woman, she wrote, should "direct her earnest interest and attention" to this part of her profession.[64] Although homemaking and, hopefully, motherhood were the highest professions to which a woman could aspire, teaching was an acceptable substitute. In a letter to the female graduates of the West Newton Normal School, however, Beecher made it clear that women who taught also had special hygienic responsibilities. "Teach all your pupils the *laws of health*, and present them as the *laws of God*," she wrote emphatically. Let your students know that they commit a sin when they violate these laws, she continued, and, "set them an example of strict obedience to them yourselves."[65]

Beecher and many of her contemporaries believed that the health of American women had deteriorated to the point that it constituted a national crisis.[66] "[There is] a terrible decay of female health all over the land," Beecher wrote in 1855, "bringing with it an incredible extent of individual, domestic and social suffering."[67] Beecher's concern over women's health may have been fueled by her friendship with Mrs. R. B.

Gleason, a hydropathic physician at the Elmira Water Cure. Gleason wrote in 1853, "So long have I sojourned in the midst of a sick and suffering sisterhood that it often seems to me as if all women were sick save myself." To correct this impression, Gleason continued, she did an informal survey of the women she met during a six-months trip. "I looked for *well women* in city, town and country and found only here and there one."[68]

Beecher viewed *Letters to the People on Health and Happiness* (1855) as the pivotal piece in her campaign to improve women's health. Although written as a physiology primer, Beecher's outrage at the ways American women mindlessly contributed to their own physical problems was quite apparent. "If a plan for *destroying* female health, in all the ways in which it could be most effectively done, were drawn up," she charged, "it would be exactly the course which is now pursued by a large portion of this nation, especially in the more wealthy classes."[69] *Letters* aimed to provide women with the physiological knowledge they needed in order to be successful health guardians, but as it included Beecher's own medical history, it carried the force of personal example. Beecher also included in it a statistical study she had undertaken that analyzed the health of American women. Although modern sociologists would argue with both her methodology and sample, Beecher seemed satisfied to conclude that the standard of health among American women was "so low that few have a correct idea of what a healthy woman is."[70]

Beecher's health reform dreams went well beyond the publication of *Letters to the People on Health and Happiness*, however. She hoped to form a national organization of women who would lend their influence to her cause. She called the organization the American Women's Educational Association, and its stated aim was to help women receive the intellectual and physiological education they needed to fulfill their appropriate profession—"the distinctive profession of women being considered as embracing the training of the human mind, the care of the human body in infancy and sickness, and the conservation of the family state."[71] Beecher hoped to achieve this goal by establishing endowed schools in major cities in the United States in which women would receive training in traditional academic subjects, domestic tasks, and physiology and exercise. She assigned the proceeds from the sale of *Letters*, and its companion volume, *Physiology and Calisthenics for Schools and Families*, published in 1856, to the association.[72]

Beecher also hoped that *Physiology and Calisthenics* would be adopted as a school textbook throughout the United States, and thus promote a great improvement in the physical training of the next generation."[73] To further this dream, and to increase book sales, Beecher organized a promotional tour to help generate interest in what she called her calisthenics system. Beecher reported on 5 February 1856, from Columbus, Ohio, that the promotional tour was at that point a great success:

> I am on a tour visiting the chief cities to introduce my system of calisthenics into the *public* schools as well as private. I find great interest excited. At Cincinnati the City School Board issued an order to have all the schools dismissed that the teachers might meet me & I had an audience of 500 teachers & friends of Common Schools. They were much interested and said the thing *should* go there—& if it does it will go all over the West. I shall do the same in Washington, Phila., N. York, Albeny [sic], N. Haven, Hartford & Boston.[74]

In a letter to her family, dated two days previously, Beecher reported that she had already visited Chicago, Galesburg, and Indianapolis on this same tour.[75]

Beecher's promotional tour would not have worked without the assistance of a network of interested women. In each town she planned to visit, Beecher tried to organize a committee of women to whom she then sent four articles for insertion in the local papers "giving an account of the plan and the books."[76] The "plan" that Beecher referred to was that after she made her own visit to the town and made her presentations, these local women would continue to act as book agents for her. If people bought *Letters to the People* and *Physiology and Calisthenics* directly from these local agents, then all profits from the sale of the books supposedly went to the American Women's Educational Association. If people bought the books from a regular bookseller, then only half the profits ended up in the Association's coffers. The two books, postage paid, sold together for one dollar.[77]

Although the tour apparently went well, and Beecher enlisted such prominent women as Lydia Sigourney, Sarah Hale, Catharine Sedgwick, and her sister Harriet Beecher Stowe to serve as members of the Board of Managers for the organization, the sales of the books did not raise enough money to endow the women's schools as Beecher had hoped.[78]

## Beecher's System of Calisthenics

Beecher's involvement with calisthenics began in 1827, the same year she finally received sufficient financial backing from the Hartford business community to construct her own school building.[79] Beecher viewed her first experience with calisthenics as an experiment in remedying physical defects. As she related the story many years later, "An English lady of fine person and manner came to us as a teacher of what then had no name, but now would be called Calisthenics." According to Beecher, this anonymous Englishwoman "gave a large number of the exercises that are in my work on *Physiology and Calisthenics*, published by the Harpers, and narrated how she had cured deformities in others by her methods."[80] Furthermore, the woman claimed that she had cured herself of a severe humpback, a fact Catharine glowingly recalled as she explained how impressed she was by the woman's grace and fine proportions. "The whole school took lessons of her," Beecher wrote, "and I added others."[81]

Although Beecher did not claim that the changes were "conspicuous," she apparently observed enough improvement in her students to believe that the Englishwoman's system had merit.[82] While Beecher's books and writings provide no other details about the Englishwoman, what constituted the exercise sessions, or the length of time the calisthenics classes continued, it seems likely, based on the fact that visible differences could be seen in the students, that the classes continued for some weeks. Beecher never named the woman who helped introduce calisthenics to the United States. The fact that Beecher didn't identify the Englishwoman may simply have been a nineteenth-century act of good manners, but it could also be a reflection of Beecher's interest in being credited with inventing calisthenics. In any case, Beecher claimed that "from this came the system of Calisthenics which I invented, which spread all over the country," despite the fact that Zilpah Grant and several British physical culturists had preceded her.[83] Although Beecher's Hartford school was not the first American school to adopt calisthenics for its students, it was admittedly one of the earliest, and it must be granted that from the time of her first meeting with the Englishwoman, Beecher maintained an interest in calisthenics as a form of remedial exercise.

It would be incorrect, however, to assume that Beecher viewed calisthenics as the best form of exercise for women during most of her active years in the field of education. In *Domestic Economy*, for instance, written in 1842, Beecher firmly pressed her hygienic stamp of approval on manual labor. She recommended that boarding schools set aside at least two hours a day in which their students could participate in cleaning, gardening, and laundry, and suggested calisthenics only as a secondary measure to improve posture and cure deformities.[84] Even when Beecher launched her women's physical culture campaign in the mid-1850s, she did not endorse calisthenics as the *best* system of exercise for women. Despite her time with Elizabeth Blackwell and George Taylor—both of whom argued against the idea that housework was adequate exercise for women—Beecher still wrote that calisthenics were "the next best thing" to domestic labor for women. [85]

In her two day schools, where there was no meaningful domestic labor for the students to perform, Catharine herself relied on "the next best thing"[86] In 1831, Beecher's last year in Hartford, calisthenics appeared on the school's daily schedule in the morning and in the afternoon.[87] In Cincinnati, Ohio, where she moved with her father in 1832, Beecher opened the Western Female Institute and, again, included two half-hour sessions of calisthenics on her new school's daily schedule.[88]

It was in Cincinnati that Beecher claimed she hit upon the idea of accompanying the exercises with music, hoping to "secure all the advantages supposed to be gained in dancing schools."[89] The musical exercises "were extensively adopted in schools, both East and West," Beecher later claimed, "but finally passed away." They failed, Beecher reported, because teachers needed a large, unfurnished room and a piano or other musical instrument. While Beecher apparently had these luxuries available to her in Cincinnati, most frontier schools did not. To bring purposive exercise to the frontier, however, Beecher arranged a system of exercises to be performed in a schoolroom without removing desks or benches. Her stated goal for these exercises—as it was for the more movement-oriented musical calisthenics—was to train young girls to "move heads, hands and arms gracefully; to sit, to stand and to walk properly, and to pursue calisthenic exercises for physical development as a regular school duty as much as their studies."[90]

## *Calisthenic Exercises for Schools, Families, and Health Establishments*

In the 1850 edition of her *Treatise on Domestic Economy*, Beecher mentioned that she had begun preparing a guidebook to calisthenics exercises "of her own invention." She wrote that parts of her system had already been used in several schools, and said that singing, "with a great variety of amusing and graceful evolutions, designed to promote health and easy manners will be incorporated into the new regimen."[91] Despite this mention of a work in progress, it was 1856 before *Physiology and Calisthenics for Schools and Families*, and *Calisthenic Exercises for Schools, Families and Health Establishments* finally appeared in one binding.[92] *Physiology and Calisthenics* was a textbook written for school use—a scaled-down version of her *Letters to the People* minus the closing chapters discussing woman's moral duties. There were no calisthenic exercises described in the manuscript despite the use of "calisthenics" in the title.

Bound in the same volume with *Physiology and Calisthenics* was *Calisthenic Exercises for Schools, Families and Health Establishments*, a pamphlet-length book that contains the only written record of Beecher's "system." She admitted on the title page of *Calisthenic Exercises* that she had "selected and arranged" her exercises from various sources.[93] Those sources no doubt included the French and English exercise texts Blackwell had loaned Beecher, the exercises she learned at Taylor's Institute, and, in all probability, Mathius Roth's *The Free Gymnastic Exercises of P. H. Ling, Arranged by H. Rothstein.* Published simultaneously in Britain and America, Roth's 1853 interpretation of Ling's system introduced many Anglophiles to the tenets of Swedish gymnastics, and it would seem likely that someone with Beecher's interest in exercise and wide-ranging contacts would have been familiar with such an important book.[94]

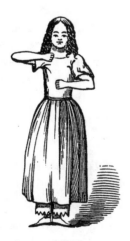

Figure 46: George Taylor's influence can be seen in the chest expansion exercise. Students filled their lungs with air and then beat along the sides of their chest with their fists to force air into parts of the lungs not normally used. From: Catharine Beecher, *Calisthenics for Schools, Families and Health Establishments* (1856).

In *Calisthenic Exercises*, Beecher divided her movements into those to be done while standing beside a desk in a classroom and those to be done in a calisthenics hall. The fifty classroom exercises were very similar to those seen in more conservative calisthenics books of the 1820s and 1830s, except that Beecher did not recommend that implements of

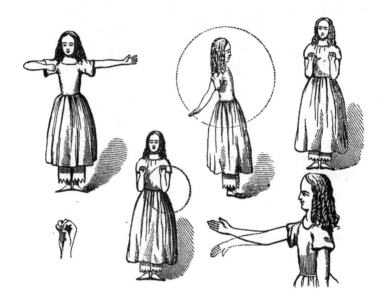

Figure 47: Upper extremity exercises from Catharine Beecher's *Calisthenics Exercises for Home, Schools and Families* (1856).

any sorts be used for her drills. Beecher included ten arm and hand exercises designed to produce "roundness of outline, grace of movement, and purity and clearness of skin," and nineteen relatively stationary lower limb exercises.[95] Among the more difficult leg and foot movements were several dips and curtseys, a deep-knee bend, knee raises, and leg extensions. There were no movements that would provide real strength to women. In fact, on the more difficult knee raises, Beecher cautioned girls to raise their knees only half as much as the boys because the weight of their skirts would balance out their difference in effort.[96] The remaining classroom exercises consisted of deep breathing, vocal exercises, and simple limb extensions.

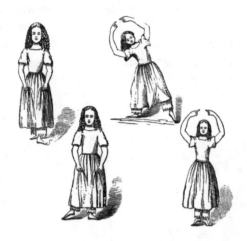

Figure 48: Lower limb exercises from Catharine Beecher's *Calisthenics Exercises for Home, Schools and Families* (1856).

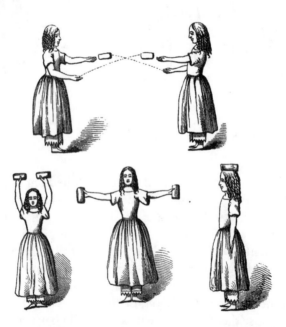

Figure 49: Weight exercises from Catharine Beecher's *Calisthenics Exercises for Home, Schools and Families* (1856).

For the calisthenics hall, Beecher included two kinds of exercises. She first described several marches to be done on an oval walking pathway inlaid in the floor of the gymnasium. As Alexander Walker had done twenty years earlier, Beecher cautioned that the marching step should never exceed the length of a foot. Beecher also demonstrated several marches using what she called "weights," which were actually small cloth sacks, six inches wide and eight to twelve inches long, filled with dried corn. With these cornbags, the students performed several isometric exercises, holding the weights overhead and out to the side as they continued to march around the room. The most vigorous exercise of the five weight exercises was what Beecher called "Weights Balancing," in which the students swung the weights up and down in time to music without moving their feet. In the final exercise of the series, the students threw cornbags back and forth between themselves.[97]

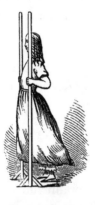

Figure 50: Upright parallel bar exercise from Catharine Beecher's *Calisthenics Exercises for Home, Schools and Families* (1856).

Finally, Beecher introduced a section on the movement cure in which she featured upright parallel bar exercises to open the chest and straighten the spine. These exercises were no doubt similar to those she did at George Taylor's institute.

### The Legacy of Catharine Beecher

Beecher's contribution in the area of exercise was not unlike that of the late-twentieth-century advertising executive. First and foremost, she was a promoter—savvy, culturally aware, and in touch with the *zeitgeist* of her America. For three decades she preached the benefits of exercise for women, but she carefully embedded her message within the socially acceptable framework of domesticity, intuitively understanding that this approach would have far greater mass appeal.

The highlight of Beecher's career as a physical educator came in the mid-1850s when she embarked on her physical culture campaign. Capitalizing on her status as a celebrity, Beecher organized what appears to have been the first true promotional campaign in the United States for any exercise system.[98] She set up a book tour, created a press packet to get her ideas and the news of her imminent visit inserted into the local papers, and involved local women in both her publicity campaign and her direct marketing scheme to sell books. For that era, it was a brilliant promotional concept.

But does Beecher deserve, as she asserted in her 1874 *Educational Reminiscences*, to be remembered as an "inventor" and innovator of American calisthenics and exercise? Let us consider the record:

(1) Beecher *was* among the first educators to argue that women needed physical education as part of their school curriculum, but she undoubtedly came to this opinion because she attended Sarah Pierce's school in Litchfield, Connecticut. Pierce required all her students to walk regularly, and she may also have encouraged her students to participate in an early form of calisthenics.

(2) It is certainly true that Beecher included calisthenics in the Hartford Female Academy's curriculum in 1827, making it one of the earliest examples of a female physical education program in the United States. However, Beecher's involvement with calisthenics came about because an Englishwoman spent time in Hartford and taught the exercise system to Beecher and the students.

(3) Beecher claimed that calisthenics were included in "all the schools" with which she was associated. While it is certainly true that she devoted much of her life to the promotion of education for women in general, she was only directly connected to three schools. Following Hartford, she served as principal/fund-raiser for a school in Cincinnati from 1833 to 1837. According to Kathryn Sklar, however, Beecher did no teaching at the new academy.[99] At Milwaukee Female College, begun in 1850, Beecher served as a fund-raiser and policy setter and made only occasional visits to the school. Again, she did no actual teaching.[100]

(4) During this same time frame, 1827–1855, the Zilpah Grant-Mary Lyon version of calisthenics enjoyed uninterrupted growth as

many of their students became teachers and moved throughout the United States.

(5) Beecher claimed that she invented a new system of calisthenics set to music while living in Cincinnati. Evidence from Mount Holyoke's archives suggests that music was also central to Grant and Mary Lyon's earlier system.

(6) Beecher's long periods of residence at different water cure establishments during the 1840s exposed her to many different types of light exercise and calisthenics and had to affect her ideas about training.

(7) It appears that Beecher became a personal convert to calisthenic-type exercise only after she spent time with Drs. Elizabeth Blackwell and George Taylor. Blackwell provided Beecher with the books and intellectual arguments in favor of exercise, while Taylor taught her how to perform the movements. Prior to her time with the movement cure, Beecher had most frequently recommended domestic labor for exercise.

(8) Beecher openly admitted her debt to Swedish calisthenics expert, Pehr H. Ling, whose system of exercises was well known in New England physical training circles prior to the publication of Beecher's book on calisthenics.

(9) Finally, there is no evidence to suggest that Beecher authored the 1832 anonymously published *Calisthenics* other than the fact that its publisher had a Hartford address.

It seems clear that, although Beecher was not an inventor of calisthenics, she was a resourceful synthesizer. She took the ideas of others, reconciled those ideas with her passion for domesticity and the subordinate nature of women, and then turned her attention to plans for promotion. That flair for promotion resulted in a considerable legacy. Although she was fully aware of the resolutions of the Seneca Falls convention and the push for gender equity begun by Elizabeth Cady Stanton, Lucy Stone, Amelia Bloomer, and others, she rejected this approach to womanhood in favor of the far more socially acceptable image of a healthy woman in the home. Women, Beecher argued, needed to understand physiology and the laws of health because they had been chosen by God as the guardians of health. While this responsibility would seem to confer a special and more liberating status on women, Beecher did not view her new women's profession as a step toward more egalitarian gender relations. To the end of her days, Beecher argued that a woman should take a "subordinate place—as the Bible and Nature both teach is her true position."[101]

It has been argued that, by linking exercise to domesticity, Beecher stymied egalitarian progress for nineteenth-century women. Contrasting Beecher's contributions to those of Thomas Wentworth Higginson, chief oracle of the muscular Christianity movement, for instance, the historian Linda Borish concluded that Beecher's interpretation of sport and exercise narrowly restricted women to the domestic sphere, while Higginson's muscular Christianity movement urged men to be "cultural participants of the world outside the home."[102] The historian Patricia Vertinsky has similarly argued that Beecher's approach to calisthenics created a dichotomy in male and female physical training that continues to negatively influence our ideas about fitness, exercise, and gender. "The direct effect" of Beecher's program, Vertinsky wrote, "was in the development and reinforcement of a specialized physical education curriculum for uniquely female needs."[103] According to Vertinsky, Beecher's was a gender-specific exercise program that reinforced cultural differences between the sexes and slowed the march toward equity. In Beecher's defense, it should be noted that *Calisthenics* contained a number of illustrations of boys performing calisthenics movements. Beecher viewed her calisthenics system as a school physical education program, not simply a female physical education program. To give Vertinsky her due, however, Beecher's advocacy of manual labor as the best form of exercise for women, and her cautions to girls to do only half the movement in the more vigorous calisthenics exercises, should be read as nothing more than what it is: gender specific exercise.

Although it was not her intention, Beecher's articulation of a relationship between purposive exercise, domestic happiness, and separate sphere ideology ironically forged a persuasive tool for the greater emancipation of women. By linking exercise with domestic felicity and ceding to women a moral responsibility in this area, Beecher opened the gymnasium doors to many women who would never have considered attempting Fowle's or Beaujeu's vigorous systems. Some of these women learned more than the exercises of the movement cure and how to hold and toss their cornbags. They also learned that they could control their bodies by the use of exercise. By suggesting that women's bodies could be "trained," Beecher enabled women to begin viewing their bodies as uniquely their own. As the historian Harvey Green put it in *Fit for America*, Beecher's assertion that a causal relationship existed between health, beauty, and happiness—a concept that seems obvious to our twentieth-century exercise sensibilities—was "a breakthrough for the nineteenth century."[104]

The historian Nancy Struna argued in an analysis of the sporting experiences of American colonial women that post-Revolutionary proponents of the Republican Mother ideal "had recognized the importance of health as the state in which women must exist," but had not been able to take the next intellectual step and link physical performance, sport, and exercise to that concept of health.[105] Catharine Beecher, although not necessarily original in her approach, provided American women with that important link. She placed in the hands of nineteenth-century women the means for their own self-improvement and gave them hope that they could live more fully and make a greater contribution to their culture. By inculcating these same ideas in the students and young teachers with whom she worked, Beecher spread her message to thousands of American students as well.[106]

Beecher's inclusion in *Letters to the People on Health and Happiness* of a line drawing of the Venus de Medici, illustrative of the ideal female body, is also significant in light of later developments in the nineteenth century. The Venus de Medici, like most Greek representations of the feminine form, is full-bodied, natural-waisted, and visibly athletic. It is, at the same time, a maternal, womanly form that by its sheer size suggests substance and importance. Contrasted with the dominant beauty ideal of the day—the wasp-waisted "steel engraving" woman described by Lois Banner—the de Medici appears majestic, much as a draft horse, does standing alongside an underfed saddlehorse.[107] Beecher, like George Taylor, equated an increase in size with an increase in health. The de Medici represented not simply an unfettered waistline and healthy reproductive organs, but larger, more physically fit women in general. Beecher's interest in increasing the size of women's bodies was yet another harbinger of a paradigm shift in the way Americans viewed the healthy/beautiful woman. Despite her insistence on domesticity, Beecher was not advocating that women should be passive, insipid, and useless. She viewed women as important to the culture, and the aim of her exercise program was to increase that usefulness.

Larger and more physically competent women could obviously be greater contributors to the life of the nation.

In deconstructing the mythology surrounding Catharine Beecher's reputation as an exercise innovator, it is important that we do not lose sight of her considerable influence on nineteenth-century women's lives. Had it not been for Beecher, Dio Lewis and the many exercise advocates who so suddenly proliferated in the late 1850s and early 1860s would have found it much harder to sell their more vigorous and socially emancipating systems to women. In addition, Beecher turned the public's attention to the need for remedial and therapeutic exercise, which both facilitated the growth of the hygienic system known as the movement cure and paved the way for the dominance of Ling's Swedish system in American physical education at the end of the nineteenth century.

Despite Beecher's campaign to promote her system, domestic labor and light calisthenics faded in popularity in the early 1860s and was replaced by vigorous systems popularized by George Barker Windship, Dio Lewis, and others. Beecher's conservatism did not allow her to embrace these new systems, however, and her eminence as a physical educator declined sharply during this decade. Beecher hated losing the limelight. As her *Educational Reminiscences* reveal, she accused Lewis of stealing her system, and she claimed for herself more credit than she deserved as an innovator of calisthenics. Twentieth-century historians, reading Beecher's claims, have been quick to credit her for the entire calisthenics movement of the nineteenth century. Future histories of physical education should pay homage to Blackwell, Taylor, Roth, and the others who showed her the way.

---

[1]Beecher's life is remarkably well documented. For a contemporary assessment of her contributions, see Sarah Josepha Hale, *Biography of Distinguished Women; or, Woman's Record, from the Creation to A.D. 1869* (New York: Harper & Brothers, 1876), 578-82. The best modern source on Beecher is Katherine Kish Sklar, *Catherine Beecher: A Study in American Domesticity* (New York: W. W. Norton and Company, 1973). For information on Beecher's legacy to education and exercise, see Kathryn Kish Sklar, "Catharine Beecher: Transforming the Teaching Profession," in Linda Kerber and Jane De Hart-Matthews, eds., *Women's America: Refocusing the Past*, 2nd ed. (New York: Oxford University Press, 1987), 158-66; Patricia Vertinsky,

"Sexual Equality and the Legacy of Catharine Beecher," *Journal of Sport History* 6 (Spring 1979): 38-49; Fred Eugene Leonard, "Chapters from the Early History of Physical Training in America: The Introduction of Calisthenics for Girls and Women (Dating from about 1830)," *Mind and Body* 13 (December 1906): 289-96; J. H. Sawyer, "Henry Ward and Catherine [sic] E. Beecher and Their Influence on the Physical Work of the Young Men's Christian Association," unpublished paper, Luther Gulick Thesis Collection, Springfield College Library, Springfield, MA; Lyman Beecher Stowe, *Saints, Sinners and Beechers* (Indianapolis: Bobbs-Merrill Company, 1934), 73-137; Linda J. Borish, "The Robust Woman and the Muscular Christian: Catharine Beecher, Thomas Higginson, and Their Vision of American Society, Health and Physical Activities, *International Journal of the History of Sport* 4 (Summer 1987): 139-54; Jeanne Boydston, Mary Kelley, and Anne Margolis, *The Limits of Sisterhood: The Beecher Sisters on Women's Rights and Woman's Sphere* (Chapel Hill: University of North Carolina Press, 1988); Marie Caskey: *Chariot of Fire: Religion and the Beecher Family* (New Haven: Yale University Press, 1978), 71-100; and Mae Harveson, "Catharine Beecher, Pioneer Educator," (Ph.D. diss: University of Pennsylvania, 1932).

[2]Whorton, *Crusaders for Fitness*, 278.

[3]Vertinsky, "Sexual Equality," 38-49; and Borish, "The Robust Woman and the Muscular Christian," 139-54.

[4]Catharine Beecher, *Letters to the People on Health and Happiness* (New York: Harper & Brothers, 1856), 112. Beecher defined "scrofulous condition" as a tendency to "humors" in the blood. Her case manifested itself in skin eruptions, swollen glands, and inflamed joints.

[5]See Chapter One for the story of Sarah Pierce's involvement with women's exercise.

[6]Catharine E. Beecher, *Educational Reminiscences and Suggestions* (New York: J. B. Ford and Company, 1874) 25.

[7]Catharine Beecher, quoted in Emily Noyes Vanderpoel, *Chronicles of a Pioneer School from 1792–1833: Being the History of Miss Sarah Pierce and Her Litchfield School*, Elizabeth C. Barney, ed. (Cambridge: University Press, 1903), 179-80.

[8]Beecher attended Litchfield from 1810 to 1816. Sklar, *Catharine Beecher*, 17.

[9]Alexander Metcalf Fisher was Yale's young, brilliant professor of Natural philosophy. See Sklar, *Catharine Beecher*, 28-39; and Stowe, *Saints*, 73-95, for the story of their courtship.

[10]Stowe, *Saints*, 95. The italics are original to the quote.

[11]"Hartford Female Seminary and Its Founder," *The American Journal of Education* 3 (1878): 81-82.

[12]Harriet Beecher Stowe wrote *Uncle Tom's Cabin*.

[13]Stowe, *Saints*, 112.

[14]Quoted in Sklar, *Catharine Beecher*, 100.

[15]Catharine Beecher, "To the Alumni of the West Newton Normal School," *The Common School Journal* 8 (15 January 1846): 22; Beecher, *Letters*, 115; and Sklar, *Catharine Beecher*, 206.

[16]Beecher, "To the Alumni," 22.

[17]Beecher, *Letters to the People*, 115.

[18]Sklar, *Catharine Beecher*, 205.

[19]Catharine Beecher, *Woman Suffrage and Women's Profession* (Hartford: Brown & Gross, 1871), 144-45; and Beecher, *Letters to the People*, 117-19.

[20]Beecher, *Letters to the People*, 117-19; Sklar, *Catharine Beecher*, 205; and Beecher, *Woman Suffrage*, 144-45. For an overview of the water cure movement, see Harry B. Weis and Howard R. Kemble, *The Great American Water-Cure Craze: A History of Hydropathy in the United States* (Trenton, NJ: Past Times Press, 1967); Susan E. Cayleff, *Wash and be Healed, The Water-Cure Movement and Women's Health* (Philadelphia: Temple University Press, 1987). See also Marshall Scott Legan, "Hydropathy in America: A Nineteenth-Century Panacea," *Bulletin of the History of Medicine* 45 (May-June 1971): 267-80.

[21]Sklar, *Catharine Beecher*, 204-205. See also Kathryn Kish Sklar, "All Hail to Pure Cold Water!" *American Heritage* 26 (December 1974): 64-70.

[22]Sklar, *Catharine Beecher*, 205; and Weis and Kemble, *Great American Water-Cure Craze*, 12.

[23]For insight into the day-to-day practice of the water cure in the nineteenth century, see *The Water Cure in America: Over Three Hundred Cases of Various Diseases Treated with Water, by Drs. Wesselhoeft, Shew, Bedortha, Schieferdecker, Trall, Nichols, and Others. With Cases of Domestic Practice; Designed for Popular as Well as Professional Reading, Edited by a Water Patient* (New York: Fowler & Wells, 1852).

[24]Bruce Haley, *The Healthy Body in Victorian Culture* (Cambridge: Harvard University Press, 1978), 16.

[25]Beecher, *Letters to the People*, 118.

[26]M. L. Shew, *Water-Cure for Ladies: A Popular Work on the Health, Diet and Regimen of Females and Children, and the Prevention and Cure of Diseases; With A Full Account of the Processes of Water-Cure; Illustrated with Various Cases* (New York: Wiley and Putnam, 1844), 114-15. The hydropathic method practiced most commonly in America evolved from the work of Vincent Priessnitz, a Silesian farmer, who cured himself with cold compresses and then began operating a water cure establishment in Grafenberg in the early 1820s.

[27]Beecher, *Letters to the People*, 143.

[28]Shew, *Water Cure for Ladies*, 115-16.

[29]Beecher, *Letters to the People*, 143. Hydropathic physician Russell Trall's, *The Illustrated Family Gymnasium*, published in 1857, included a lengthy section of calisthenic exercises designed for use by women that were, undoubtedly, similar to the exercises Beecher saw in the water cures. Russell

T. Trall, *The Illustrated Family Gymnasium; Containing the Most Improved Methods of Applying Gymnastic, Calisthenic, Kinesipathic, and Vocal Exercises to the Development of the Bodily Organs, the Invigoration of Their Functions, The Preservation of Health, and the Cure of Diseases and Deformities.* (New York: Samuel R. Wells, [1857] 1873). See also Russell T. Trall, "Exercise-pathy," *The Water Cure Journal and Herald of Reforms*, 24 (October 1857): 74-76. For other views on the hydropathic approach to exercise at mid-century, see Joel Shew, M.D., *The Water-Cure Manual: A Popular Work Embracing Prescriptions of the Various Modes of Bathing, The Hygienic and Curative Effects of Air, Exercise, Clothing, Occupation, Diet, Water-Drinking, & C. Together With Descriptions of Diseases and the Hydropathic Means to be Employed Therein. Illustrated With Cases of Treatment and Cure* (New York: Fowler & Wells, n.d.), 113-15; *Fowler's and Wells's Water-Cure Library*, Vol. 3 (New York: Fowler & Wells, n.d.), 145-53; and Joel Shew, M.D., *Consumption: Its Prevention and Cure by the Water Treatment* (New York: Fowler &Wells, 1855), 208-19.

[30]Beecher's least favorite treatment was a six-week "mucus cure." The physician told Beecher that an accumulation of mucus in her lower intestines caused her weak limb. What she needed, he told Beecher, was a "mucus crisis" in which the excess mucus would be drawn from her body. One can only imagine the relief Beecher felt when the physician died before he completed her treatments. Beecher, *Letters to the People*, 118.

[31]Beecher, *Letters to the People*, 119.

[32]Blackwell's school, the Central Medical College of New York, was considered an "eclectic" school. Part of the regular curriculum was a course of lectures on hydropathy given by Dr. S. O. Gleason. Alex Wilder, M.D., *The History of Medicine* (New Sharon ME: New England Eclectic Publishing Company, 1901).

[33]Harveson, "Pioneer Educator," 214. Beecher tells the story of her chronic ill health in most of her post-1850 publications. The details appear for the first time, however, in Beecher, *Letters*, 112-20. Several water cures followed Taylor's lead and began offering movement cure treatments by the end of the 1850s. A "Kinesipathic Institute," operated at 52 Morton Street in New York City in 1859, for instance. Run by physician Charles Shepard, it advertised that patients could take advantage of either Kinesipathy, or Swedish Movement Cure, combined with the Water Cure. "Kinesipathic Institute," *The Water Cure Journal and Herald of Reforms* 28 (August, 1859): 29.

[34]Blackwell's father died soon after the family moved to Cincinnati. Forced to support themselves, the three older Blackwell sisters opened a boarding school for young women. Blackwell's version of these years is reported in her autobiography, *Pioneer Work in Opening the Medical Profession to Women* (London: Longmans Green and Company, 1895; reprinted by Source Book Press, New York, 1970). See also Hale, *Woman's Record*, 584-85.

[35]Ishbel Ross, *Child of Destiny: The Life Story of the First Woman Doctor* (New York: Harper & Brothers, 1949), 81-82.

[36]According to Ross, it was Catharine Beecher's example that inspired Blackwell to pursue a professional life. Ross, *Child of Destiny*, 66.

[37]Blackwell, *Pioneer Work*, 26-27.

[38]Ibid., 31.

[39]For details of Blackwell's professional life, see Regina Markell Morantz-Sanchez, *Sympathy and Science: Women Physicians in American Medicine* (New York: Oxford University Press, 1985); Mary Ruth Walsh, *Doctors Wanted: No Women Need Apply: Sexual Barriers in the Medical Profession, 1835–1975* (New Haven: Yale University Press, 1977); William K. Beatty, *Women in White* (New York: Charles Scribner's Sons, 1972); and Ruth J. Abram, *Send Us a Lady Physician: Women Doctors in America, 1835–1920* (New York: W. W. Norton and Company, 1985 ). For a contemporary account of her pursuit of a medical degree, see "Dr. Elizabeth Blackwell," *Litell's Living Age* 58 (1858): 231-34.

[40]Ross reports: "Elizabeth went frequently to the consulting rooms of Dr. George Henry Brandt in Picadilly to take lessons from Professor Heinrich Georgii, professor of kinesipathy who had introduced into England, Professor Henry Ling's system of medical gymnastics. Here she learned healthful exercises . . ." Although Ross refers to him as "Heinrich, the person with whom Blackwell took lessons," he was probably Carl Augustus Georgii who, according to sport historians Fred Eugene Leonard and Emmett Rice, introduced Ling's exercise system to London in late 1849 or early 1850. Emmett A. Rice, *A Brief History of Physical Education* (New York, A. S. Barnes and Co., 1927), 121; Fred Eugene Leonard, *A Guide to the History of Physical Education* (Philadelphia: Lea and Febiger, 1927), 266-67; and: Ross, *Child of Destiny*, 164.

[41]Beecher, *Letters to the People*, 119.

[42]Ross, *Child of Destiny*, 172.

[43]Ibid., 173.

[44]Blackwell, *Opening the Profession*, 194. Following the lectures, a group of Quaker women, who had been her most faithful listeners, assisted Blackwell in finding patients.

[45]Elizabeth Blackwell, M.D., *The Laws of Life With Special Reference to The Physical Education of Girls* (New York: George P. Putnam, 1852).

[46]Elizabeth Blackwell, *The Laws of Life*, 15.

[47]Born in Williston, Vermont, in 1821, George Taylor became a common school teacher at age eighteen. He was such a success in the classroom that at the end of his first year of teaching, his superiors appointed him superintendent of all the Williston schools. Ill health forced him to retire two years later, however, and he remained an invalid for nearly a decade. In searching for a cure to his problems, Taylor became interested in medicine. He enrolled in Harvard's Medical School and then attended New York Medical

College, from which he graduated in 1852. In 1858, Taylor traveled to Stockholm and studied at Ling's school. "Taylor, George H.," *The National Cyclopedia of American Biography*, vol. 5 (New York: James T. White and Company, 1907), 494. To understand Taylor's methods, see George H. Taylor, *An Exposition of the Swedish Movement-Cure, Embracing the History and Philosophy of this System of Medical Treatment, with Examples of Single Movements, and Directions for Their Use in Various Forms of Chronic Disease, Forming a Complete Manual of Exercises; Together with a Summary of the Principles of General Hygiene* (New York: Samuel R. Wells, 1868).

[48]George H. Taylor, *An Illustrated Sketch of the Movement Cure: Its Principles, Methods and Effects* (New York: published at the Institute, 1866), 6-7.

[49]In the late nineteenth century a new scientific discipline based on bodily measurements—Physical Anthropometry—became a significant part of institutional physical education.

[50]Beecher, *Letters to the People*, 120.

[51]Taylor, *Illustrated Sketch*, 36.

[52][George H. Taylor] *A Brief Sketch of the Principles Involved in Dr. George H. Taylor's Remedial Methods* (New York: Drs. Taylor and Patchen, 1887), 1-5.

[53]Taylor, *Illustrated Sketch*, 11.

[54]Taylor, *Exposition*, 125-26.

[55]*Brief Sketch*, 6.

[56]Taylor used a mechanical massager for "kneading" the abdomens of his patients, a treatment deemed especially useful for constipation; employed the "Lifting Couch for gynecological problems and hernias, and invented a "Chest Developer" consisting of a free-swinging weight attached to a handlebar. As the patient pushed against the bar, the weight swung backward. When the patient returned the bar to its original position, the weight swung forward again. Taylor believed this device would stretch the diaphragm, expand the chest, and cure spinal curvatures. The pictures of it in Taylor's book are strikingly reminiscent of modern bench press machines seen in bodybuilding gyms. George H. Taylor, *Mechanical Aids in the Treatment of Chronic Forms of Disease* (New York: George W. Rodgers, 1893), 20-24.

[57]Beecher, *Letters to the People*, 120-21.

[58]Ibid., and Harveson, "Pioneer Educator," 128.

[59]She later recovered $500 from the Boston Grocer's Bank. Beecher, *Educational Reminiscences*, 207.

[60]Beecher's, *A Treatise on Domestic Economy for the Use of Young Ladies at Home and at School* (Boston: T. H. Webb and Co., 1841) contained a condensed physiology text, a general discussion of the Laws of Health, and a chapter entitled "On Domestic Exercise," which discussed the healthful benefits of doing one's own housework. In 1843, Harper and Brothers took over *Domestic Economy*'s publication and issued new editions every year until 1856. Sklar, *Catharine Beecher*, 151. All page citations in the present volume are taken from the 1850 "revised edition" published by Harper & Brothers.

[61]Catharine E. Beecher, *Suggestions Respecting Improvement in Education* (Hartford, CT: Packard and Butler, 1829).

[62]See Whorton, *Crusaders for Fitness*, for an excellent discussion of the moral reform movement of the early nineteenth century and how hygiene became part of that campaign.

[63]Beecher, *Suggestions*; quoted in: "Calisthenics," 190-191.

[64]Beecher, *Letters to the People*, 186.

[65]Beecher, "To the Alumni, 22.

[66]Beecher, *Letters to the People*, 121. For information on women's health in antebellum America, see Patricia Vertinsky, *The Eternally Wounded Woman: Women, Exercise and Doctors in the Late Nineteenth Century* (Manchester, England: Manchester University Press, 1990); Martha Verbrugge, *Able-Bodied Womanhood: Personal Health and Social Change in Nineteenth-Century Boston* (New York: Oxford University Press, 1988); Carrol Smith-Rosenberg and Charles Rosenberg, "The Female Animal: Medical and Biological Views of Women and Her Role in Nineteenth-Century America," *Journal of American History* 60 (September 1973): 332-56; Ann Douglas Wood, "'The Fashionable Diseases': Women's Complaints and Their Treatment in Nineteenth-Century America," *Journal of Interdisciplinary History* 4 (1973): 25-52; Sklar, "All Hail to Pure Cold Water," 64-70; and Regina M. Morantz, "Making Women Modern: Middle Class Women and Health Reform in Nineteenth-Century America," *Journal of Social History* 10 (1977): 490-507.

[67]See Beecher's chapter, "Statistics of Female Health, *Letters to the People*, 121-33.

[68]R. B. Gleason, "Hints to Women," *The Water-Cure Journal and Herald of Reforms* 15 (January 1853): 7.

[69]Beecher, *Letters to the People*, 7.

[70]Ibid, 122. Beecher's survey is not only referred to by most modern historians examining the issue of women's health in the nineteenth century, but references to it frequently appeared in the nineteenth century. See, for instance, D[aniel]. H. Jacques, "Physical Perfection," *The Water-Cure Journal and Herald of Reforms* 23(April 1857): 78.

During her extensive travels throughout the northeastern quarter of the United States, Beecher asked her women friends and others she met at several health establishments to list ten married women acquaintances by initials only and then to describe in several words the state of their health. The report of a woman in Milwaukee was typical. She had among her acquaintances one healthy woman, three "delicate or diseased" ones, and six habitual invalids. Beecher, *Letters to the People*, 130. Conscious of the class issue, Beecher also attempted to survey women from rural and lower socioeconomic levels. Her findings here "pained and surprised me the most," for rather than finding the great contrast one might have expected, "such has not been the case."

In Beecher's eloquent address to the American Association for the Advancement of Education, she provided additional statistics documenting the problems of women. She visited one city school with 148 pupils, and reported that 3/4 of the students suffered from headaches, and 35 had some stage of lateral curvature of the spine. At a country boarding school, she examined 109 students and found that 50 of them had spinal curvature, while the rest suffered from flat chests, round shoulders, and bent bodies. Catharine E. Beecher, "Health of Teachers and Pupils," *The American Journal of Education* 2 (September 1856): 404.

[71]Beecher, *Letters to the People*, 189.

[72]Ibid., 191.

[73]Ibid., 192.

[74]C. E. Beecher to Mr. Phillips, personal letter, 5 February 1856. Ch. A. 9.48. Boston Public Library, Boston MA. [Several commas were added by the author for clarity.] Sklar makes no mention of Mr. Phillips or any similar literary agent in her biography of Beecher.

[75]Catharine Beecher to her family, 3 February 1856. White Collection, Stowe Day Foundation, Hartford, CT.

[76]Beecher to Phillips.

[77]Ibid.

[78]Sklar claimed that Beecher planned to build a home on the site of the new college she was building in Milwaukee with the profits. Sklar, *Catharine Beecher*, 216.

[79]See "Hartford Female Seminary," *American Journal of Education* 2 (April 1827): 252-53, for details of Beecher's curriculum and the formation of the Board of Trustees.

[80]Beecher, *Educational Reminiscences*, 42.

[81]Ibid., 43.

[82]Ibid.

[83]Ibid.

[84]Beecher, *Domestic Economy*, 56, 247, 251-52. Beecher especially favored gardening: "No father, who wished to have his daughters grow up to be healthful women, can take a surer method to secure this end."

[85]Beecher, *Letters to the People*, 129.

[86]Beecher, *Educational Reminiscences*, 66.

[87][Catharine Beecher], *The Annual Catalogue of the Hartford Female Seminary, Together with an Account of the Internal Arrangements, Course of Study and Mode of Instructing the Same* (Hartford: 1831).

[88]"Western Female Institute," *American Annals of Education and Instruction* 3(August 1833): 380-81.

[89]Beecher, *Educational Reminiscences*, 84 ; and "Hartford Female Seminary," *American Journal of Education*, 83.

[90]Beecher, *Educational Reminiscences*, 84.

[91]Beecher, *Domestic Economy*, 56.

[92]Catharine E. Beecher, *Physiology and Calisthenics for Schools and Families* (New York: Harper and Brothers, 1856); and Catharine E. Beecher, *Calisthenic Exercises for Schools, Families and Health Establishments* (New York: Harper and Brothers, 1856).

[93]Ibid., title page. Beecher later claimed that the exercise system presented in *Physiology and Calisthenics* resulted from her Cincinnati experiments. "Hartford Female Seminary and Its Founder," *American Journal of Education*, 83.

[94]M[athius]. Roth, *The Free Gymnastic Exercises of P. H. Ling, Arranged by H. Rothstein* (London & Boston: Groombridge & Sons, 1853). Roth's book represented the first English translation of Ling's ideas. It spurred the movement cure enthusiasm of the 1850s and undoubtedly influenced Blackwell and Taylor who both claimed allegiance to Ling's ideas regarding physical training. Roth's influence is discussed in Roberta J. Park, "Biological Thought, Athletics, and the Formation of a 'Man of Character': 1830–1900"; J. A. Mangan and James Walvin, eds. *Manliness and Morality: Middle-Class Masculinity in Britain and America: 1800–1940* (New York: St. Martin's Press, 1987), 15.

[95]Beecher, *Calisthenics*, 14-19.

[96]Ibid., 35.

[97]Beecher, *Calisthenics*, 44-47.

[98]The only competitor for this title is Theodore Weld who, in the early 1830s, tried to foster the manual labor movement as a form of physical education. See Robert H. Abzug, *Passionate Liberator: Theodore Dwight Weld and the Dilemma of Reform* (New York: Oxford University Press, 1980).

[99]Sklar, *Catharine Beecher*, 131.

[100]Ibid., 221-23.

[101]Catharine E. Beecher to Leonard Bacon, 9 March 1872. Reprinted in Boydston, Kelley, and Margolis, *Limits of Sisterhood*, 257.

[102]Borish, "Robust Woman," 148.

[103]Vertinsky, "Sexual Equality," 39.

[104]Harvey Green, *Fit for America: Health, Fitness, Sport and American Society* (New York: Pantheon Books, 1986), 300.

[105]Nancy Struna, "'Good Wives' and 'Gardeners', Spinners and 'Fearless Riders': Middle and Upper-Rank Women in the Early American Sporting Culture," in *From 'Fair Sex' to Feminism: Sport and the Socialization of Women in the Industrial and Post-Industrial Eras*, J. A. Mangan and Roberta J. Park, eds. (London: Frank Cass Ltd., 1987), 249.

[106]By 1846, the number of female teachers in the United States was nearly twice that of males. Only ten years earlier, the *Common School Journal* reported that there were 3,591 female teachers to 2,370 male teachers. In 1846, the *Journal* reported there were 4,997 females to 2,585 males. "Female Teachers," *The Common School Journal* 9 (March 1847): 96.

[107]Lois Banner, *American Beauty* (New York: Alfred A. Knopf, 1983), 45-66.

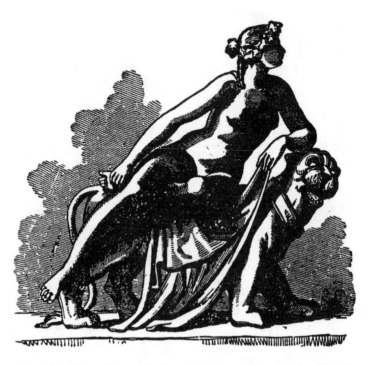

Figure 51: According to Orson Fowler, this image of the Goddess Una illustrated "a perfect female pelvis and form throughout." From Orson Fowler's *Creative and Sexual Science* (1870).

# Chapter 7
# Bigger Bodies, Better Brains:
# Phrenology and the Health Lift

American phrenologist Orson Squire Fowler examined the question of women's exercise in 1870. "Dio Lewis's light gymnastics are excellent," Fowler wrote, "especially for sedentary women." But, he cautioned, Lewis's system was not nearly as beneficial as Butler's Lifting Cure. The New Gymnastics fatigued a person before "giving the muscle-developing exercise demanded," he explained, while "just five minutes of Butler-style lifting, will yield more and better exercise than an hour in any other form."[1]

Orson Fowler's phrenologically-based interest in physical training and his ultimate advocacy of the form of heavy weightlifting known as the Health Lift comprise one of the most interesting chapters in the history of exercise for American women. Although best known for his attempts to read character from the conformation of the head and face, Fowler and his phrenological colleagues also paid attention to the contours and size of the body—particularly women's bodies. Phrenology's endorsement of exercise not only provided a culturally acceptable rationale for women to train and grow fitter; it encouraged women to become stronger and larger, physical attributes that fostered the development of the ideal of Majestic Womanhood. The present chapter begins by exploring phrenology's influence on women's attitudes toward exercise and the powerful physical ideal Fowler promoted. It concludes with an examination of the phrenologically-endorsed exercise system known as the Health Lift.

## Orson Fowler and American Phrenology

The historian John Davies has suggested that phrenology's influence on nineteenth-century America is best understood in comparison to Freudianism's hold on the twentieth century. Like Freudianism in this century, phrenology was a system of beliefs that underlay nineteenth-century social thought. It was regarded by many doctors, scientists, and educators as a serious, inductive discipline, yet it also exerted a significant influence on popular culture.[2] America's fascination with the pseudoscience began in the fall of 1832 when European phrenologist Johann Gaspar Spurzheim, hailed by Ralph Waldo Emerson as one of the world's great minds, arrived in New England.[3]

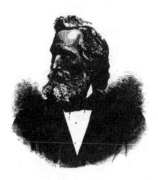

Figure 52: Orson Fowler in an engraving from *Private Lectures on Perfect Men, Women and Children* (1883).

In Boston, Spurzheim delivered a highly publicized series of lectures explaining the facets of his scientific theory and addressing phrenology's implications for education. The lectures proved a resounding success. *The Boston Medical and Surgical Journal* reported that Spurzheim's lectures had drawn "our most distinguished physicians, lawyers and divines, and citizens best known for their scientific and literary attainments."[4] Yale Professor Benjamin Silliman reported that his colleagues were "in love" with Spurzheim and his ideas.[5] Harriett Martineau, visiting the United States at the time, recalled that the "great mass of Americans became phrenologists in a day."[6]

In 1838, phrenology got a second boost when Scotsman George Combe, brother of the famous physiologist Andrew Combe, began an American lecture tour. Author of the hugely successful phrenology/ physiology text, *Constitution of Man*, George Combe delivered 158 speeches in eighteen months, receiving as much as $750 per lecture.[7] As Spurzheim had done, Combe posited his ideas for personal reform around one main theme: phrenological improvement was only possible when allied with physiological improvement. Combe's Scottish Common Sense approach to the question of mind and body particularly appealed to Horace Mann, first Secretary of the State Board of Education for Massachusetts and an early champion for public education.[8] Mann's phrenological conversion was a significant step in linking the pseudoscience to physical education. Following his conversion, Mann began a campaign to promote the idea that physical education should be part of the standard curriculum in all schools.[9] In his *Sixth Annual Report as Secretary of the Massachusetts Board of Education*, Mann devoted more than one hundred pages to discussions of health, physiology, and bodily improvement, all of which directly echo Combe's sentiments.[10] A lifelong believer, Mann claimed near the end of his life that he was "a hundred times more indebted to phrenology than to all the metaphysical works I ever read."[11]

Although Combe's and Spurzheim's brand of phrenology found acceptance among New England's leading intellectuals, the science quickly degraded in the hands of the American entrepreneurs who succeeded them.[12] Often referred to as "practical" phrenologists because they offered personal advice and tried to apply phrenology to the problems and decisions of everyday life, these itinerant head examiners fanned out through the United States during the 1830s, 1840s, and 1850s, aiming their pitches at the middle and lower classes.[13] Two former divinity students, Orson and Lorenzo Fowler, became the most popular practical phrenologists in antebellum America.[14]

Phrenology was both a philosophical crusade and an extremely lucrative business for the Fowler brothers. Orson poured his enthusiasm for the pseudoscience into a series of hyperbolic bestselling books that, coupled with their earnings as lecturers, allowed the brothers to establish their own publishing house and open a museum in New York City.[15] Nelson, less enamored with the written word, served as phrenologist in residence at the Fowler Brothers Phrenological Cabinet and helped to manage their rapidly expanding publishing house; their phrenological school where they trained more than three hundred people for the profession; and their lecture circuit, which at one point employed twenty-six itinerant phrenologists.[16] By 1846, the Fowler brand of phrenology was so popular that their *Phrenological Almanac* sold more than ninety thousand copies. Their magazine, *The American Phrenological Journal*, begun in 1837, had more than fifty thousand subscribers in the early 1850s.[17] All of which suggests, of course, that when Orson Fowler began discussing body ideals and exercise, it mattered. Through his lectures, books, and articles in the *Phrenological Journal*, Fowler's theories reached thousands of Americans.

### Better Brains via Exercise

Although phrenology left us the phrase "reading the bumps on your head," Orson Fowler and his fellow phrenologists actually measured the brain's thirty-seven different "faculties" by drawing imaginary lines from the spinal axis, in the medulla oblongata, to the surface of the head. In the beginning, they believed that the brain consisted of a mass of long fibers, fanning outward from the center, and that these fibers lengthened or contracted depending upon the degree of activity in that area of the brain. The right sort of behavior caused

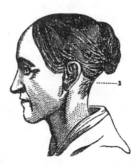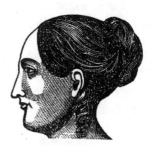

Figure 53: Illustrations from Orson Fowler's *Perfect Men, Women and Children* (1883) demonstrating women possessing "conjugal love-deficient" on the left and "conjugal love-large" on the right.

the fibers to expand, enlarging the organ and molding the skull above it.[18] The large, well-developed skull thus came to represent both intelligence and a person whose moral faculties were fully developed.[19]

By the 1850s, the phrenological community had concluded that another factor also contributed to these brain changes. Fowler's partner and brother-in-law, Samuel Wells, explained the new phenomenon as a "nervous" fluid or vital force that "strengthens and develops any part of the body or brain in proportion as it is brought to bear upon it." There were particles in this vital fluid, Wells continued, that, if exercise was regular, would collect in the area being exercised. Study and reflection would summon this vital fluid to the forehead and thus help the frontal lobes to protrude gradually. Similarly, a young woman in love with her husband would find her organ of amativeness enlarging at the base of her skull. Physical exercise, the phrenologist contended, worked in exactly the same manner. The repetitive movements of exercise caused the particles to bulge the blacksmith's biceps and swell the dancer's calf.[20]

Orson Fowler soon moved past this original position to argue that physical exercise and its concomitant muscular enlargement would actually enhance brain size and improve intellectual function. He called it the "law of increase by action and decrease by inaction" and further claimed that "good muscles are more useful than anything . . . ." Fowler believed that the brains of muscularly fit, physically active individuals were physiologically different than the brains of those who took no exercise. The nervous tissue was more clearly defined or "stringy" in the muscular individual, he argued, and their brains subsequently functioned more efficiently and quickly. "Hence," he wrote, "the stronger the muscles the more efficient and impressive all the mental operations." Women were also subject to this law, he concluded, and were perhaps its greatest transgressors. "Female muscular inertia," he warned, is "the great modern mind-paralyzer."[21]

Dozens of other phrenologists, physical culturists, and a surprisingly large number of regular physicians took Fowler's message to heart and began to preach the brain-expanding virtues of vigorous exercise. New England physician George Capron even went so far as to argue that physical exertion "feeds the muscles," acting as a kind of "fertilizer." In fact, Capron continued, the brain of a laboring man "is as much larger and stronger than the brain of the inactive man, as his muscles are larger and stronger."[22] Body size, skin tone, muscularity, vigor, and carriage must come under scrutiny in every phrenological examination, Fowler argued[23] Ever ready to play on patriotic sentiments, Fowler claimed that this insight had come to him as he made busts of Benjamin Franklin, Patrick Henry, George Washington, and Thomas Jefferson for inclusion in his phrenological museum. The Founding Fathers were larger than average men, Orson wrote, a fact that accounted for their larger brain size and greater intelligence. "Without exception," he continued, they had "amply developed chests, and superior muscular and nervous organizations."[24]

Fowler's theory presented a radical departure from early nineteenth-century ideas about the mind and body. Earlier experts, largely proponents of the theory of vitalism, had argued that the body had finite resources and that these were used up during a person's lifetime. Excessive exercise, such as German-style gymnastics, should be shunned, early vitalists had argued, because it placed too great a demand on the body's vital reserves. The fear, of course, was that the exertions of exercise and the enlarged muscles caused by that exercise used up the body's vitality, drained the brain of intelligence, and hastened one's death.[25] Fowler and his phrenological followers believed exactly the opposite. They argued that exercise increased intelligence, and that the brain could continue to grow and improve until age sixty-five[26] They further believed that the larger body created by exercise could not use up its vital forces because their use increased the body's vital reserves. For both sexes this new interpretation of vitalism provided a powerful argument for the inclusion of exercise in an adult's daily schedule. For phrenologically-minded women, the fear that vigorous exercise would use up their body's vitality and hamper their ability to have healthy children now seemed groundless. Fowler argued that vigorous exercise—true musclebuilding exercise—would make women healthy, increase their brain size, improve their intelligence, and enhance their maternal capacities. That his message had an impact can be seen in the comment of radical health reformer Harriet Austin: "Healthy well developed muscles are the basis for healthy brains."[27]

Fellow women's rights advocate Eliza Farnham also affirmed the law of increase, suggesting that women had a moral duty to use the physical gifts God had given them. "Woman is no exception to this beautiful law," Farnham wrote, even in "muscular vigor."[28] Orson Fowler liked to put such matters more graphically for his readers. "Soft hands belong to soft brains and soft and weak intellects," he declared, arguing further that a great man or a great woman without a broad, deep foundation in hard labor or vigorous physical exercise would be a "monstrosity—a being not governed by the laws of life or health."[29]

## Bigger Bodies, Better Brains

As a confirmed Lamarckian who believed that traits acquired in one's lifetime could be passed on to future generations, Fowler had reasons other than brain function for advocating exercise to women. He feared for the next generation unless women remade themselves on a new, phrenological model. Fowler's approach to womanhood placed a high value on size, substance, and physical strength. Exercise would not just make women fitter and childbirth easier, Fowler contended. It would also make their offspring stronger, larger, and more intelligent. A mother, he warned, must "EXERCISE her muscles habitually, not merely in light work, such as sewing, walking about the house, etc., but in something which requires her to put forth much strength, and that often." He wondered rhetorically how deficient American women were in this respect and claimed that "the muscular feebleness of most American women is...disgraceful."[30] Sarah Hale concurred. In "Hints about Phrenology," Hale told her readers that women should not be surprised if God punished them for not obeying these divine orders. People of great talents, she claimed, came from exceptional mothers, not exceptional fathers.[31]

Fowler's belief in the anabolic powers of exercise allowed him to suggest that it enlarged internal organs such as the womb and digestive tract just as it did the brain and the muscles.[32] Small bodies meant small brains to Fowler, but small waistlines presented an even greater danger as they represented "feeble vital organs, a delicate constitution, sickly offspring and a short life." In 1842, he adopted the phrase

"Natural Waists or No Wives" as a eugenic campaign slogan, urging men "who wish healthy wives and offspring to shun small waists and patronize full chests."[33]

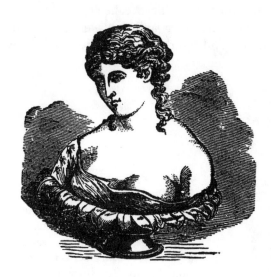

Figure 54: Plumpness on a pedestal: Orson Fowler's image of "the perfect female bosom" from *Sexual Science* (1870).

Surprising as it may seem by our modern standards, Fowler's advocacy of the large waist was in vogue among certain groups of reform-minded Americans. In an article discussing Elizabeth Cady Stanton, for instance, Harriet Austin recounted an exchange between a friend of Stanton's and one of her detractors: "My idea of a perfect woman, nobly planned," declared the male opponent of women's rights, is a pleasant face, a bright eye, a graceful figure with a good sized waist, arrayed in clean well-fitting calico . . . with a broom in her hand." "For the edification of this man, and the world at large," rejoined Stanton's friend, "allow me to say that Mrs. Stanton has a pleasant face, a good figure, a sizable waist—sometimes wears calico . . . and is said to be as thorough and systematic a 'sweepist' as she is a 'talkist.'"[34] Similarly, Dio Lewis described as a "priceless treasure" a healthy young woman of his recent acquaintance who possessed a "fine large waist and a muscular arm."[35] Even conservative-minded Catharine Beecher took pride in reporting that the six-week movement cure she took at George Taylor's establishment had increased her waistline by two inches and her chest measurement by three inches.[36]

Fowler's campaign went beyond simple dress reform, however. He wanted more than the waistlines of women to be large. "Good size is important in wives and mothers," Orson Fowler wrote in 1842. "Little women usually have too much activity for their strength ... feeble constitutions, hence they die young, and . . . suffer extremely as mothers."[37] Larger women, he continued, were "better in every way." Their larger brains indicated greater intelligence, he explained, and a more highly developed moral character; and they were more self-reliant, less prone to hysterics, and could be taken more seriously by their peers.[38]

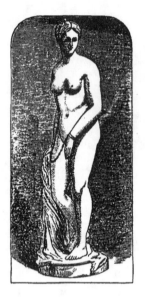

Figure 55: "The perfect Female Form" according to Orson Fowler belonged to Hiram Power's statue, The Greek Slave. Fowler wrote: It "shows large breasts, thighs, calves and arms ... with a perfect proportion of all to all ... therein illustrating our mediumistic doctrine." *From Perfect Men, Women and Children* (1883).

Fowler wanted his women to be muscularly large and fit, but he also wanted them to be well padded. "Lean, lank women cannot possibly be good looking," Fowler wrote, "while a full, plump form, with all its hollows filled up, and slopes well smoothed by adipose matter ... becomes an element of female beauty."[39] The effectiveness of this aspect of Fowler's campaign can be seen in the personal ads of the *Water Cure Journal*. In the "Matrimonial Correspondence" column, men specified their phrenological and physiological preferences in women.[40] The ads indicate a decided preference for women of medium size or larger. The words "slender," "thin," "lean," and "trim"— words frequently used in the late-twentieth century to describe desirable female bodies—are startlingly absent in these ads from the mid-nineteenth century. As one Massachusetts correspondent put it, he sought a woman who was "medium sized, well developed, erect and plump (not gross, but full and round)."[41] Other ads used similar words to describe the correspondent's preference for large women. "Still-Alone—I Want a Wife," began an 1859 ads, "with auburn hair, full form, warm heart and reform principles."[42] "I wish to become acquainted," read another "with a lady ... possessing a sound and healthy constitution.... I do not admire skeletons."[43] "My life companion should be physically, intellectually and morally well developed," read one from 1855, "of good size, healthy and industrious.[44] Fowler also provided clues as to where to find such large, desirable women. The women of Vermont, he claimed, possessed the largest heads and best bodies to be found in the Union. "If I mistake not," he told the readers of the *American Phrenological Journal*, "they will make better wives and mothers than girls in any other section of the country."[45] Fowler was not alone in championing larger women. Phrenological convert Daniel H. Jacques's influential work, *Hints Toward Physical Perfection*, preached precisely the same message. There could be no beauty without substance, Jacques asserted; leanness might indicate an abnormal development of the mental temperament or outright disease.[46] Jacques's book ran in its entirety in the *Water Cure Journal* and thereby influenced thousands of women who would never have purchased it as a single tome.[47] That the message began to be heard and believed can be seen by the accompanying illustration from reform-minded physician Wooster Beach's *Family Physician and Home Guide* extolling the desirability of the obviously larger, stronger, and uncorseted woman on the right.[48] Other advice on how to achieve the new strong, yet plump physique appeared in William Milo's book, *Notes on Beauty, Vigor and Development; or How to Acquire Plumpness*

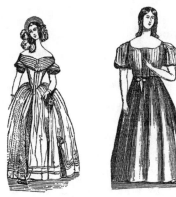

Figure 56: Illustration from Dr. Wooster Beach's *Family Physician and Health Guide* (1862) demonstrating the move toward a larger ideal for womanhood within the health reform community.

*of Form, Strength of Limb, and Beauty of Complexion, With Rules for Diet and Bathing, nd a Series of Improved Physical Exercises.* [49]

Fowler's influence on this matter also spread to women themselves, creating a concern among women with their size and weight. With the invention of a smaller and more accurate platform scale in 1857, it was suddenly possible for women to weigh themselves on a regular basis. Those who fell below the desirable ideal of 130 to 160 pounds worried about their thinness.[50] As the Reverend David McRae observed just prior to the Civil War, "The American girls, themselves, I think, are nervous about their thinness, for they are constantly having themselves weighed and every ounce of increase is hailed with delight . . . Every girl knows her own weight to within an ounce or two, and is ready to mention it at a moment's notice. It seems to be a subject of universal interest."[51]

Dr. Augusta Fairchild of the Western Hygeian Home in St. Anthony, Minnesota, was certainly interested in weight. She used it as an indicator of the success of her treatment methods and gleefully wrote to the editors of the *Herald of Health* that a young woman in her care had gone from 80 to 160 pounds and was now a "healthy, strong woman" after following hydropathic treatments and regular exercise.[52] In the 1870s, at least one women's school began tracking the weight of its students as an indication of their relative health. Mills College, in California, reported pridefully that its female students gained more than fourteen hundred pounds in a year, and gave special mention to one young woman who put on twenty-five pounds in six months.[53]

## Women of Strength

From the beginning of his writing career, Fowler's interest in body size also related to his fascination with physical strength. "So exalted is my idea of the constitutional muscular power of man," Fowler wrote in the *Phrenological Journal* in 1844, "that I believe . . . man was made to be the strongest animal created. I believe man capable of taking the best part of a ton upon his back and carrying it as easily as our horses draw it on carts."[54] Fowler frequently made reference to professional strongmen in his writings and to his eighteenth-century ancestor, Jonathan Fowler, an exceptionally large man known for unusual strength.[55] Jonathan Fowler's mother had reportedly weighed close to three hundred pounds, and Orson argued that her size and vigor had influenced her son and the next several generations of Fowlers.[56] Orson Fowler's interest in the strength of both sexes helped pave the way for the more rigorous exercise and physical training systems that appeared in the 1850s. By linking the size and strength of the brain to the size and strength of the body, Fowler helped make it possible for women, as well as men, to view muscular strength as a desirable entity rather than as a badge of shame. Fowler ungendered strength, size, and muscularity by turning on its head the stereotype that claimed these attributes as masculine. He linked these traits first to intelligent humankind and then to femininity and maternity through a phreno-logically-based eugenics campaign arguing that these traits were actually more important in the female than the male because it was from the mother that a child received its physical attributes.

Although Fowler's interest in female strength was primarily eugenic, his assertion that strength and health should be attributes of humankind and not just mankind provided a rallying point for women's rights advocates who came to view strength as a facilitator of female independence in daily life and the culture at large. Mrs. R. B. Gleason warned the readers of the *Water Cure Journal* that "something must be done quick," for "women need physical strength as much as men do." Women's rights activist and hydropathic physician Harriet Austin agreed, writing, "Women are not only entitled to have strong muscles and robust health as truly as men are, but without these their lives may be in larger or lesser measure lamentable failures."[57] Writing from the feminist agricultural commune, Home of the Free, Delos Dunton argued that changes in women's status would only come to pass when they fulfilled their physical potential. "If women were as healthy and strong in proportion to their weight . . . as men are . . . changes would be far-reaching and wide, and would all tend to human improvement and happiness."[58] The physician Elizabeth Blackwell went even further. She held up as exemplars of ideal womanhood such physically powerful women as "the beautiful Cymburga, wife of the stalwart Duke Ernest of Austria, who could crack nuts with her fingers, and drive a nail into a wall with her hand as far as others with a ham-mer," and "Brinhilda," who bound her offending lover with her girdle and hung him from a beam in the ceiling. In these turbulent times, Blackwell warned her readers, "we should ponder the question whether . . . we have not lost much stout virtue, with the failure of our bodily powers."[59] Leading women's rights activist Elizabeth Cady Stanton agreed. In an article for *The Lily*, Stanton wrote, "Let us now consider man's claim to physical superiority. Methinks I hear some say surely you would not contend for equality here." But, Stanton continued, we "must not give an inch . . . We cannot accord to man even this much, and he has no right to claim it . . . " "Even the difference in the relative size of the sexes would level out with proper training, Stanton argued, adding that it must be remembered in any case, she continued, that even if women were ultimately smaller, this was no excuse for women to be weak. "Bodily strength depends much on the power of the will. The sight of a small boy, thoroughly thrashing a big one, is not rare. Now would you say the bigger fat boy whipped was superior to the small active boy who conquered him?" We simply cannot say, Stanton continued, "what the woman might be physically, if the girl were allowed all the freedom of the boy." However, she wrote, "physically as well as intellectually, it is use that produces growth and development."[60]

### Fowler on Exercise

Fowler's beliefs about the types of exercise suitable for women substantially changed over time. In his early books, his recommendations primarily centered on manual labor and domestic work. With the publication in 1848 of *Maternity, or the Bearing and Nursing of Children*, however, he came out strongly in favor of gymnastic training in addition to domestic occupations. "Oh, I do wish some of this prim, sedate, stiff-jointed, inert, ladified, starched-up artificiality, could be shook out of women," Fowler wrote. "Come women, snap these fashionable restraints, and give yourselves that freedom so promotive of the specific foundations of your sex."[61] Fowler contrasted the vigor of American women to that of their British cousins, reporting, "English women—those of rank included—often take walks of eight and twelve miles, just for exercise, and ride much, and practice gymnastics . . . . "If American women hoped to stem the tide leading to the debility of an entire generation, he warned, girls needed more romping and more vigorous exercise. "Scarcely anything would do more for either mothers or children, than the general practice of gymnastic exercises by females."[62]

By the late 1850s, inspired by the stories of George Barker Windship, Fowler gave his strongest endorsements to several systems of heavy weightlifting. His message that "bigger is better" when it came to American womanhood provided precisely the rationale needed to justify for women as well as men what became generically known as the "Health Lift." In stark contrast to calisthenics, which promised to produce grace and a sense of lightness in a woman's bearing, the acquisition of measurable physical strength was the most important consideration of a Health Lift workout. That the workouts also increased the body's size was a phrenological bonus.

## II
### A Mid-Century Enthusiasm for Strength

Fowler's theories fostered the mid-century enthusiasm for strength and body size, but a steady stream of European immigrants and an increasing number of touring circuses also contributed to the fascination with heavy weight lifting that struck Americans in the 1850s.[63] Inspired by reports of the physical transformations made at Hippolyte Triat's upper-class Parisian gymnasium—where men trained with heavy dumbbells and what may well be the first true barbells—there was on the Continent a newfound enthusiasm for greater muscular size and the incremental measurement of strength.[64] Germans arriving as part of the great migration of 1848 brought that enthusiasm with them to America as they established Turner societies and revived interest in the flips and turns of their vigorous gymnastics system, a system that had always included dumbbell training.[65] Scottish immigrants also brought a love of strength sports to their new homeland. Although the Scots did not train as systematically as the Germans, they organized Caledonian Clubs and sponsored contests in which the traditional highland events of stoneputting and caber tossing attracted considerable interest. In fact, more than four thousand people turned out to watch the New York Caledonian Club's Twelfth Annual Games in 1868.[66]

The European fascination with heavy lifting also affected, and was affected by, the circuses. By 1860, nearly every circus had some kind of strength act.[67] When one considers that on just one day, in 1847, more than seventeen thousand people paid to enter the big top in Pittsburgh, Pennsylvania, alone it is not difficult to understand how the circus could be an influential transmitter of cultural ideals and images. It stands to reason that at least some of those seventeen thousand spectators left the circus that day inspired by the strength and acrobatic acts and excited by the prospect of what their own body might be capable of with proper training.[68] That such excitement could influence women as well as men can be proven by the 1835 memoir, *Notes of Travel and Life*, written by Miss Mendell and Miss Hosmer. According to that work, these two single women began a regular physical training program after watching the strength and acrobatic feats performed at the local circus.[69]

By mid-century, Americans who wished to train for strength and size had a number of options. Private gymnasiums opened in many large urban centers prior to the Civil War, and in many of these gyms heavy dumbbell training played an important role in the physical transformation of the customers. Men and women who could not

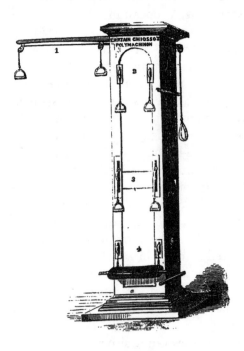

Figure 57: James Chiosso built his first, crude weightlifting device in 1829. Over the next several decades he continued to refine his machine, enclosing the weights and pulleys in a column, and building interior compartments so that the weights could move up and down smoothly. With this model, marketed in 1855, Chiosso demonstrated curling movements, squats, chest work, leg extensions and a variety of other resistance exercises still in modern use. From: Captain James Chiosso's *The Gymnastic Polymachinon* (1855).

train at a gym could buy dumbbells and Indian clubs or order James Chiosso's latest version of the Gymnastic Polymachinon and train in the privacy of their own homes.

As seen in the illustration, Chiosso's versatile Polymachinon allowed both sexes to work their entire body using resistance exercise. Chiosso considered his machine "elegant and ornamental" and suitable for prominent display in the dining room, library, or boudoir of anyone's home.[70] To check their progress, and to see how they compared to their neighbors, people could try the strength testing machines that appeared on many street corners and at fairs. These machines allowed a person to test his "main strength"—meaning the strength of his back, hips, legs, and hands—by moving a large weight a short distance. It was from lifting on a machine such as this that the Harvard-trained physician George Barker Windship, who became the most visible spokesperson for heavy lifting, began his career in physical culture.

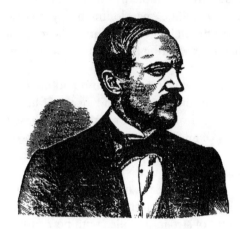

Figure 58: Dr. George Barker Windship, the "American Samson" or "Roxbury Hercules" as he appeared in the *Phrenological Almanac* for 1859.

### George Barker Windship
### "Strength is Health"

George Barker Windship entered Harvard University in 1850 as a sixteen-year-old freshman standing five feet tall and weighing a hundred pounds. Although not quite a ninety-seven pound weakling, Windship was not far off the mark until he resolved, after tiring of the jeers of his classmates, to build himself up by doing gymnastic training. According to his own account, "Autobiographical Sketches of a Strength-Seeker," published in the *Atlantic Monthly* in 1862, he spent part of every evening training in the Harvard gym until, by graduation time, he was known as the strongest man at Harvard.[71] In the summer of 1854, on a trip to Rochester, New York, Windship discovered a crowd surrounding a lifting machine on the town's main street. Windship managed to lift only 420 pounds in what we would today describe as a partial deadlift, or hand-and-thigh lift. This failed to impress the crowd, and the experience wounded his young male ego. Apparently, Windship's gymnastic work had primarily strengthened his upper body, whereas the lifting machine tested the large muscles of the trunk and lower body. Upon returning to Roxbury, he devised a similar lifting machine in his backyard by sinking a hogshead in the ground and placing inside it a barrel filled with rocks and sand, to which he attached a rope and handle. Then, standing on a platform constructed above the barrel, he mimicked the movement of the lifting machine he had tried in Rochester. Windship progressed rapidly and became fascinated with the great weights he could hoist in this partial movement. Although the weight he lifted moved no more than several inches, he found it both physically and emotionally satisfying to watch his strength grow in measured increments. Abandoning his gymnastic training, he continued to increase the weights he used in his workouts. As he trained, he studied medicine, graduating from Harvard's medical school in 1857.[72]

For the remainder of his short life, Windship's mind and medical practice seem to have centered around his love and advocacy of heavy weightlifting. As earlier exercise advocates had done, Windship based his physical ideals on the statuary of ancient Greece, although he chose as his inspiration not the finely-made Apollo Belvedere but the Farnese Hercules, a massively-muscled statue on display in the Boston Athenaeum. The statue was precursor of today's modern bodybuilders, and Windship believed it displayed a bodily outline "compatible with the exercise of the greatest amount of strength." Filled with new enthusiasm, Windship wanted his now 5'7" and 140-pound body to resemble more closely this larger-than-life ideal, so he began heavy dumbbell training in addition to his partial deadlifts.[73] He apparently succeeded. *The Philadelphia Inquirer* reported after one of Windship's lecture/demonstrations, on "the volume of muscle which swelled and trembled in his full arm."[74] Windship's advocacy of lifting drew additional force from his belief that it was an efficacious form of medical therapy. "I discovered that with every day's development of my strength," he wrote, "there was an increase of my ability to resist and overcome all fleshly ailments, pains and infirmities." In simplest terms, Windship wrote, he had discovered that "Strength is Health."[75] As he put it in The Massachusetts Teacher in 1860, "Lifting, if properly practiced, was the surest and quickest method of producing harmonious development; while it was also the most strengthening of all exercises, and consequently the most healthful."[76] *Harpers Weekly* agreed. Windship's methods, the prestigious magazine reported, "could make any man strong, and in many cases . . . cure him of disease."[77]

Billing himself as the "Roxbury Hercules" and the "Strongest Man in the World," Windship spread his message through a series of well-received lectures and exhibitions.[78] He also invented and patented several machines that helped standardize his favored exercise. Following the Civil War, he moved to new quarters in the Park Street Church Building and opened a combined gymnasium and medical practice.[79] The new gymnasium was much larger than his previous establishment and had a "separate apartment for ladies," although no evidence has been found to suggest how many women were members.[80] We can be certain, however, that those who came did the Health Lift. At least one women's school in the New England area had already adopted Windship's Health Lift as its school exercise program. One teacher later reported that the girls became bored wih the program after the novelty wore off, adding that the system was "better than no exercise at all."[81]

Windship created many converts to the principles of heavy exercise, including Orson Fowler, who offered his readers the cheapest solution for partaking of the new fad. Get about thirty feet of cod line or other cotton cord that slightly stretched, Fowler wrote, "twist and double, then twist and double again, tie the ends, and attach two sections of a broom-handle, or any round stick adapted to lift by . . . adjusting its length to your height." Once these handles were attached, Fowler instructed, the person should stand on the bottom handle and pull upward as hard as possible, holding the pull for several seconds. In just five minutes, Fowler claimed, a person could perform several of these all-out pulls and get all the exercise he or she needed.[82]

### David P. Butler: Bringing the Health Lift to Women

Windship's lectures and exhibitions did initially popularize the Health Lift, but it was David P. Butler, Windship's Boston rival, who possessed the entrepreneurial skills to take the Health Lift to the masses. During the 1860s, Butler ran a gym in Boston, but he devoted much of his spare time to decreasing the size of Health Lift machines in order to make them more suitable for home use.[83] By 1870, Butler's business had grown to the point that he manufactured several models of Health Lift machines and franchised his system, offering Health Lift converts a chance to open gyms using his name, his equipment, and his approach to exercise.[84] It appears that Butler was the first gymnasium owner in the United States to hit upon this particular promotional scheme. Furthermore, and unlike Windship, Butler published a detailed account of his methods entitled *Butler's System of Physical Training: The Lifting Cure.*[85]

It was Butler's system that so excited Orson Fowler, who saw in it the scientific tool he had been searching for in his quest to help men and women find appropriate health, strength, and increased size.

Fowler had reason to praise Butler's ideas—they were essentially his own. For one thing, Butler argued that his system produced "brain-power" in two ways. Indirectly, it enhanced brain function through the generalized vigor it created in the whole body. Directly, the Health Lift enhanced mental acuity by calling into play the mental organs for self-reliance, firmness, "concentrativeness," hope, courage, and faith. Butler and Fowler also agreed on the idea that perfect physical development was the key to mental and physical excellence. Physical culture, Butler argued, again echoing Fowler, could be an important tool of social reform through the bearing of fitter citizens; marriage should not be entered into unless both partners had trained for physical perfection.[86] Although it might take more than one generation to see substantial changes in the American people, Butler argued, beneficial changes would come if men and women—particularly women—would see to their strength and physical development. "How important is this culture to every prospective mother in America!" he exclaimed. "How potent must be its influence upon coming generations."[87] Again, like Fowler, Butler argued that women must be physically stronger and larger, with an amply developed waistline.[88]

Butler's special concern was that growth be symmetrical, and that it affect the vital organs, the brain, and the external muscles simultaneously. His machines, he claimed, could do just that. They allowed both the body and the brain to be naturally and harmoniously developed and were "at the basis of a true system of phrenology."[89] Like Windship, Butler centered his system on heavy, partial movements, writing that "perfect lifting, is perfect exercise."[90] Butler's lifting machines, however, had springs underneath the platform so that as the weight was being pulled upward, the floor gave way slightly, which he believed allowed the strain to be gradually absorbed by the body, making the lift safer and more stimulating to the internal organs. It brought "the whole body into action," he wrote, and not just the muscles themselves.[91]

Although Butler argued that lifting on his machine was the most beneficial exercise known to mankind, a full workout at a Butler studio consisted of four distinct types of exercise. The first of these was pulley work, with which both men women began their exercise sessions. On the back edge of a small wooden platform Butler had installed a number of upright posts with attached pulleys. Whether these pulleys were exactly like Chiosso's column is not known, but the principle appears to have been the same. In the center of the platform, he placed and secured another post against which the person would press his back

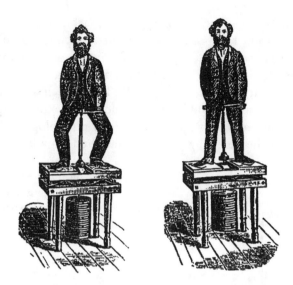

Figure 59: Butler's called this technique "center-lifting," and argued, incorrectly, that it was safer for the spinal column than other versions of the Health Lift. Wooden machines such as this sold for between $225 and $250. Note the springs separating the two layers of the platform. Illustration from the sixth edition of Lewis Janes's *Health-Exercise: The Rationale and Practice of the Lifting-Cure or Health Lift* (1871).

and hips while performing the pulley exercises. For the first exercises of the workout, the trainer grasped the wooden handles of the pulleys and pushed them forward while simultaneously executing a partial squatting motion. Four attempts with successively heavier weights were to be made each day on this machine as a warm-up exercise, and Butler advised increasing the maximum weight each day.

The second exercise in the series was the Health Lift itself. The machine consisted of a substantial table through the center of which passed an upright rod, on which weights rested. This rod could be adjusted for height so that the handle rested at the thighs with the knees only slightly bent. Butler believed that by grasping the handle with one hand in front of the body and the other behind the body, the spine stayed absolutely upright and was protected from strain.[92] "The position," he explained, "brings the body as nearly as possible into perfect shape; the manner of lifting distributes the weight cooperatively over the whole body, giving each muscle and organ its proper action, and developing the whole harmoniously."[93]

In contrast, Windship's machine was referred to as a "dead-weight" machine; it had no springs or buffers to soften the force of the exertions. Between all the joints on Butler's machines, however, springs and pieces of rubber helped cushion the lift. A complete cooperation of all parts of the body, Butler argued, could only be attained by lifting in this manner. Again, Butler recommended beginning with a light weight and making four attempts at the Health Lift in each workout. Butler believed that patients should gradually increase the total weight lifted. When it seemed as if they had reached their physiological limit, they should reduce the weight by fifty to one hundred pounds and begin the

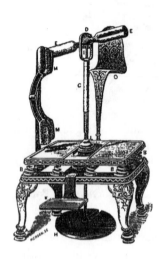

Figure 60: "The most perfect form of apparatus for the application of the Health Lift," and the most expensive, was this cast iron model with springs located between the layers of the platform and at the end of the four legs. It sold for $300. Although suggested for home use, the machine, alone, weighed seven hundred pounds. Fifty pound iron weights were added to the rod underneath the platform. The seat on the rear of the platform allowed the lifter to rest between attempts. Illustration from the sixth edition of Lewis Janes's *Health-Exercise: The Rationale and Practice of the Lifting-Cure or Health Lift* (1871).

ascent again. Butler recognized that maximum weights should not be approached in every workout. He advised taking some workouts that were below one's absolute limits, trying the heaviest weights only every couple of weeks.[94] It is worth noting that at no place in Butler's exercise manual did he suggest that there should be any limits on the amount of weight lifted in this method by men or women.

Following the completion of the Health Lifts, the trainer went to heavy dumbbell exercises. Butler warned that dumbbell work should not be performed as was done in the ordinary gymnasium, although the only exercise he gave instructions for was the overhead "jerk," one of the most common dumbbell exercises of this era. Perhaps it was the speed of the lift which concerned him, for in his instructions he suggested lifting the bell slowly to the shoulder. In the final phase of the overhead lift, however, he recommended a "thorough motion of the whole body, moving upon the hips and ankles" until the dumbbell was at full arm's length overhead, a recommendation that suggests a sudden, explosive movement. In any case, four progressively heavier attempts were to be made with each arm, with gradual weight increases over time.[95]

The final exercises of the session were a series of light dumbbell movements. Women's dumbbells, Butler noted, should weigh between two and six pounds (which was considerably heavier than other exercise advocates of the 1860s recommended for women), while men and boys should use weights from six to fourteen pounds. With these dumbbells, Butler had his pupils do squatting movements while simultaneously pressing the weights overhead, leg and arm extensions, and several circular motions reminiscent of Indian club work.[96] Butler considered this light dumbbell work "of least importance," and he warned that in many cases it was injurious instead of beneficial. He also argued that invalids, women, and children rarely needed such light exercises unless they were phlegmatic or overly stout.[97]

Butler claimed to be particularly successful in treating female diseases and weaknesses such as uterine hemorrhage, falling wombs, and sterility.[98] He had cured a "number" of women patients who had been "unable to perform the maternal function," he wrote, adding that he had also helped bring about the birth of healthy children in women who had not previously been able to bear a living child. Accordng to Butler, his maternity patients lifted during their pregnancies, and "after a few months of this preparation, during the period of pregnancy, labor has, in all cases, been comparatively easy and of short duration, and the children have, in every instance, been healthy and strong."[99] Butler believed that his success with women clients derived from the fact that "women and girls are unaccustomed to the use of nearly or quite all their power." Women made faster gains than men did, he argued, because manual labor had made the male of the species less responsive to any sort of exercise. But woman's greater sensitivity and her peculiarly feminine temperament made her more easily invigorated by proper training, according to Butler.[100] He taught that healthy women should train three times a week, those unwell, only twice.[101]

Butler vigorously opposed the growing popularity of Dio Lewis's New Gymnastics, a system of movements employing light appparati such as wooden dumbbells and Indian clubs that was especially popular with women. Lewis's system was ineffective and potentially dangerous, Butler argued. "Were it only a harmless amusement," he wrote, "we should pass it by as such; but . . . we have reason to know from abundant testimony and personal experience that it is doing a vast amount of injury."[102] Light weights actually created more injuries

and accidents than heavy weights, he warned, because Lewis's system
was too "social" and enervating.[103] Butler also warned that, when combined with walking, Lewis's system created too much muscular
development in the lower limbs "at the expense of vitality and true
symmetry." Exercise for women, according to Butler, should first and
foremost increase the size of the contracted waist and chest, and
thereby enhance the power of the vital organs inside the abdominal
cavity. Butler wanted the body to be larger and muscular, of course, but
he wanted the increase to be symmetrical. He claimed that Lewis's system created too much muscle on the body's appendages and spoiled
the body's balance.[104] Despite his sniping at Lewis's methods, Butler's
own system of training also would have produced considerable muscle
in the "appendages," as well as great strength. The prime movers of the
Health Lift were the large muscles of the legs and hips. The heavy
dumbbell presses would have increased the size of the arms and shoulders. Current training theory suggests that by doing relatively few
repetitions with heavy weights, Butler's clients could have added considerable muscular size and bulk to the body. After all, the amount of
weight he prescribed was not insignificant; even his home use machine
adjusted as high as 1,250 pounds.

### Marketing the Health Lift

By 1871, the Butler Health Lift Company had five different
branches in New York City, four of them on Broadway.[105] Lewis G.
Janes headed up the New York arm of the company from its main
offices on the second floor of the Park Bank Building at 120 Broadway.
Women could partake of Butler's Health Lift at all locations, but special
accommodations were made for women at 830 Broadway, where
Caroline E. Young supervised their training sessions, and at 158
Remsen Street, in Brooklyn, where Caroline Branson taught. Two "low-
rate" studios also bore the Butler name. One was at 348 Broadway in
the New York Life Insurance Building, and the other was on the second
floor of the Equitable Insurance Building, at 214 Broadway. In addition, John W. Leavitt operated a Health Lift studio at 113 Broadway in
the heart of Wall Street.[106] Leavitt and Lewis Janes had started in New
York as partners after studying with Butler in Boston. Their move to
New York in 1868 proved such a financial success, however, that Leavitt
soon left the firm and opened his own gym where he preached the
"efficiency" of the Butler system and continued to use Butler's
machines.[107]

In Boston, women could work out at Butler's original studio on West Street or at physician Elizabeth Branson's gymnasium at 784 Washington Street. Another Butler studio, again advertising "low rates," operated at 53 Temple Place in Boston. Butler Health Lift studios also operated in San Francisco, and in Providence, Rhode Island.[108]

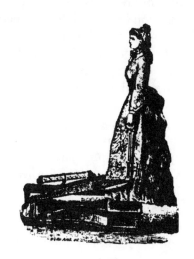

Figure 61: Mann's Reactionary Lifter was a side-lifting machine sold for home and gymnasium use. Its ads promised "Disease and Weakness Supplanted by Health and Strength." Courtesy Todd-McLean Collection, The University of Texas at Austin.

Other Health Lift entrepreneurs also took into consideration the special needs of women. The Health Lift Company of New York, for instance, marketed Mann's Reactionary Lifter, a cast iron lifting machine suitable for home or gym use.[109] Although relatively small, the Mann Reactionary Lifter still adjusted from twenty to twelve hundred pounds. Two handles attached to the weighted lever arm so that by standing on the machine's base, with a handle in each hand and the knees slightly bent, the lifter could simply straighten the legs to move the weighted arm a few inches. Prominently displayed in the advertising for this machine was a fashionably dressed young woman complete with bustle and corset.[110]

Side lift machines, such as Mann's Reactionary Lifter, were actually designed with women in mind. Having two handles, rather than the one used by Butler and Windship, made it unnecessary for a woman to change out of her street clothes to take a workout. Side lifting could be done in a full length dress, without even loosening the corset. Butler, and no doubt Windship as well, preferred their women clients to don gymnastic dress. But Mann's machine made the Health Lift—already touted for its time-saving efficiency—even more abbreviated. With Mann's machine, a woman could walk in off the street, do her required pulls, and be on her way again in minutes. Lewis G. Janes, however, a leading proponent of Butler's center-lifting method, voiced his opposition to side lifting for women in vehement tones, "No lady, dressed in the ordinary combination of close-fitting corsets, and garments supported about the hips, can attain a thorough exercise, without danger of congestion or visceral displacements as an effect of this compression . . ." If women would simply take time to loosen their corsets, Janes advised, they could do center-lifting wearing their regular street clothes, "as many of our lady patrons will testify."[111] Janes, it would seem, preferred his customers to skirt impropriety rather than risk the dangers of side lifting.

At least three gyms featured Mann's side lift machines. Besides the Health Lift Company's New York studio, side lifting establishments also opened in Cincinnati and Chicago. Other Health Lift entrepreneurs appeared as the fad for heavy lifting escalated. J. Fletcher Paul, also in Boston, promised that men and women could double their strength in just three months by training at his health studio[112] A much lighter approach was taken by Dr. Barnett, an early pioneer of the home equipment industry, who advertised a Health Lifting machine using rubber "wands" on each side of a platform. Barnett also sold a rowing machine and a "parlor gymnasium"—a rubberized cable with attached handles that today we would call an expander. Barnett's small book on the parlor gymnasium showed both men and women using the appliances.[113] The Goodyear Company copied Barnett's device in the 1880s and sold it as the "*Pocket Gymnasium or Health Pull.*"[114]

### Women and the Health Lift

In *Fit for America*, the historian Harvey Green wrote of the Health Lift craze of the 1860s: "Windship's brand of 'physical culture' . . . was something in which women—allegedly because of their constitution and reproductive system—could not participate. More important, they were not allowed to do so."[115] Green's obvious error is understandable, although lamentable. Most other historians of this epoch also neglected to examine the involvement of women in the Health Lift movement of the 1860s. But, as this chapter has demonstrated, women not only participated in the vigorous lifting Windship popularized, they undertook the regimen for the same basic reasons as men—greater strength, enhanced muscularity, and an increase in body size.

Orson Squire Fowler, the most successful practical phrenologist of the nineteenth century, paved the way for the women's Health Lift movement of the Civil War era, when, early in the 1840s, he began linking exercise, muscularity, and body size to brain improvement. In his many bestselling books and hundreds of popular articles, Fowler reinterpreted the classical theory of *Mens sana in corpore sano* into the phrenological language of self-improvement and physical perfectionism. In both men and women, argued Fowler, a large, powerful body was an indication of greater intelligence and increased mental efficiency: the bigger the body—the better the brain.

Fowler approached his women's campaign from both phrenological and Lamarckian perspectives, promising his followers that they could attain physical and mental perfection and that the desirable traits they acquired through exercise would subsequently be passed along to the next generation. Fowler's primary motivation in this campaign was, of course, eugenics. He did not personally champion the cause of women's rights, even though his phrenological theories provided women with a model for empowering themselves.

Despite Fowler's lack of philosophical commitment to the cause of women's rights, his phrenological endorsement of vigorous exercise and larger bodies directly contributed to the development of an alternate ideal of womanhood, called elsewhere in this text Majestic Womanhood. With Fowler's pseudoscientific backing to support them, many members of the women's rights campaign—and many other reform-minded Americans such as the male readers of the *Water Cure Journal*—embraced his notion of the larger, stronger, female body. Women of size and substance, the argument went, were less likely to be regarded as childlike and dependent; they were seen as more serious, more competent, and as possessing greater authority.

By far the most interesting aspect of the phrenological model of womanhood was the newfound importance of physical strength. Earlier in the century, "strength"—when applied to women—generally referred to simple good health, reproductive capacity, and the ability to carry out the duties of the household. Fowler, however, used "strength" quantitatively. He reveled in the stories of professional strongmen and frequently speculated on the physiological limits of mankind. When he urged women to try David P. Butler's new exercise system, he did so with the full knowledge that he was encouraging women to lift as much weight as they could manage.

It is impossible, of course, to know how many women truly practiced the type of heavy lifting advocated by Fowler, Windship, and

Butler. A stroll down Broadway in the late 1860s, however, would have taken a pedestrian past six different Health Lift studios, which suggests that, at least in New York City, and at least for a time, the Health Lift was a popular exercise method. But the Health Lift was not done only in New York. Boston, Chicago, Cincinnati, and San Francisco all had studios, and at least one women's school adopted Health Lifting as an exercise program. Further indication of the popularity of Health Lifting can be found in the publishing record of Lewis Janes's 1869 book on the Butler system; two years later it was in its sixth edition. Proof that the Health Lift continued to be regarded as an acceptable form of exercise for women can be found in health reform physician John Harvey Kellogg's *Ladies Guide in Health and Disease*. Published in 1888, Kellogg's book called the method "too important to overlook" and "an exceedingly valuable measure."[116]

Despite the fact that Dudley Allen Sargeant later recalled seeing lifting machines spring up "in parlors and offices and schools everywhere," the Health Lift was not without detractors.[117] When Windship died unexpectedly at his home on 12 September 1876, advocates of lighter systems of exercise claimed the Health Lift killed him.[118] Windship's death did effectively mark the end of the Health Lift movement of the mid-nineteenth century. However, the movement's health had already been considerably compromised by the anti-lifting campaign waged by exercise experts such as homeopathic physician and exercise revolutionary, Dr. Dioclesian Lewis. Lewis also promised women strength, health, and vigor, but he argued that such physiological changes would come about through his New Gymnastics, not through Health Lifting. Lewis's system would touch far more women's lives because of its adoption by public schools, private academies, and many colleges and universities for women. It was also the first physical education program specifically designed to elevate women beyond their separate sphere of duties. Thus it was that Lewis's system also provided a lift, albeit one of a more democratic kind.

[1]Orson S. Fowler, *Human Science: or, Phrenology; Its Principles, Proofs, Faculties, Organs, Temperaments, Combinations, Conditions, Teachings, Philosophies, etc. etc., as Applied to Health, Mental Philosophy, God, Immorality, Intellect* ... (Philadelphia: National Publishing Company, 1870), 578-79.

[2]John D. Davies, *Phrenology: Fad and Science* (New Haven: Yale University Press, 1955), x. Phrenology claimed its basis as a "science" because of its reliance on the Baconian method of scientific inquiry. A lengthy discussion

of Baconianism as applied to phrenology occurs in Andrew Boardman's "Essay on the Phrenological Mode of Investigation," included in George Combe's *Lectures on Phrenology,* 3rd ed. (New York: Fowler & Wells, 1882), 2-25. See also Orson S. Fowler, *Religion; Natural and Revealed; or the Natural Theology and Moral Bearings of Phrenology and Physiology* (New York: Fowler & Wells, 1844), viii.

[3]Charles Caldwell was probably the first person to bring phrenological information to the United States. On a trip to Europe in 1806, he met Franz Josef Gall, the founder of the science and purchased a phrenological bust. Upon his return to the United States, he gave several lectures on phrenology, but his views did not receive wide circulation. Nelson Sizer, *Forty Years in Phrenology; Embracing Recollections of History, Anecdote and Experience* (New York: Fowler & Wells, 1892), 383-84.

Spurzheim arrived in New York on 4 August 1832, and delivered a series of lectures there before traveling on to Boston. Davies, *Phrenology: Fad and Science*, 16. Biographical information on Spurzheim may be found in J. G. Spurzheim, *Phrenology, in Connection with the Study of Physiognomy; to Which is Prefixed A Biography of the Author by Nahum Capen* (Boston: Marsh, Capen & Lyon, 1834); "Biography of Dr. Spurzheim," *The American Phrenological Journal and Miscellany* 3 (1840): 1-2; and Anthony A. Walsh, "The American Tour of Dr. Spurzheim," *Journal of the History of Medicine* 27 (1972): 187-205.

[4]*Boston Medical and Surgical Journal* 7 (1832): 162.

[5]Davies, *Phrenology: Fad and Science*, x.

[6]Quoted in: Dwight L Young, "Orson Squire Fowler, To Form a More Perfect Human," *The Wilson Quarterly* 14 (Spring 1976): 121.

[7]Like Spurzheim, George Combe circulated in New England's social stratosphere. His well-regarded book, *The Constitution of Man Considered in Relation to External Objects* (New York: William H. Colyer, 1844 [1828]), was a combination of phrenology, physiology, and Scottish Common Sense philosophy. Combe acknowledged his debt to Adam Smith and Thomas Reid on page one, explaining that his own work was a "humble attempt to pursue the same plan, with the aid of new lights afforded by Phrenology." Harriett Martineau observed that Combe's *Constitution of Man* ranked with the Bible, *Pilgrim's Progress,* and *Robinson Crusoe* in popularity. More than one hundred thousand copies of the book had been sold in Britain and Ireland alone, she believed, adding that "it is in almost every home in the United States." "Harriett Martineau on George Combe," *The Phrenological Miscellany; or, the Annuals of Phrenology and Physiognomy from 1865–1873, Revised and Contained in One Volume* (New York: Fowler & Wells, 1882), 280. According to historian Arthur Wrobel, Combe's book sold more than 70,000 copies between 1828 and 1838. Wrobel, "Orthodoxy and Respectability," *Journal of Popular Culture* 9 (1975): 43.

Combe's views on physical education can be found in George Combe, *Lectures on Phrenology: Including its Application to the Present and Prospective Condition of the United States*, 3rd ed. (New York: Fowler & Wells, 1882), 312-32.

[8]"Phrenology shows us that to improve the human mind, we must begin by improving the condition of the brain," Combe observed in 1841, "to attain success in this object, all moral, religious, and intellectual teaching, must be conducted in harmony with the laws of physiology." George Combe, *Notes on the United States of North America During a Phrenological Visit in 1838-39-40*. 3 vols. (Edinburgh: Maclachlan, Stewart and Company, 1841) 3:428-29.

[9]*Phrenological Miscellany*, 117; Merle Curti, *The Social Ideas of American Educators: With New Chapter on the Last Twenty-five Years* (Totawa NJ: Littlefield, Adams & Co., 1966), 117, observed that Mann "regarded phrenology as the greatest discovery of the ages, recommended its study to teachers, referred to it constantly in his lectures on education, and modified some of his own attitudes as a result of its influence on him." See also Combe, Notes on the United States, 1: 64.

For further information of Mann's views on health and exercise, see Horace Mann, "Prospectus," *The Common School Journal* 1 (November 1838): 10-11; and Horace Mann, *Lectures on Education* (Boston: Wm. B. Fowle, 1848). See also Curti, *Social Ideas of American Educators*, 101-38.

[10]Horace Mann, *Sixth Annual Report as Secretary of the Massachusetts Board of Education* (Boston: January 1843). See Edward Mussey Hartwell, School *Document No. 22-1891. Report of the Director of Physical Training, December 1891* (Boston: Rockwell and Churchill, 1892), 30-31, for other details of Mann's advocacy of physical education.

[11]Sizer, *Forty Years*, 14.

[12]Combe's three-volume *Notes on the United States*, published in 1841, is filled with references to meetings with presidents, professors, governors, and clergymen.

[13]Many distinguished Americans continued to believe in the merits of phrenology. Henry Ward Beecher, for instance, one of America's most well-known and influential ministers, defended phrenology from the pulpit on at least twenty occasions. Sizer, *Forty Years*, 14.

[14]The Fowler brothers dropped out of Amherst Theological Seminary in 1843 to pursue their new career. For information on the lives of these men, see Davies, *Phrenology: Fad and Science*; and Young, "Orson Squire Fowler, To Form a More Perfect Human," 120-24.

[15]Orson's first two books, *Love and Parentage and Amativeness*, had gone through forty editions by 1844, according to *Dictionary of American Biography*, vol. 6 (New York: Charles Scribner and Sons, 1931), 566.

[16]Samuel Wells became the Fowler brothers's partner and business manager through marriage to their sister, Charlotte, in 1844. The publishing firm was

known thereafter as Fowler(s) and Wells. The plural form of Fowler was not always used. Robert J. Joynt, "Phrenology in New York State," *New York State Journal of Medicine* 73 (1 October 1973): 2383.

[17]Ibid. *The American Phrenological Journal* ran from 1837 to 1911.

[18]Sizer, *Forty Years*, 385-86.

[19]Paul Broca, for instance, became fixated on this aspect of what he called craniometry. He collected brains, weighed and measured them, and used his skewed data to prove to his own satisfaction the intellectual superiority of the Caucasian race. See Stephen Jay Gould, *The Mismeasure of Man* (New York: W. W. Norton & Co, 1981), 84-107.

[20]Samuel R. Wells, *New Physiognomy or Signs of Character, as Manifested Through Temperament and External Forms, and Especially in the Human Race Divine* (New York: Samuel R. Wells, 1868), 656.

For an early nineteenth-century interpretation of the relationship of phrenology to vitalism, see John Harrison Curtis, *Observations on the Preservation of Health in Infancy, Youth, Manhood and Age with the Best Means of Improving the Moral and Physical Condition of Man, Prolonging Life and Promoting Human Happiness* (London: Henry Renshaw, 1838), 39-42.

[21]Orson S. Fowler, *Creative and Sexual Science or Manhood, Womanhood and Their Mutual Inter-Relations, Love, Its Laws, Power, Etc.* (New York: by the author, 1870), 694-95.

[22]George Capron, M.D., and David B. Slack, *New England Popular Medicine* (Providence: J. F. Moore, 1846), 244-45.

[23][Orson Fowler], "Practical Phrenology—No. 1: Directions for Making Examinations with Rules for Finding the Organs," *American Phrenological Journal* 4 (1 January 1842): 14-16. See also Orson Fowler, *The Illustrated Self-Instructor in Phrenology and Physiolgy* (New York: Fowlers and Wells, 1854), 32-35.

Orson worked at forging strong links with the popular health reform movement. His publishing house, Fowlers and Wells, became the leading printer of hygiene and health reform texts in the United States. Fowler also took over the financially ailing *Water Cure Journal and Herald of Reforms*, an editorial change that helped its subscription list soar to more than twenty thousand names. He quickly introduced regular features on phrenology to its readers. Madeline Stern, *Heads and Headlines: The Phrenological Fowlers* (Norman OK: University of Oklahoma Press, 1971), 51, 63-68.

In the mid-1840s, a new editorial thrust in his own *Phrenological Journal* stressed the links between phrenology and physiology. The six issues of the *Phrenological Journal*, which appeared in 1845, for instance, contained sixteen articles dealing with aspects of physiological living, out of a total of fifty-one regular articles. The "Miscellany" at the end of each issue always contained references to the water-cure, nutrition, and hygiene. *The American Phrenological Journal and Miscellany* 6 (1845): i.

[24]Orson S. Fowler, *Phrenology and Physiology Explained and Applied to Education, and Self-Improvement; Including the Intellectual and Moral Education and Government of Children: Mental Discipline & The Cultivation of Memory; and the means of Regaining and preserving the Health By Pointing Out the Methods of Increasing and Decreasing the Phrenological Organs in Children and One's Self* (New York: O. S. & L. N. Fowler, 1842), 11.

[25]See Patricia Vertinsky, *The Eternally Wounded Woman: Women, Exercise, and Doctors in the Late Nineteenth Century* (New York: Manchester University Press, 1990), 69-88, for more complete information on the effect of vitalism on antebellum women.

[26]Sizer, *Forty Years*, 393.

[27]Harriett N. Austin, "Thoughts About Health. Extracts from an Address Delivered at a Health Convention in Cooper Institute, New York, Thirty-One Years Ago," *The Laws of Life* 32 (September 1886): 260.

[28]Eliza W. Farnham, *Woman and Her Era*, vol. 2 (New York: A. J. Davis & Co., 1864), 331.

[29]Fowler, *Phrenology and Physiology Explained and Applied to Education*, 22.

[30]Orson S. Fowler, *Maternity; or the Bearing and Nursing of Children, Including Female Education and Beauty* (New York: Fowler and Wells, 1848), 87.

[31][Sarah Hale], "Hints About Phrenology," *The Ladies Magazine and Literary Gazette* 6 (April 1833): 174.

[32]Fowler, *Maternity*, 52-53.

[33]This phrase is printed on the title page of several Fowler texts, including Orson S. Fowler, *On Matrimony: Or, Phrenology and Physiology Applied to the Selection of Congenial Companions for Life; Including Directions to the Married for Living Together Affectionately and Happily* (New York: O. S. and L. N. Fowler, 1842).

[34]Eleanor Kirk, "Two Women of the Present," *The Phrenological Journal and Life Illustrated* 51 (July 1870): 57-58.

[35][Dio Lewis], "Miss Beecher and her Western College," *Lewis's New Gymnastics for Ladies, Gentlemen and Children and Boston Journal of Physical Culture* 1 (August 1861): 155.

[36]Beecher, *Letters to the People*, 120.

[37]Fowler, *Matrimony*, 62.

[38]Ibid.

[39]Orson S. Fowler, *Sexual Science; Including Manhood, Womanhood, and Their Mutual Interrelations; Love Its Laws, Power, Etc. . . . As Taught by Phrenology* (Philadelphia: National Publishing Company, 1870), 172.

[40]Many ads requested that phrenological readings be sent as character references, and some specifically advertised for women with certain phrenological traits. See "Matrimony," *The Water-Cure Journal and Herald of Reforms* 22 (February 1856): 47; and "Matrionial," *The Water-Cure Journal and Herald of Reforms* 27 (April 1859): 63. In one example, "Anna," a twenty-

five-year-old Massachusetts teacher, included in her self-description the fact that she had high marks for amativeness, inhabitiveness, combativeness, approbitiveness, firmness, and benevolence.

[41]"Matrimonial," *The Water-Cure Journal and Herald of Reforms* 19 (December 1855): 89.

[42]"Matrimonial: Still Alone—I Want a Wife," *The Water-Cure Journal and Herald of Reforms* 27 (February 1859): 31.

[43]"Matrimonial Correspondence," *The Water-Cure Journal and Herald of Reforms* 19 (May 1855): 113.

[44]"Matrimonial Correspondence, *"The Water-Cure Journal and Herald of Reforms* 19 (August 1855): 42.

[45]"Miscellany: The Green Mountain Boys," *The American Phrenological Journal and Miscellany* 6 (February 1844): 46.

[46]D[aniel]. H. Jacques, *Hints Toward Physical Perfection: Or the Philosophy of Human Beauty; Showing how to Acquire and Retain Bodily Symmetry, Health and Vigor, Secure Long Life, and Avoid the Infirmities and Deformities of Age* (New York: Fowler & Wells, 861 [1859]), 223.

[47]Jacques's serial in the *Water Cure Journal* began with vol. 23 (April 1857), 77.

[48]Wooster Beach, M.D., *Beach's Family Physician and Home Guide for the Treatment of the Diseases of Men, Women and Children of Reform Principles, Forty-fifth thousand* (Cincinnati: Moore Wilstach, Keys & Co., 1862), 123.

[49]William Milo with "Additions, Alterations, Notes, and Illustrations by Handsome Charles, the Magnet," *Notes on Beauty, Vigor and Development; or How to Acquire Plumpness of Form, Strength of Limb, and Beauty of Complexion* (New York: Samuel R. Wells, n.d.. This book was advertised in Russell Trall, *The Illustrated Family Gymnasium; Containing the Most Improved Methods of Applying Gymnastic, Calisthenic, Kinesipathic, and Vocal Exercises to the Development of the Bodily Organs, the Invigoration of their Functions, the Preservation of Health, and the Cure of Diseases and Deformities* (New York: Samuel R. Wells, 1873), 219.

[50]Hillel Schwartz, *Never Satisfied: A Cultural History of Diets, Fantasies and Fat* (New York: Anchor Books, 1986), 164, 59.

[51]David McRae, *The Americans at Home*, rev. ed. (Glasgow, 1860) 29; quoted in Schwartz, *Never Satisfied*, 58.

[52]M. Augusta Fairchild, M.D., "The Fitness of Things," *Herald of Health* 4 (July 1864): 37.

[53]Rosalind A. Keep, *Four Score and Ten Years: A History of Mills College* (California: 1946) 81; quoted in Paul Atkinson, "The Feminist Physique: Physical Education and the Medicalization of Women's Education," in Park and Mangan, *From "Fair Sex" to Feminism*, 51.

[54][Orson S. Fowler], "Health—Its Value and Conditions; Including the Means of Preserving and Regaining It," *The American Phrenological Journal and Miscellany* 6 (May 1844): 137.

[55]The phrenologist cited circus performers such as Giovanni Belzoni, the Ravel Family, and J. A. J. Bihin, known as the Belgian Giant, as models of what the human body could do with proper training. O. S. Fowler, *Hereditary Descent; its Laws and Facts Appled to Human Improvement* (New York: Fowler and Wells, 1848), 37.

[56]Orson Fowler retells the Jonathan Fowler story in a number of places. See, for example, Fowler, *Hereditary Descent*, 38-43; [Fowler], "Health.—Its Value and Conditions," 137-38; Fowler, *Physiology, Animal and Mental*, 229-30; and Orson Fowler, Human Science or, Phrenology; Its Principles, Proofs, Faculties, *Organs, Temperaments, Combinations, Conditions, Teachings, Philosophies, etc. etc., as Applied to Health* . . . (Philadelphia: National Publishing Company, 1868), 568.

[57]Austin, "Thoughts About Health", 260-61.

[58]Delos Dunton, "Items from Home of the Free, *The Herald of Health* 4 (September 1864): 103.

[59]Elizabeth Blackwell, M.D., *The Laws of Life With Special Reference to The Physical Education of Girls* (New York: George P. Putnam, 1852), 20-21. Others apparently shared her views. An article in the *Atlantic Monthly* copied Blackwell's examples of women of great strength and added to Cymburga and Brinhilde, tales of the extraordinary strength of Oberea, Queen of the Sandwich Islands, and of seventy-four-year-old Lady Butterfield of Essex, England, who advertised, "This is to give notice to my honored masters and ladies and loving friends, that my Lady Butterfield gives a challenge to ride a horse, or leap a horse, or run afoot, or hollo, with any woman in England." Quoted in "Physical Training of Girls," *Lewis's Gymnastic Monthly for Ladies, Gentlemen and Children and Boston Journal of Physical Culture* 1 (April 1861): 99.

[60][Elizabeth Cady Stanton], "Man Superior—Intellectually—Morally—and Physically," *The Lily* 3 (1851): 31-32. Stanton's article also chronicled feats of exceptional strength and endurance by indigenous females.

[61]Fowler, *Maternity*, 166-67.

[62]Ibid., 87.

[63]Historian Lois Banner credits the circuses and German Turner societies of the mid-nineteenth century for the dissemination of the idea of dress reform and exercise in general. Lois Banner, *American Beauty* (New York: Alfred A. Knopf, 1983), 91. For insight into the growing popularity of heavy weight lifting at mid-century, see Ed James, *How to Acquire Health, Strength and Muscle, Including Treatment for Free Livers and Sedentary People, About Air, Clothing, Food and Stimulants; Also Best Mode of Exercise for all Ages, Cures and Preventives for Various Diseases, Proportions of a Perfect Human Figure; Sketches of Dr. G. B. Windship's and R. A. Pennell's Methods, Remarkable Feats of Strength, Measurements of Noted Athletes, The Muscular System, Tables of Nutrition and Digestion*, 12th ed. (New York: Ed James, 1878).

[64]Hippolyte Triat opened a school of physical culture in Brussels in 1840. In 1849, he moved to Paris and attracted many of the Paris *haute monde* to his establishment. Triat was among the first to manufacture and sell iron dumbbells and barbells in a variey of sizes. Edmund Desbonnet, *Les Rois de la Force* (Paris: Berger-Levrault, 1911) 58-60.

[65]In the United States, Turner societies were among the first associations formed by the German immigrants. Established to help maintain their heritage, there were, by 1861, approximately nine thousand registered members of the national American organization Socialist Turnerbund and more than 150 different, individual Turner societies. In 1865, this group changed its name to the Nordamerikanisher Turnerbund, and by 1886, it included 231 societies and some 23,823 members—5,562 of whom were listed as active athletes. See Robert K. Barney, "German Turners in America: Their Role in Nineteenth Century Exercise Expression and Physical Education Legislation," in: *A History of Physical Education and Sport in the United States and Canada,* Earle F. Ziegler, ed. (Champaign IL: Stites Publishing, 1975) for other information on the German Turner Societies in the United States.

[66]David Webster, *Barbells and Beefcake: An Illustrated History of Bodybuilding* (Irvine, Scotland: by the author, 1979), 18-20.

[67]Although the professional strongman was the norm, there were several European women who performed strength acts in the nineteenth century. Madame Gobert at various times billed herself as the French Female Hercules and the Strongest Woman in Europe. A handbill announcing her appearance at the Bartholomew Fair in London on 4 September 1818, advertised that she would "lift with her teeth a table five feet long and three feet wide, with several persons seated upon it . . . carry thirty-six weights, fifty-six pounds each, equal to 2,016 lbs. . . . carry a barrel containing 340 bottles; also an anvil 400 lbs. weight, on which they will forge with four hammers at the same time she supports it on her stomach." For the finale of her show, she lifted by ropes tied to her hair an anvil supposedly weighting four hundred pounds. In the 1860s, the Frenchwoman, Mademoiselle Doublier, did an act of dumbbell and barbell work that concluded with her shouldering a zinc cannon and setting it off. Other strongwomen such as Madame Ali Bracco; Olga, the 'Mulatto Strongwoman"; her partner Kaira; and "Mademoiselle Cora" played the European music hall circuit. Jan Todd, "The Strongwoman and the Police Gazette," unpublished paper, presented at North American Society for Sport History, Clemson University, 1989; and Jan Todd, "Legacy of Strength: The Cultural Phenomenon of the Professional Strongwoman," unpublished paper, presented at North American Society for Sport History, Columbus, Ohio, 1987.

[68][Horace Mann],"Circus," *The Common School Journal* 9 (1 October 1847): 18.

[69]Miss Mendell and Miss Hosmer, *Notes of Travel and Life* (New York: Mendell and Hosmer, 1835), 54-55. Harriet Martineau also spoke favorably

of circus performers, particularly a troupe of Stockbridge, Massachusetts, female acrobats whom she saw perform while on tour in America during the 1830s. Quoted in Josephine Robinson, *Circus Lady* (New York: Thomas Y. Crowell, 1926).

[70]Chiosso claimed that he made the first version of the Polymachinon in 1829. The 1855 version of the machine is remarkably similar to our modern Universal machines. James Chiosso, *The Gymnastic Polymachinon* (New York: H. Balliere, 1855), 9. Dumbbells and ndian clubs could be purchased in many hardware stores or through gyms. See, for instance, the advertisement, "Bodily Exercise the Best Medicine," *Water Cure Journal and Herald of Reforms* 25 (August 1857): 46.

[71]George Barker Windship, "Autobiographical Sketches of a Strength-Seeker," *Atlantic Monthly* 9 (January 1862): 102-103. For other information on Windship, see Joan Paul, "The Health Reformers: George Barker Windship and Boston's Strength Seekers," *Journal of Sports History* 10 (Winter 1983): 41-57; Jan Todd, "Strength is Health," 3-14; and Terence Todd, "The History of Resistance Exercise and Its Role in United States Education" (Ph.D. diss., University of Texas at Austin, 1966), 40-48.

[72]Details of Windship's strength training methods and his personal best lifts can be found in James, *How to Acquire*, 54-57; and Jan Todd, "Strength is Health," 6-9.

[73]Windship, "Autobiographical Sketches," 108. Windship began with fifty-pound dumbbells, but was soon able to put 141 pounds over his head with one hand, a creditable feat even by today's standards for a man his size.

[74]Quote included in "To Lecture Committees," Handbill for Windship's lectures from 1860, Windship Collection, Massachusetts Historical Society, Boston MA.

[75]Ibid., 105.

[76]George Barker Windship, "Physical Culture," *The Massachusetts Teacher* 13 (April 1860): 128.

[77]"Physical Training," *Harpers Weekly* 4 (22 September 1860): 594.

[78]Jan Todd, "Strength is Health," 3-10.

[79]Windship's patients included such distinguished men as the actor Edwin Forrest. "George Barker Windship," Obituary notice, fragment in the Commonplace Book of G. B. Windship. Massachusetts Historical Society, Boston MA.

[80]Advertising Section, *Boston Directory* (Boston: Sampson, Davenport and Co., 1870).

[81]Mrs. Taylor, "Physical Training for Young Ladies," *Lewis's New Gymnastics for Ladies, Gentlemen and Children and Boston Journal of Physical Culture* 1 (February 1861): 54.

[82]Fowler's version of the Health Lift made it into a form of isometric contraction. Fowler, *Human Science or Phrenology*, 579.

[83]Butler opened a gymnasium in Boston at 19 Temple Place in 1867, but it is highly likely—since he claimed that he had been experimenting with Health Lifting for more than ten years—that he had an exercise studio prior to this time. He patented his first lifting machine on 6 June 1865, another on 19 June 1866, and claimed two more patents in 1869. John W. Leavitt, Exercise a *Medicine; or, Muscular Action as Related to Organic Life* (New York: J. W. Leavitt, 1870), 7.

[84]Butler offered several models of Health Lift machines, and all were expensive. His "Standard Iron Machine," with six hundred pounds of weight, sold for $300, or $250 if a gym owner purchased three at the same time. A simpler, wooden version sold for $250 or $225 for three. Second-hand versions of the Wooden Machine cost $200. A spring machine, preferred for home use because it required no additional iron weights, sold for $100. Parties interested in introducing the Health Lift into other cities signed a contract with the Butler Health-Lift Company giving them rights to the use of Butler's name. Lewis G. Janes, *Health-Exercise: The Rationale and Practice of the Lifting-Cure or Health Lift*, 6th ed. (New York: Lewis G. Janes, 1871), 37-38.

Windship also ran a gym and had taken out patents on exercise devices, but he didn't franchise his name as Butler did.

[85]David P. Butler, *Butler's System of Physical Training: The Lifting Cure. An Original Scientific Application of the Laws of Motion or Mechanical Action to Physical Culture and the Cure of Disease. With a Discussion of True and False Methods of Physical Training* (Boston: by the author, 1868). Historian Leonard reported that a book by Windship was scheduled for release by Ticknor and Fields in 1862. However, no record can be found of its publication. Fred Eugene Leonard, *A Guide to the History of Physical Education*, R. Tait McKenzie, ed., 2nd ed. (Philadelphia: Lea and Febiger, 1927), 58.

[86]Butler, *Butler's System*, 80.

[87]Ibid., 81.

[88]Ibid., 79.

[89]Ibid., 75-77.

[90]Ibid., 88.

[91]Ibid., 89.

[92]In actuality, such a position slightly twists the spine and makes it more susceptible to back injuries. A similar lift, using barbells, is known as the Jefferson Lift.

[93]Butler, *Butler's System*, 94.

[94]Ibid., 95-96.

[95]Ibid., 97.

[96]Ibid., 99-100.

[97]Ibid., 100.

[98]Ibid., 27. Butler's lifting cure would supposedly remedy a variety of chronic ailments as well. Dyspepsia, catarrh, neuralgia, liver and kidney

disease, ruptures, hernias, constipation, cancer, consumption, and even toothaches and fevers had all disappeaed, he suggested, after practicing the Health Lift. Butler, *Butler's System*, 71-73.

[99]Ibid., 80.

[100]Ibid., 71-73.

[101]Ibid., 88.

[102]Ibid., 23.

[103]Ibid., 15.

[104]Ibid., 30-31.

[105]Leavitt, *Health a Medicine*, i-v.

[106]Leavitt claimed to have seventy-five prominent bankers, brokers, lawyers, and merchants from the Wall Street area among his clients. Leavitt, *Health a Medicine*, iv.

[107]Health Lifting was ideally suited for modern times, Leavitt wrote, as one could get a full, vigorous workout in just a few minutes a day. Ibid., iii-iv, 10.

[108]Janes, *Health-Exercise*, i. The San Francisco studio was under the direction of Dr. Swain.

[109]The Health-Lift company had its showroom/exercise salon at 178 Broadway. It is not known whether "Mann" was in any way a reference to Horace Mann.

[110]Harvey Green, *Fit for America: Health, Fitness, Sport, and American Society* (New York: Pantheon Books, 1986), 199.

[111]Janes, *Health-Exercise*, 44.

[112]*Boston Directory*, Reel 8 (1875): 1363.

[113]S. M. Barnett, *Barnett's Patent Parlor Gymnasium* (New York: J. Becker and Co., 1871) 36.

[114]*Peck and Snyder's Price List of Outdoor and Indoor Sport and Pastimes* (New York, 1886) 205.

[115]Harvey Green, *Fit for America*, 202.

[116]J. H. Kellogg, M. D., *Ladies Guide in health and Disease, Girlhood, Maidenhood, Wifehood , Motherhood.* (Des Moines IA: W. D. Condit & Co., 1888), 240.

[117]Dudley Allen Sargent, *An Autobiography* (Philadelphia: Lea and Febiger, 1927), 98.

[118]At forty-two years of age, Windship suffered a massive stroke and died instantly. Windship Biographical File, Harvard University Archives, Cambridge MA. The publicity surrounding Windship's death made many people afraid to keep lifting. In fact, for some years afterwards, Windship's unexpected death was mentioned negatively in exercise books. See, for instance, Edwin Checkley, *A Natural Method of Physical Culture Training* (New York: Harpers, 1894), 29.

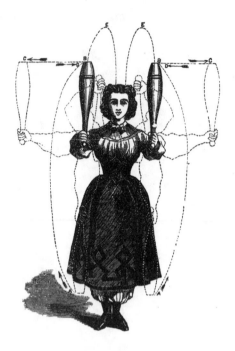

Figure 62: Woman with Indian clubs in an illustration from Sim D. Kehoe's *The Indian Club Exercise* (1864). The inclusion of female images in a text such as Kehoe's can be traced to Dio Lewis's influence.

# Chapter 8
## Dio Lewis and the New Gymnastics:
### Birth of a System

More than 130 years after the reformer-physician Dioclesian Lewis introduced the purposive training system that Thomas Wentworth Higginson called "the most important step yet taken for the physical education of American women," Lewis remains an enigmatic figure.[1] Here is a man who can count among his contributions the popularization of an influential exercise system known as the New Gymnastics, the authorship of one of the bestselling nineteenth-century texts on physical training, and the founding of the first normal college for physical educators in the United States–a man who engineered, through the force of his personality, the endorsement of a virtually unknown exercise system by the American Institute of Instruction; who began an experimental school to prove his belief that with proper exercise and challenging intellectual education women could become fully participating members of society; and whose lectures sparked the formation of the Women's Christian Temperance Union. Yet, despite all these contributions, Lewis has received only cursory scholarly attention.[2] The broad outlines of Lewis's contributions to the field of physical education are, of course, familiar to every student of the history of physical education.[3] Lewis's personal history, however, and his assertion that once women's bodies were larger, stronger, and more enduring, women would be able to participate as man's equal in the world outside the home have not received the attention they deserve.

In 1862, *The Massachusetts Teacher* glowingly observed, "It is not too much to say that to him [Lewis] more than to any other man must be attributed the deep practical interest now manifested by educators throughout the country, in reference to the proper culture of the human body."[4] By the end of the century, however, Lewis's advocacy for women's rights, combined with his often overly-enthusiastic approach to life in general, apparently caused some physical educators to dismiss Lewis and his contributions.[5] Harvard's director of physical education, Dudley Allen Sargent, spoke to this point with a group of students at Springfield College in 1903. Lewis fell into "bad repute," according to Sargent, because he "took up the temperance question and attempted the Carry Nation act." Sargent also told the young

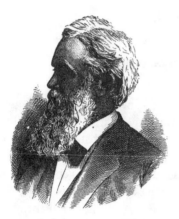

Figure 63: Dioclesian (Dio) Lewis
from: *In a Nutshell: Suggestions to
American College Students* (1883).

physical education students, "We have failed to give Dr. Lewis the credit
which he deserves."[6] Helen Cecilia Clarke Lewis, Dio's widow, agreed.
In a letter to Springfield College physical educator Luther Halsey
Gulick—who began collecting material for a biography of Lewis in
1898, which he apparently never completed—Mrs. Lewis wrote, "I am
greatly pleased that you are doing this work and hope you can do my
husband justice. He has not had it."[7] By focusing on Lewis's involvement with women's purposive training, this chapter and the following
two attempt to "do justice" to at least a part of Lewis's cultural legacy.

## Dio Lewis:
### The Early Years

Dioclesian Lewis was born in Cayuga County, in the small town of
Throopsville, near Auburn, New York, on 3 March 1823.[8] He stood
apart from the first, according to his brother Loran, who ascribed to
young Dio an unmatched energy and enthusiasm for work and living.
Reportedly precocious in both intelligence and strength, by age twelve,
Dio "was as large and mature as ordinary boys of fifteen," Loran
recalled. He continued to grow until he stood just under six feet tall,
weighed more than two hundred pounds, and had a phrenologically
near-perfect twenty-four-inch skull.[9] With his auburn hair, blue eyes,
and full beard, Dio Lewis, the man, appeared to be the very embodi-
ment of health and vigor.

Like Orson Fowler, Lewis attributed his physical strength and har-
diness to an unusually large and strong ancestor. In Lewis's case, the
revered figure was his maternal grandfather who, at three hundred
pounds, was "well proportioned, of erect carriage, and of great strength
of body and mind."[10] The daughter of this paragon, Delecta Barbour

Lewis, served as Dio's moral compass throughout his life. "From my earliest recollection," Lewis wrote late in his life, "I have had the greatest confidence in women. My remarkable mother inspired and deepened this faith."[11] Besides rearing five children, Lewis's mother became a successful tailor with several hired assistants when her husband's financial reverses brought the family close to economic ruin. As a convert to the principles of the evangelical Church of the Disciples, Delecta also possessed a strong sense of Christian mission. Well before the Washingtonian Temperance Movement of the 1840s or the advent of the Women's Christian Temperance Union in the 1870s, she organized many of the women of Auburn and nearby Clarksville into a staunch temperance band and successfully closed all the saloons and grog shops in the area.[12] Throughout his career as a lecturer, Lewis told this story as an example of the beneficial power women could exert upon society if they could learn to unite and work together to have access to the world outside the home.[13]

The financial setbacks that forced his mother into tailoring also forced Dio out of school at age twelve. His large size helped him find work at a cotton factory, however, and six months later he took a job in a hoe and scythe factory where the speed with which he carried out his work became a local curiosity.[14] At age fourteen he went to work on a construction gang helping to wheelbarrow earth for a dam. At this job, too, Dio outworked all the grown men at the site, according to his brother. Apparently, Lewis's energy was one of the most singular aspects of his character. "He could do anything he desired to do with more rapidity than any person I ever knew," Loran recalled.[15]

Dio's energy, intelligence, and resourcefulness led to an invitation to take over the new school at Jennett Center, a small community adjoining Auburn. Only fifteen years old, with no training and no real education, Dio nonetheless made a success of teaching. The fact that he could "read a page in a book once, close the book, and repeat it all" quickly made up for the lapses in his own education.[16] Unconventional even then, Lewis found that by giving the students frequent breaks during the day for recreational activities such as singing, games, and nature hikes, school discipline took care of itself. Criticized initially by fellow Cayuga County residents for this unorthodox, joyful approach to education, Lewis soon became even more famous in his community as his pupils made faster progress than they had under stricter regimes.[17]

Word of his success soon spread outside Auburn, and Dio received several job offers, one of which, on the lower Sandusky River, he accepted in 1841. At this new school, Dio expanded his course offerings to include Latin, Algebra, and Geometry, yet he retained his interest in recreation as an emotional and physical release for the students. As the small town of Fremont grew, the citizens agreed to incorporate the school and erect a stone building to house Lewis and his pupils. As a testament to the esteem with which Lewis must have been regarded by his Fremont neighbors, the new school was named the Dioclesian Institute.[18] Few men at age nineteen have been so honored.

Lewis's first teaching career ended abruptly in 1842 when he developed an "ague" and had to return to Auburn to convalesce. But when the next school term began, he was still unwell and finally abandoned his plans of returning to the Dioclesian Institute. Instead, he decided to study medicine and apprenticed himself to a local, regular physician for a three-year period. In 1845, he briefly entered Harvard's medical school where he tried to earn enough to offset his tuition and boarding expenses by editing a religious paper called *The Genius of Christianity*. According to his brother, Loran, however, the magazine could not sustain his economic needs, and Dio left Harvard and joined the practice of Dr. Lewis McCarthy, a homeopathic physician, from nearby Port Byron, New York.[19] Although he had no diploma, Lewis hung out his own shingle. From that day forward, he was Dr. Lewis.[20]

### Helen Cecilia Lewis and the Consumption Cure

Three years later, twenty-five-year-old Dio moved to Buffalo, New York. He opened his own homeopathic medical practice—one of the first in western New York State—and began a new monthly magazine, *The Homeopathist*, which stressed preventive medicine, health reform, and homeopathic medical theory. Although he later admitted that he had prescribed traditional medications early in his career, Dio's time with Dr. McCarthy convinced him of the error of such conventional therapies. By the time he moved to Buffalo, Dio had become a staunch proponent of the health reformers' creed of fresh air, pure water, rest, and exercise.[21]

These beliefs were severely tested when his new wife, Helen Cecelia Clarke-Lewis, developed consumption in the spring of 1851 and rapidly dropped in weight from 116 to 80 pounds.[22] Dio was in agony over the possible loss of his young bride, for he knew that two of Helen's sisters had already died from consumption. After reading everything he could find on the disease, Dio proposed a radical course of treatment centered around vigorous exercise. His decision to turn to exercise as a remedy for consumption was unusual, but certainly not unprecedented. Philadelphia physician Benjamin Rush had suggested a similar course in his writings at the turn of the century, and Dio quoted extensively from Rush in *Weak Lungs, and How to Make Them Strong*, his 1864 exercise manual for the treatment of consumption.[23] Although Rush and other authorities provided Lewis with a philosophical justification for choosing exercise, Lewis and Rush differed significantly on the question of the severity of the exercises a patient should perform.[24]

Dio began Helen's movement cure with a visit to the proprietor of the Buffalo gymnasium. Prior to this time, the gym did not allow women to become members, but at Lewis's urging the owner agreed to set aside a few hours each week for Helen and several of Dio's other female patients who suffered from similar problems. No record exists of what the women actually did at the Buffalo gymnasium, although Eastman reported that the gym owner selected "some of the lightest exercises," only a few of which were considered "helpful to such an invalid as Mrs. Lewis."[25]

Although Helen had long since discarded her corset, the Lewises made further changes in her dress at this time. She let out the waistlines of all her skirts and added suspenders to free her breathing. She began work on a new wardrobe, made all in flannel, in order to keep her chest and arms warm, and she purchased a pair of heavy-soled men's boots so that she could be outdoors in sun, rain, or snow. With these changes in her dress, Helen began accompanying Dio on his medical rounds. Although they owned a horse and buggy, they walked whenever possible, to make sure Helen received adequate exercise.[26]

All of these lifestyle changes helped, Helen Lewis later reported, especially one change—Dio's decision that she should begin sawing wood. "It proved helpful," Helen recalled, "for it did drive the air through the air cells of the lungs . . . [and] from being able to saw only a few sticks as large as my wrists at a time, resting after each stick, I became able before the winter was over to saw all the wood needed for two fires." While Helen sawed, Dio split the wood and provided companionship and encouragement.[27] Dio later claimed that he had chosen sawing as a remedial exercise because it (1) specifically worked the muscles of Helen's upper body, (2) increased her rate of respiration, and (3) got her outdoors into fresh, clean air. These three principles, Lewis believed, constituted a consumptive's best chance for surviving the dread disease.[28]

While Helen Lewis sawed her way to health, Dio measured her physical transformation, as Orson Fowler might have done, through the increase in the size of her waistline. "At the outset a finger's length had been added to my skirt-bindings to insure plenty of room for exercise," Helen recalled. "In six months I put in another finger's length, and again a third time, and it took two years to bring my waist to the proportions adapted to the width of my shoulders."[29] Other physical changes also showed that the exercise regimen had been effective. Prior to Helen Lewis's bout with consumption, she suffered from a spinal curvature that left her with uneven hips, according to Eastman, and a right shoulder so much larger than her left that she wore padding to conceal the deformity. Eastman claimed that Helen's new hygienic regimen, especially the "daily systematic exercise," restored her to perfect health and allowed her to regain the "natural erectness and symmetry of shoulders and hips." Helen's physical transformation held, too. Eastman reported that at seventy-three years of age, "[Helen Lewis] finds herself with no tendency to colds, headaches, or other pains, and with the thrill of health in every nerve, and its flush in her cheeks; in short a perfectly healthy and vigorous woman, to whom a walk of five miles is a pleasure and causes but little fatigue."[30]

### A New Career

Although Helen made good progress in Buffalo, the Lewises finally decided that a milder climate might prove helpful.[31] Dio placed his Buffalo medical practice for sale, and in the fall of 1853, the couple moved to Fredericksburg, Virginia, where, for a time, they lived on their savings.[32] After giving hygienic lectures in several local girls schools, Dio concluded that the citizens in his new area were remarkably ill-informed regarding physiology, hygiene, and temperance, and that he might be able to make a living as a lecturer on such topics. If he could make it work, he reasoned, such a career offered him more free time to spend with Helen and her cure, as well as the potential for greater pecuniary rewards than he could expect from practicing medicine alone.

It was also while he was in Fredericksburg that Dio decided to formally join the Sons of Temperance. Long committed to the cause of temperance, and having his mother, Delecta, as an example of the eminent suitability of women for such work, Dio was stunned to discover that the Sons of Temperance did not allow women to become members or assist with their work. Furious at the group's policy, he decided to attack the Sons of Temperance membership regulations in a public lecture. Entitled "The Influence of Christian Women in the Cause of Temperance," the lecture attracted considerable local attention and brought him invitations to speak elsewhere. His new career had begun.

For the next six years, Dio earned his living as an itinerant lecturer on health reform, temperance, and exercise. With Helen at his side still fighting consumption, Dio lectured extensively in New York, and in Virginia, Kentucky, and other southern states. In February 1855, he decided that cold air might prove beneficial to Helen's cure, and soon the two were off on a lecture tour of southern Canada.[33] Newspaper accounts of his lectures, included in the Lewis Scrapbook and elsewhere, indicate that during this six-year period he traveled as far west as Iowa City and as far east as Providence, Rhode Island.[34] As Dio moved from town to town, he generally delivered a six-lecture series on health reform. The hygienic lectures, with a heavy emphasis on exercise and the health needs of women, generally ran from Monday through Saturday nights and paid his bills. Then, on Sunday evenings, he delivered free of charge a lecture on women and temperance.[35] Lewis was by all accounts a mesmerizing speaker, and his "personal magnetism" brought frequent comment in press reports of his lectures.[36] Nathaniel T. Allen, who worked closely with Dio in Boston, claimed, "Whether in Schoolroom, Town Hall, Tremont Temple in Boston or Cooper Inst. in New York, he held an audience to the end as few persons are able to."[37] In Virginia, there developed such a demand for his services that in one five-week period he delivered seventy-three lectures. Half of these, according to Lewis, were delivered in women's academies. Testimonials, resolutions, and gifts poured in, acknowledging his efforts.[38]

Dio's eloquence in the cause of temperance sometimes presented him with a moral dilemma. On several occasions, his temperance lectures excited his audience to such an extent that women took immediately to the streets to march against the local saloons. In Dixon, Illinois, Dio recalled, a committee of fifty women formed at the end of a temperance lecture he delivered in 1858, and "in six days time not even a glass of beer could be bought in the town."[39] But Dio could not stay and watch this drama unfold. He had a lecture series scheduled in another town and could not remain behind. "I shall never forgive myself, " he wrote years later, "for not remaining [in Dixon]." Had he been able to stay there, he explained, "the woman's crusade would have been fairly inaugurated," and would have succeeded more than a decade before it finally got off the ground.[40]

As time passed, Dio's involvement with Helen's illness and the "prevalence of pale faces, underdeveloped and distorted bodies, and nervous debility" that he found crowding into the lecture halls to hear his speeches convinced him that the greater good of the nation would be served by a narrowing of his focus. By concentrating his advocacy on exercise and health reform, Lewis believed he could make a real contribution to the American people. Thus, in the late-1850s, he decided that his "life-work" lay in physical education, and he began formulating plans for a system of physical training to be used in the schools of America.[41] The evidence of the neglect of physical education was everywhere, he argued, and it was ludicrous to assume that young people would get enough exercise on their own. "It is our duty," he wrote, "to see that both boys and girls get an all-sided development, and this no one game or set of games, no one avocation can give."[42]

## The New Gymnastics

In 1856, the year Catharine Beecher published her books on calisthenics, Lewis visited Paris, France, to acquire "illustrative apparatus of the best sort for use in his lectures on physiology."[43] During his time there, Lewis visited two movement cure establishments where he saw Ling's treatment methods in use.[44] He also visited craniologist Paul Broca, toured several Parisian gyms, and purchased the latest European books on exercise.[45]

This trip was an important step in the formalization of Lewis's thoughts on exercise. What he saw there, particularly at the two Swedish-style movement cure facilities, convinced him that the American approach to therapeutic exercise was inferior to that of the European movement cures. Americans placed too much emphasis on the development of strength, Lewis argued, and not enough on flexibility and speed of movement.[46] Following his European trip, Lewis resolved to try to adapt Ling's therapeutic exercises to a general exercise program that would benefit men and women, boys and girls. How closely his system really mimicked the popular Swedish system is difficult to assess since it is not possible for modern historians to see the exercises performed. At least one Boston physician, however, who was personally familiar with Ling's methods, argued that the systems were not especially close since Ling's system relied on "slow, steady movements" and Lewis's on rapid, brisk ones.[47] Whatever the case, Lewis's use of Ling's name helped to sell the scientific nature of his new system. For example, one group of women with whom he worked wrote at the end of their sessions together, "We rejoice that Ling, the distinguished Swedish philanthropist, ever evolved his scientific system of Gymnastic, and that you, sir, have introduced the best points in his system to our acquaintance."[48] Nathaniel T. Allen, with whom Lewis enjoyed a long and profitable professional association, claimed that Lewis was "a pioneer in introducing the Swedish System of gymnastics into schools in this country."[49]

Based on an article in the Lewis Scrapbook entitled "Proceedings of the Iowa City Gymnastics Club," it appears that Lewis did more than merely lecture when he visited some communities. In Iowa City, Lewis taught a "useful and scientific system of Gymnastics" to both the male and female members of the Iowa City Gymnastics Club during a two-week stay in 1858. Fifty Iowa City women "enjoyed the benefits of his instructions" and apparently adopted most aspects of Lewis's physiological theories, voting at the end of their classes with Dio and Helen to unanimously adopt five resolutions praising Lewis's teaching methods and pledging as a group to follow his hygienic precepts. The first, fourth, and fifth resolutions acknowledged Lewis's value as a teacher and lecturer on hygiene and wished him well in his campaign to spread his gymnastics system throughout the United States. The second resolution read: "That we regard his mode of training the physical system, and especially his mode of educating and developing the female form, of the highest practical value, and worthy of attention from all who desire robust and active constitutions." The third resolution stated: "That as a proof of our concession to his reforms, we mean henceforth to adopt his advice, whatever the world may say, and we sincerely trust that no maukish [sic] sensitiveness, nor fear of ridicule will deter others from pursuing a similar course."[49b] What the women had agreed to do, of course, was to pursue exercise that would make their bodies stronger, larger, and more enduring; to discard their corsets; to wear shortened skirts for outdoor work and exercise; and to follow Lewis's basic tenets of the Laws of Health.

In 1860, after eight years on the road, Dio and Helen decided they needed a permanent home. Eastman claimed that their decision to settle in the Boston area resulted from Dio's desire to establish an institution for physical training.[50] Boston was, obviously, the logical place to try out a new system of purposive exercise because no other section of the country had such a sustained fascination with physical training. What made the Lewis's move possible, however, was the offer of a job for Dio at Nathaniel T. Allen's English and Classical School in West Newton, Massachusetts, a Boston suburb.

Having met earlier, Nathaniel Allen and Dio Lewis found they had much in common. Like most members of the health reform community, they shared a dedication to temperance, women's rights, and abolition. According to Allen, their dedication to the latter cause went beyond simple lip-service. Allen recalled that he and Lewis "sat on Music Hall Platform Sunday after Sunday to defend the freedom of speech of Wendell Phillips, during 1860 and 1861." Many times, Allen explained, "Dio Lewis carried two loaded pistols in his pockets," a fact that worried Allen almost as much as the hecklers did.[51] On one occasion, Allen reported, Lewis protected Wendell Phillips as he walked home from one of his lectures on abolition through a "howling mob." Allen recalled that years later he could still see Lewis's "erect . . . stalwart, and noble presence. His bearing was always commanding, but never more so than then."[52]

According to Allen, it was his sister-in law, Mrs. Joseph Allen, a music teacher, who first suggested to Dio "that the movements would be improved if accompanied by music." This suggestion was made in 1859, in Syracuse, New York, Allen said, when his brother, a member of the school board, had brought Dio Lewis in to lecture to the schools. Apparently, Dio heeded this suggestion. "This was done," Allen wrote, "and ever after music and Swedish gymnastics went together."[53] In the same letter, Nathaniel Allen explained that by giving Lewis a teaching position, he had also played a pivotal role in the formulation of Lewis's system. According to Allen, Dio came to him with a letter of reference from Allen's brother, Joseph, and was immediately hired, working through 1868 as a "permanent teacher of Gymnastics and lecturer upon health with us." It was at his school, Allen recalled, that "the first drills & lectures were made in Mass.," adding that he found Lewis to be an interesting and "instinctive teacher [whose] noble form & handsome make up, powerful yet melodious voice, drew eye and ear to him."[54] Lewis was only thirty-seven when he moved to West Newton and began his friendship with Allen, who remembered him as a "unique and remarkable character . . . an enthusiast, a true type of the Reformer, such as we call *Cranks*." But we must not forget, Allen cautioned, that the "world is uplifted & improved by such cranks] . . . Garrison, Phillips, Alcott, H. B. Blackwell, Lucy Stone were all termed Cranks."[55]

Following their move to West Newton in June 1860, Dio and Helen explored Boston and its growing suburbs, visited schools, and tried to devise plans for spreading his gospel of physical culture. Foremost among their concerns was making enough money to cover their living expenses. Dio's job with Allen, though considered "permanent," apparently did not pay a full teacher's salary.[56] So, Lewis approached the headmistress of Lasell Seminary for Young Women in Auburndale, Massachusetts, and she agreed to let him offer gymnastic classes to her female scholars. Soon, the headmistress, Mrs. M. L. Taylor, became an outspoken proponent of the Lewis system and claimed in an article published less than a year after his arrival in Boston that she could already see a real difference in her scholars. She wrote that it was her earnest belief "that any school of young ladies will accomplish, in the course of a year, twice as much with these exercises as they possibly could do without them, beside having a well-developed, beautiful, and healthful physique."[57]

Lewis also affiliated himself with the McLean Asylum at Somerville that summer, instituting an exercise and recreational program for the mentally ill, which was one of the first of its kind in the United States.[58] In the evenings, he picked up a few extra dollars by offering classes in gymnastics. Nathaniel Allen reported: "In our village, Dr. Lewis formed large classes which met for drill and instruction in our town hall . . . where tossing of bean bags small and large É etc., kept up a great interest."[59] Apparently, Dio offered evening classes in other small communities as well. Elizabeth Weir recalled that "Dr. Lewis had a class for physical training at one time in Concord, but I did not attend it. I simply went in as a spectator now and then, and was much pleased with his methods and success." Continuing her reminiscence, Weir wrote, "I remember that Louisa Alcott was a leading member of the class" and that one of our "young ladies, Una Hawthorne, attended his school at Lexington, and we always enjoyed the accounts of it that she brought home from time to time."[60]

Less than two months after settling in West Newton, Lewis and a group of gymnasts from his evening classes in West Newton appeared before the American Institute of Instruction at Tremont Temple in Boston. This event formally launched what Lewis had begun calling his New Gymnastics.

## The American Institute of Instruction

The members of the American Institute of Instruction, the nation's largest professional society for educators, arrived in Boston for their annual convention in August 1860. On the afternoon of 21 August, the Institute's members settled down to hear Thomas W. Valentine deliver one of the featured lectures of the convention: "Is it Expedient to Make Calisthenics and Gymnastics a Part of School Training?" Following Valentine's address, the Reverend Bridey G. Northup asked that Dio Lewis, who was neither on the program nor a member of the Institute, be allowed to speak. According to reports—including his own—Lewis kept the audience spellbound for two hours with his forceful oratory on the "new system" being taught in West Newton.[61] Intrigued by his novel ideas, the Institute sent over a six-man committee to watch Lewis's classes that evening. The West Newton gymnasts trained hard that night, and the committee, impressed by what they saw, invited Lewis to return the next day and put on a demonstration for the entire convention. Lewis recalled the scene. "The next morning was foggy and dark, but the hall was full, and they passed over their important business and gave me nearly two hours more, and at noon another hour. With such an opening as this, it is not remarkable that the interest spread over the entire country."[62] Edward Mussey Hartwell reported of these exhibitions, "The exercises consisted of club-swinging and class exercises with bean-bags and with wands, together with a variety of free movements. A number of gentlemen from the audience took part in the exercises and there was much merriment among the actors as well as amusement for the audience.'"[63] At the close of these exhibitions, the members passed a unanimous resolution, acknowledging that the New Gymnastics was one of the "most important and practically valuable subjects which has come before the meetings of this Institute . . . and . . . we believe it eminently worthy of general introduction into all our schools, and into general use."[64]

Lewis's system of New Gymnastics thus became the first exercise system to receive the endorsement of a national group of educators. Although Horace Mann had argued for such a move in the 1840s, and Catharine Beecher had tried for national acceptance of her calisthenics program in the 1850s, it took Lewis and his charismatic personality to convince the educators that his system was adaptable to all schools and both sexes.[65]

Having won the endorsement of the Institute, however, Lewis faced a number of serious problems. Suddenly, Lewis had a great many people interested in his plan for physical reform, but he had no text-book or articles with which to instruct them, and no gymnasium or school in which to train them. What he did have in abundance, however, were energy, desire, and intelligence, and he quickly got to work to find the means through which he could capitalize on the Institute's endorsement.[66]

## The Essex Street Gymnasium

One of Lewis's first steps was to open a public gymnasium at Number 20, Essex Street, Boston. A public ceremony held on 2 October 1860 inaugurated the new business. Following a demonstration of exercises, John D. Philbrick, Superintendent of the Boston Public Schools, took the floor. Philbrick praised Lewis for undertaking a subject "highly important to the public welfare," and for training men, women, and children in the laws of life, calisthenics, and gymnastics. Philbrick argued that the opening of this public gymnasium symbolized something even more important than the health of the public, however. "Its doors are open to both sexes," he wrote. "This is a feature which I believe has not been embraced in the gymnasium's plan of the institutions for physical training heretofore existing among us." Suggesting that Lewis's gymnastics marked the beginning of a "new era in education," Philbrick strongly concluded his thoughts on the need for female exercise by declaring, "The[re] can be no doubt but that in a system of education designed for females, more attention should be devoted to bodily culture, than in that intended only for the hardier sex. And yet, as a matter of fact, this essential branch of education has been almost wholly neglected in the training of females."[67]

The Essex Street gym quickly differentiated itself from its Boston competitors. Instead of having a single exercise studio and allowing customers to walk in as it suited their schedule, Lewis organized exercise classes and housed several different entrepreneurial operations under the same roof.[68] Lewis occupied the top two floors of the spacious building on the corner of Essex and Harrison Streets. There were two gymnastic halls, filled with a variety of exercise apparati, in which men and women trained together under the supervision of drill masters. The exercise areas were sixty-five feet long, with eighteen-foot ceilings.[69] Off of these large halls were dressing rooms for both sexes and a special space where clients could work with Lewis's new antituberculosis devices, the Spirometer and the Blow Gun.[70] Edward Hitchcock, director of the physical education program at Amherst College from 1861 to 1911, took lessons at the Lewis gymnasium that

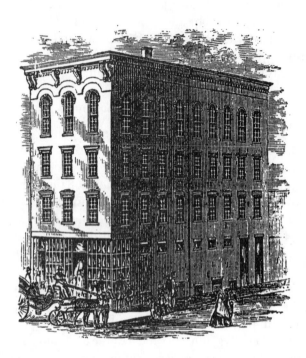

Figure 64: This Essex Street building housed Dio Lewis' gymnasium, his Normal School, and his medical offices. From *Lewis's Gymnastic Monthly and Journal of Physical Culture* (October 1862).

fall and described his classroom as a "small hall in an upper story & I should think there were from fifty to seventy-five pupils of both sexes."[71] A year-long membership, which included four exercise classes a week, cost twenty dollars.[72]

Also in the building was Lewis's medical office where he saw patients and prescribed hygienic movement cures.[73] This part of the Essex Street gym opened on 18 November 1860. Lewis advertised for patients with paralysis, curvature of the spine, and stiffened joints, and specialized in the treatment of spinal disorders.[74] Ever the optimist, he promised to completely cure any lateral curvature of the spine that women might have as the result of tight corsets, unhygienic living, or insufficient exercise.[75] He employed several female assistants and his wife, Helen, to work individually with his female clients, just as personal trainers do in the late twentieth century. Like George Taylor and other movement cure physicians, Lewis met with the patients, assessed their physical condition, and then prescribed a series of exercises—or a routine—to effect two ends: (1) the overall improvement of the patient's fitness and (2) specific remedial adjustments. He also made suggestions regarding diet, dress, and the amount of sleep people needed. Sarah Ashley, a former movement cure patient, described her "treatment" as a combination of massage, exercise, and lifestyle modifications. Ashley recalled, "He did not believe in drugs at that time, and had some radical notions about food, dress, habits, etc. He advocated short street dresses for ladies, and the swinging of the arms when walking, morning bathing in cold water, early hours for retiring, abstinence from tea, coffee and liquors of all kinds, pies and cake."[76] Although a large number of men came to study gymnastics with Lewis, most of his movement cure patients were females, and his medical practice grew at such a rapid rate that he could not accommodate all the people who came to him for help. In 1864, he established a sanitarium in nearby Lexington, to treat chronic invalids who needed long-term care and greater supervision than he could provide at the gym.[77]

## The Normal Institute for Physical Education

As Lewis attempted to ride the wave of enthusiasm generated by his presentations at the American Institute of Instruction, the most glaring problem he faced was the lack of trained teachers ready to go out into the public schools and begin teaching his New Gymnastics. Following the exhibitions at the American Institute, Lewis reported that "a number of teachers" wrote to him saying they had implemented his system in their schools. Lewis worried about the inadequate preparation of these teachers and about whether anyone "can learn to teach the system by witnessing two or three brief exhibitions." Anxious to prevent his system from being bastardized before it was fully born, Lewis decided to train and certify teachers who could understand and implement his physiological philosophy and exercise methods. In November 1860, Lewis reported that he had "five assistants, thoroughly drilled, and prepared to give full instruction in one hundred and fifty gymnastic exercises."[78] During the winter of 1860–1861, he apparently had four other students studying with him to become teachers.[79] In the April issue of his magazine, he announced the imminent graduation of Charles S. Royce of Norwalk, Ohio, the first person Dio officially certified as a teacher of the New Gymnastics.[80] In a second article in that same issue, he announced the formal opening of a normal school for the training of teachers in the New Gymnastics, with tuition set at seventy-five dollars for men and fifty dollars for women.[81] Lewis lowered the tuition for women to encourage more women to enter the normal school and because of what he described as the "unjust disparity of compensation which everywhere obtains between male and female labor." He expected the training program to take about three months.[82]

During that same winter, he met with leading educators, ministers, and physicians in Boston to obtain their endorsement for a normal school for the training of teachers of gymnastics. The Essex Street Gym was also to house this new enterprise. The letters of incorporation, finally signed on 4 June 1861, gave Lewis nearly complete control of the school and one hundred percent of its profits. The board of directors, whose input came primarily through their approval of teachers recommended by Lewis, consisted of Alanson Hawley, S. E. Sewell, T. C. Severance, J. C. Burrage, Otis Clapp, and Lewis himself. The papers of incorporation also reveal that Cornelius C. Felton, then the president of Harvard University, would serve as the first president of the Normal College. Lewis was named treasurer, and T. C. Severance was secretary.[83]

Lewis's Normal Institute for Physical Training was the first school in the United States that exclusively trained teachers of physical education. It was also one of the earliest professional schools to admit male and female students to the same course of study and to grant them the same diploma. As Philbrick noted in his speech at the opening of Lewis's public gymnasium, Dio Lewis viewed both the practice and the profession of physical education as eminently suitable for women. Though his egalitarian stand was not totally original, it was, nevertheless, extremely important. Lewis advertised that "men and women of enterprise and industry, will find in this field *health, usefulness* and *large profit.*"[84] In an advertisement in the *Gymnastic Monthly*, Lewis argued that the compensation paid teachers of the New Gymnastics "is much larger than teachers of our public schools receive." Indeed, Lewis argued, in the northern states, where there was a great demand for gymnastics teachers, a trained "Gymnastiarch" should receive five times the salary of a regular school teacher. "Were there five thousand competent laborers to begin the good work to-day," he told his readers, "the number would have to be doubled next year." Furthermore, he enthused, the financial rewards were only part of the benefits of the profession. "A teacher would have to manage very badly not to make three or four hundred dollars per month, and besides the pecuniary return, would be sure to acquire splendid health."[85] Lewis's assessment of what a trained female gymnastics teacher could earn was almost surely optimistic. In the Minutes of the School Board for the City of Boston, on 22 December 1874, for instance, a salary of four hundred dollars a year was proposed to hire a "woman for the teaching of gymnastics in the Latin School." In the same meeting, a salary of five hundred dollars was suggested for teachers of German and French.[86] In other meetings of the Board that same year, proposed salaries for academic teachers were occasionally as high as eight hundred dollars.[87]

In any case, during its seven years of operation, Lewis's school drew students from nearly every state in the Union and graduated 421 gymnastics teachers, approximately half of whom were female.[88] Many of these women, Lewis wrote in 1883, came to him "in broken health, seeking in the new profession a better means of living."[89] A number were also former schoolteachers seeking to make a professional shift. According to Lewis, these women found both a new profession and the return of their health. In the beginning, he wrote, the health of his female pupils was poorer than that of his male students. "But with the removal of the corset and the long, heavy skirts, and the use of those exercises which a short and very loose dress renders easy," he wrote, "a remarkable change ensued." Not only did the women become fitter, they surpassed the men at gymnastics: "In every one of ten classes of graduates, the best gymnast was a woman. In each class there were from two to six women superior to all the men." In his annual exhibitions at Tremont Temple, Lewis regularly placed women in the front of the stage, "not because they were women, but because they were the finer performers."[90]

The school ran two courses per year; the first began on 4 July 1861. The first class after incorporation consisted of nineteen students, although only five men and eight women graduated that first year. Six of those graduates were from Massachusetts, two from Virginia, and one each from the District of Columbia, Michigan, Rhode Island, New Hampshire, and Connecticut.[91] They were trained not just to teach regular exercise classes but to prescribe the Swedish movement cure as well.[92] When he opened his girl's school in Lexington, Massachusetts, summer sessions were held there to escape Boston's heat.

Lewis again proved successful in attracting the support of Massachusetts's most prominent citizens and leading intellectuals. Members of the Harvard faculty such as Walter Channing, who "spoke with great enthusiasm of the superiority of the women," helped teach some of the traditional subjects at the normal college. Transcendentalist A. Bronson Alcott gave a series of lectures on philosophy. Vocal culture came under the guidance of T. E. Leonard, a noted expert.[93]

Love Brown attended Lewis's normal school in the summer of 1866. A Mount Holyoke student, Brown had grown increasingly dissatisfied with the seminary's approach to education. In a letter to her friend, Helen Savage, Brown wrote:

> Oh Helen—words cannot express the joy and gratitude I feel at being through the tiresome discipline (almost drudgery) we have been under-go [sic] at the Sem.—the studies I delight in but it does seem to me there is something absolutely wrong about the system socially and physically—if not mentally and morally. I have puzzled my poor brain over it to decide *what* the radical defects were & *how* they might be remedied . . . if I ever found a Mt. Hol. Sem. there shall be a different state of things in many respects—else there shall be no system at all.[94]

What Love wanted, she explained to Helen, was an education that would "unite physical and mental culture." Which was why, she reported, "I came here, to attend Dr. Lewis's Normal class,—in order to learn his complete system of the New Gymnastics in the most approved style."[95] A former teacher, Love claimed she "never will be guilty of teaching again & neglect to do all in my power, so far as my knowledge extends, to educate my scholars in a physical point of view."[96]

Contrasting the physical program of Mount Holyoke to the New Gymnastics she learned from Lewis, Love Brown declared that gymnastics as taught at Mount Holyoke did not amount to a "dime's worth of culture physically." In fact, she explained, "I don't see what muscles are benefited except of the limbs, the same we get in walking." Mount Holyoke girls, she continued, "don't know that *every* set of muscles in the whole body can be educated & developed & strengthened by gymnastic exercise . . . I wish you could see his class practice as trained by him."[97]

During the seven years of the Normal School's operation, Lewis used his twice-yearly graduation exercises as a chance to hold public exhibitions and gain further acceptance for his ideas on purposive exercise. The Tremont Temple, seating two thousand people, filled to capacity for these gymnastic extravaganzas. Eastman reported, in fact, that Lewis and his board of directors decided to charge admission— the proceeds of which were then donated to charity—as a way to limit the number of spectators. A contemporary report of one of these shows revealed that the program consisted of gymnastics and singing. "The class consisted of about forty, many of whom were ladies, and they represented nearly every state in the Union. They were dressed in costume, that of the ladies being conspicuous because of its shortness. The gymnastics performances were varied and interesting and were warmly applauded."[98] Of the twenty-seven graduates on this particular evening, twenty were single women, two were married women, and five were men.[99]

By March 1861, Lewis and his system of New Gymnastics were apparently well established in Boston. Colonel Thomas Wentworth Higginson surveyed the trend toward gymnastics in March of 1861 for the *Atlantic Monthly*, writing,

> It would be unpardonable in this connection not to speak a good word for the hobby of the day,—Dr. Lewis and his system of gymnastics or, more properly, calisthenics . . . Dr. Lewis [is] so hale and hearty, so profoundly confident in the omnipotence of his own methods and the uselessness of all others [that he can] flood any company, no matter how starched or listless, with an unbounded appetite for ball-games and bean-games.[100]

Although Higginson meant to offer praise, he sounded amused, and Lewis was not altogether happy with the article. For one thing, he objected to Higginson's suggestion that his presence was necessary for the sessions to be successful: "I am very much surprised," Lewis replied in his journal, "that any observing person, living in Boston or [its] neighborhood, should not have learned that the success of classes engaged in the practice of my system does not depend at all upon my personal presence." Indeed, Lewis countered, some of the most successful experiments with his exercises were occurring in places he had never visited, such as Mobile, Alabama, "and with results so happy that hundreds of teachers are impelled to write me letters all aglow with gratitude." Concluding, Lewis wrote, "I simply . . . wish that the writer could at least have seen *one* of my classes before writing the article. It is evident from the essay itself that he had never seen one."[101]

Lewis did not really need to worry that his system would be misunderstood. Ever the promoter, he had already started his own magazine and begun working on a book explaining his system. He had little time in his hectic schedule for writing, but the time he spared proved worth his effort. *Lewis's New Gymnastics for Men, Women and Children* became a bona fide bestseller, stayed in print for more than thirty years, and spread his system throughout the world.

[1][Thomas Wentworth Higginson], "Gymnastics," *The Atlantic Monthly* 7 (March 1861): 301.

[2] No scholarly work, with the exception of Fred Eugene Leonard's "The 'New Gymnastics' of Dio Lewis (1860–1868)," *American Physical Education Review* 11 (June 1906): 83-95, and 11 (September 1906): 187-98, has published a detailed monograph assessing Lewis's life and contributions. Physical educator Luther Gulick did attempt to gather materials for a book on Lewis in the late 1890s, and donated his scrapbook on Lewis to Springfield College's Babson Library. Gulick, however, did not publish the planned biography, nor is there a known manuscript.

To this day, in fact, Lewis's only biography appears to be the one produced by Mary F. Eastman—at the request of Mrs. Lewis—in 1891. While fascinating in many respects, Eastman's book is lacking in historical objectivity and, unfortunately, focuses more on Lewis's work with temperance than it does on his ideas of physical culture. Mary F. Eastman, *The Biography of Dio Lewis, A.M., M.D.* (New York: Fowler & Wells, 1891).

There is no record of any doctoral dissertation on this important reform figure. Three student papers on Lewis are housed in archives. At Springfield College, see Alfred Albert Smith, "Dio Lewis: Physical Educator" (master's thesis, International Young Men's Christian Association College, 1914); and Alanson L. Fish, "Life, Work, and Influence of Dio Lewis, A.M., M.D" (master's thesis, Springfield College, 1898, Gulick Thesis Collection). A far more useful analysis is Paul David Natterson, "Dio Lewis and Physical Fitness: A Social Innovator in a Scientific Sphere" (senior honors thesis, Harvard University, 1985), on deposit at University Archives, Harvard University, Cambridge, MA.

[3]Lewis's New Gymnastics are discussed in varying detail in the following studies: Frances B. Cogan, *All-American Girl: The Ideal of Real Womanhood in Mid-Nineteenth-Century America* (Athens: University of Georgia Press, 1989), 45- 48; Martha Verbrugge, *Able-Bodied Womanhood: Personal Health and Social Change in Nineteenth-Century Boston* (New York: Oxford University Press, 1988), 38-41, 44-48; Arthur Weston, *The Making of American Physical Education* (New York: Appleton-Century-Crofts, 1962), 30-31; James Whorton, *Crusaders for Fitness: The History of American Health Reformers* (Princeton NJ: Princeton University Press, 1982), 275-82; Allen Guttman, *Women's Sports: A History* (New York: Columbia University Press, 1991), 112-14; Harvey Green, *Fit for America: Health, Fitness, Sport and American Society* (New York: Pantheon Books, 1986), 185-90.

[4]Quoted in Eastman, *The Biography of Dio Lewis,* 130.

[5]See, for instance, Edward Hitchcock, *Report of the Director of Physical Training, December, 1891* (Boston: Rockwell and Churchill, 1891), 36. "In short Dio Lewis was a revivalist and agitator, and not a scientist in any proper sense. His originality has been much over-rated,—very few of his

inventions, either in the line of apparatus or of methods of teaching, being really new."

[6]Dudley Allen Sargent, "The Achievements of the Century in Gymnastics and Athletics Together with Notes and Questions," Lecture Delivered to the Students of Springfield College, 1903, ts. pp. 3-4 of attached notes. Rare Books Room, Babson Library, Springfield College, Springfield, MA.

[7]Mrs. Dio Lewis to Dr. Luther Gulick, 8 March, 1898. Lewis Scrapbook, Rare Book Room, Babson Library, Springfield College, Springfield, MA. (Note: The term "Lewis Scrapbook" shall be used hereafter to refer to this scrapbook put together by Dr. Luther Halsey Gulick in 1898. Entitled "Dio Lewis Mss and Miscels, 1853–1898," this scrapbook consists of letters, newspaper clippings, and ephemera related to the life of Dio Lewis).

[8]"Dio Lewis: A Noted Son of Auburn Dies Today," *The Auburn Bulletin*, 21 May 1886.

[9]Eastman, *Biography*, 29.

[10]Ibid., 19.

[11]Ibid., 48.

[12]Ibid., 27.

[13]Ibid., 48.

[14]Ibid., 30-31.

[15]Ibid., 30-31.

[16]Ibid., 29.

[17]Ibid., 34.

[18]Ibid.

[19]Ibid., 36. McCarthy was the Lewis family physician at this time.

[20]Homeopathic medicine had arisen in response to the widespread dissatisfaction with traditional medical care. Extremely popular with the upper classes, homeopathy centered around the belief that the body was capable of curing itself and argued against the use of most medications. So widespread did homeopathy become, especially in the Northeast, that several medical colleges quickly opened to teach its methods. Alhough Lewis never attended, he received an honorary degree in 1851 from the Homeopathic Hospital College in Cleveland, Ohio. For information on homeopathy, see Harvy Green, *Fit for America*, 7-8; and William B. Walker,"The Health Reform Movement in the United States: 1830–1870" (Ph.D. diss., Johns Hopkins University, 1955), 17-22.

[21]Dio Lewis, *Weak Lungs, and How to Make them Strong. Or Diseases of the Organs of the Chest, With Their Home Treatment by the Movement Cure* (Boston: Ticknor and Fields, 1864), 1.

[22]The Lewises married on 11 July 1849. "Lewis Dioclesian, M.D.," handwritten m.s., Lewis Scrapbook. Helen's father was a physician in New York City. She met Dio while on a summer vacation to upstate New York where her family had a summer home.

[23]Lewis also read Galen, Bacon, Rousseau, Hufeland, Sydenham, Dr. Chisholm, and Plato on the value of therapeutic exercise in treating respiratory diseases. See Lewis, *Weak Lungs*, 222-23, 236.

[24]Conservative on many aspects of medicine, Rush recommended a slow, six-step movement cure for advanced cases of consumption. Beginning with passive exercise such as rocking in a cradle or riding "on an elastic board commony called a chamber horse," the patient would, when able, move on to swinging, then to sailing, then to riding in a carriage, then to walking, and finally to running and dancing, according to Rush's plan. Ibid., 243-44.

[25]Eastman, *Biography*, 43.

[26]Ibid., 44-45.

[27]Ibid.

[28]Lewis, *Weak Lungs*, 248.

[29]Quoted in Eastman, *Biography*, 43-44.

[30]Ibid., 51-52.

[31]It was widely believed that one of the few effective treatments for consumption was to travel in the southern states. See Robert F. Speir, M.D., *Going South for the Winter With Hints to Consumptives* (New York: by the author, 1873) for a look at this early travel phenomenon.

[32]Eastman, *Biography*, 42-43.

[33]Ibid., 50.

[34]The full extent of the Lewises' travels in this era is unknown.

[35]Lewis Scrapbook; and Eastman, *Biography*, 62.

[36]See, for instance, the newspaper clipping "Dio Lewis Coming," in the Lewis Scrapbook; and Thomas Wentworth Higginson, "Gymnastics," 300.

[37]Nathaniel T. Allen to Luther Gulick, 24 February 1878, Lewis Scrapbook.

[38]Quoted in Eastman, *Biography*, 50, 53. The women's guild of Fredericksburg Baptist Church presented Lewis with a silver tea set, and he received similar presents from women's groups in Paris, Lexington, and Georgetown, Kentucky.

[39]Ibid., 66-68. A similar committee, consisting of 116 women, formed in Battle Creek, Michigan, and within six weeks had closed all forty-nine drinking establishments in the town.

[40]Quoted in Eastman, *Biography*, 67.

[41]Ibid., 67.

[42]Ibid., 70.

[43]Ibid., 62.

[44][Dio Lewis], "Movement Cure in Boston," *Lewis's New Gymnastics For Ladies, Gentlemen and Children and Boston Journal of Physical Culture* 1 (November 1860): 12.

[45]Ibid.

[46]Ibid.

[47]Quoted in Edward Mussey Hartwell, *School Document No. 22—1891, Report of the Director of Physical Training* (Boston: Rockwell and Chruchill, 1891) 34-35.

[48]"Proceedings of a Meeting of the Iowa City Gymnastic Club, held Oct. 1st, 1858," Lewis Scrapbook.

[49]Nathaniel. T. Allen to Luther Gulick, 24 February 1878, Lewis Scrapbook.

[49b]"Proceedings,", Lewis Scrapbook.

[50]Eastman, *Biography*, 75.

[51]Ibid.

[52]Ibid., 114.

[53]Nathaniel T. Allen to Luther Gulick, 24 February 1898, Lewis Scrapbook.

[54]Ibid. Mrs. Lewis told Luther Gulick that Dio continued working at the Allen School ten or twelve years. Mrs. Dio Lewis to Luther Halsey Gulick, 21 February 1898, Lewis Scrapbook. Eastman claimed that he worked for Allen until 1875. Eastman, *Biography*, 76.

[55]Nathaniel T. Allen to Luther Gulick, 24 February 1898, Lewis Scrapbook.

[56]Allen told Gulick that Lewis was listed as a teacher of gymnastics and lecturer on health in the school's catalog. Allen to Gulick, 24 February 1898, Lewis Scrapbook.

[57]Mrs. Taylor, "Physical Training for Young Ladies," *Lewis's New Gymnastics for Ladies, Gentlemen and Children and Boston Journal of Physical Culture* 1 (February 1861): 54.

[58]Eastman, *Biography of Dio Lewis*, 77. Previous to this, Lewis had worked with the mentally ill at the State Lunatic Asylum at Utica, New York. Lewis discussed his work at the McLean Insane Asylum in "Teachers of the New Gymnastics," *Lewis's New Gymnastics for Ladies, Gentlemen and Children and Boston Journal of Physical Culture* 1 (December 1860): 30.

[59]Nathaniel T. Allen to Luther Gulick, 24 February 1898, Lewis Scrapbook.

[60]Elizabeth J. Weir to Luther Gulick, 25 February 1898, Lewis Scrapbook.

[61]No transcript of Lewis's remarks was made. However, in a two-part article, Dio Lewis, "Physical Culture," in *The Massachusetts Teacher* 13 (October, November 1860): 377, 404, Lewis summarized his lecture and discussed the response he received from the Institute. See also Board of Censors, *Lectures Delivered Before the American Institute of Instruction, Boston, Massachusetts, August 21, 1860* (Boston: Ticknor and Fields, 1861), 19-21, 23-25, 45-46, 77, for the official version of his demonstrations and comments. See also "American Institute of Instruction, Interesting Proceedings. Gymnastics in Schools—Lectures and Discussions—Educational Movements in Different States—Closing Scenes," *New York Times*, 27 August 1860, 2.

[62]Dio Lewis, Lecture to the Graduates of the Normal Institute for Physical Education, 18 March 1863. Lecture, quoted in Fred Eugene Leonard, *A Guide to the History of Physical Education*, 256.

[63]Hartwell, *Report of Physical Training*, 34.

[64]Dio Lewis, "Physical Culture," *Massachusetts Teacher* 13 (October, November 1860): 377, 404.

[65]See Peter J. Wosh, "Sound Minds and Unsound Bodies: Massachusetts Schools and Mandatory Physical Training," *The New England Quarterly* 55 (March-December 1982): 42, for a discussion of Lewis's impact at the convention. See also Hartwell, *Report of the Director*, for a discussion of the impact of the Civil War on the question of military drill training for men and how this conflicted with the spread of Lewis's gymnastics.

[66]Newspaper reports of Lewis's lectures and exhibitions before the American Institute of Education also appeared in the *New York World*, 25 August 1860; *New York World*, 27 August 1860; *New York Times*, 27 August 1860; *New York Tribune*, 27 August 1860; the *Boston Evening Atlas*, 3 August 1860; and the *Boston Daily Courier*, 24 August 1860. Quoted in [Dio Lewis], "Gymnastics Before the American Institute of Instruction, at Its Recent Meeting in Tremont Temple, Boston, Mass.," *Lewis's New Gymnastics for Ladies, Gentlemen and Children and Boston Journal of Physical Culture* 1 (November 1860): 15-16.

[67]"John D. Philbrick at the Inauguration of Lewis's New Gymnasium. Essex St. Boston. Oct. 2," Lewis Scrapbook.

[68][Dio Lewis], "Boston Gymnasia," *Lewis's New Gymnastics For Ladies, Gentlemen Children and Boston Journal of Physical Culture* 1 (November 1860): 11. At this time, apparently, neither Butler nor Windship had opened gyms. Lewis's competitors in 1860 were Mr. Doldt, owner of the Tremont Gym on Eliot Street, and Mr. Stewart, "long identified with gymnastics in Boston," who ran a German-style gym in Chapman Place. See "Mistakes in Gymnastics" in the same issue for details on the organization of the exercise classes.

[69]Dio Lewis, *The New Gymnastics for Men, Women and Children*, 4th ed. (Boston: Ticknor & Filelds, 1862), 96.

[70]The Spirometer was sufficiently beautiful, Lewis advertised, to adorn any parlor. It consisted of a long tube, attached to a dial, that measured the amount of air being forced through the machine when the patient blew into the tube. Harvard's president C. C. Felton endorsed the spirometer in Lewis's advertising. The blow gun consisted of a slender copper tube, a specially fitted arrow, and a target. To increase their lung expansion, patients made a game out of target practice. See Lewis, *The New Gymnastics*, 272-74, for other details.

[71]E. Hitchcock to Luther Gulick, 24 March, 1898, Lewis Scrapbook.

[72]"Lewis's New Gymnasium," *Lewis's New Gymnastics for Ladies, Gentlemen and Children and Boston Journal of Physical Culture*. 1 (November 1860): 16.

[73]Eastman suggested that Lewis relied on diet, exercise, baths, sunlight, and "cheerful home-life" in these medical prescriptions. Eastman, *Biography*, 89.

[74]"Lewis's New Gymnasium," *Lewis's New Gymnastics for Ladies, Gentlemen and Children and Boston Journal of Physical Culture* 1 (November 1860): 16.

[75][Dio Lewis], "Spinal Curvature," *Lewis's New Gymnastics for Ladies, Gentlemen and Children and Boston Journal of Physical Culture* 1 (February 1861): 48.

[76]Sarah Ashley to Luther Gulick, 18 February 1898, Lewis Scrapbook.

[77]Eastman, *Biography*, 89.

[78][Dio Lewis], "Teachers for Gymnasia," *Lewis's New Gymnastics for Ladies, Gentlemen and Children and Boston Journal of Physical Culture* 1 (November 1860): 9.

[79][Dio Lewis], "Normal School for Gymnastics," *Lewis's New Gymnastics for Ladies, Gentlemen and Children and Boston Journal of Physical Culture* 1 (April 1861): 91. The four students came from Ohio, Maryland, Maine, and New Hampshire.

[80][Dio Lewis], "Teachers of Gymnastics," *Lewis's New Gymnastics for Ladies, Gentlemen and Children and Boston Journal of Physical Culture* 1 (April, 1861): 87.

[81][Lewis], "Normal School," 91.

[82]Advertisement for Lewis's Normal Institute for Physical Education, *Lewis's Gymnastic Monthly and Journal of Physical Culture* 2 (October 1862): inside cover.

[83]"Lewis's Normal Institute for Physical Education: Articles of Association," Lewis Scrapbook. By 1862, the Board of Directors had expanded to include twenty-five men. Advertisment for Lewis's Normal Institute for Physical Education, *Lewis's Gymnastic Monthly and Journal of Physical Culture* 2 (July 1862): inside cover.

[84]Lewis, *New Gymnastics for Men, Women and Children*, 269.

[85]Ibid. Shortly after the graduation of his first group of graduates, Lewis reported that all were employed and that one man, working only three hours a day, expected to make about three thousand dollars in the next year as a gymnastics teacher. [Dio Lewis], "The First Graduates of the Normal Institute for Physical Education," *Lewis's New Gymnastics for Ladies, Gentlemen and Children and Boston Journal of Physical Culture* 1 (October 1861): 188.

[86]*City of Boston School Records, 1873–1874*, 509. On deposit in: Rare Books and Manuscripts, Boston Public Library, Boston, MA.

[87]Ibid., 509-10. No gender was specified for these positions.

[88]Dio Lewis, *In a Nutshell: Suggestions to American College Students* (New York: Clarke Brothers, 1883), 173.

[89]Ibid.

[90]Ibid.

[91]See "Commencement Exercises at the Normal Institute for Physical Education," *Lewis's New Gymnastics for Ladies, Gentlemen and Children and Boston Journal of Physical Culture* 1 (October 1861), 178; and "First Graduates of the Normal Institute for Physical Education," 188.

92"This special use of muscle-culture," Lewis wrote, "has won a reputation so world-wide, that a course of instruction in physical education which should omit its development, would be seriously defective." [Dio Lewis], "Second Course of Lewis's Normal Institute for Physical Education," *Lewis's New Gymnastics for Ladies, Gentlemen and Children and Boston Journal of Physical Culture* 1 (October 1861): 190.

93Eastman, *Biography of Dio Lewis*, 80-81. An 1862 letter on Lewis's stationary indicates that the faculty included Anatomy—Thomas Hoskins, author of *What We Eat*; Physiology—Dr. Josiah Curtis; Hygiene—Dr. Walter Channing; and Gymnastics—Dr. Dio Lewis. Dio Lewis to "Dear Sir," 10 March, 1862, Massachusetts Historical Society, Boston MA.

94Love Brown to Helen Savage. 11 August 1866, Mount Holyoke College Archives, South Hadley, MA.

95Ibid.

96Ibid.

97Ibid.

98"Graduating Exercises of Dr. Dio Lewis's Training School," newspaper clipping, Lewis Scrapbook.

99Ibid. The marital status of the men was not indicated.

100[Thomas Wentworth Higginson], "Gymnastics," *Atlantic Monthly* 7 (March 1861): 300.

101[Dio Lewis], "Gymnastics in the Atlantic Monthly," *Lewis's New Gymnastics for Ladies, Gentlemen and Children and Boston Journal of Physical Culture* 1 (March 1861): 74-75.

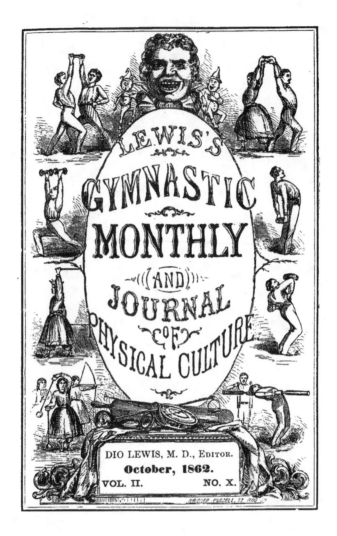

Figure 65: Front Cover, *Dio Lewis's Gymnastic Monthly and Journal of Physical Culture.*

# Chapter 9
## Textbooks for Majestic Womanhood:
## The Literary Legacy of Dio Lewis

Three of Dio Lewis's many books bear directly on the question of appropriate women's exercise: *The New Gymnastics for Men, Women and Children*, published in 1862; its completely rewritten tenth edition, published in 1868; and a lesser-known book entitled *Our Girls*, published in 1871. These three works reveal the nature and evolution of Lewis's exercise system in the 1860s, and, of equal importance, reveal his attitudes toward women's sphere, women's rights, and women's physical and intellectual capacities.

### Dio Lewis Enters the World of Publishing

One of the largest problems Lewis faced after receiving the endorsement of the American Institute of Instruction in August 1860 was the lack of a written description of his system. Lewis knew that if the Institute's endorsement was going to have any meaning, he quickly had to provide the public and America's educators with written instructions about the New Gymnastics.

Lewis began codifying his system with a two-part article entitled "Physical Culture," published in the *Massachusetts Teacher*.[1] In November 1860, he also published the first issue of a monthly periodical called *Lewis's New Gymnastics for Ladies, Gentlemen and Children and Boston Journal of Physical Culture*. This journal appears to be the first magazine in the United States whose central mission was to disseminate information on exercise as an aspect of physical culture.[2] In the early issues of his new journal, Lewis attempted to lay the philosophical and physiological groundwork for the exercise regimen he was apparently still formulating.[3] But, rather than relying on his own ideas for the first issue, he gave the cover to an article titled "Physiology and Calisthenics," a series of excerpts from Catharine Beecher's book of that title.[4]

The first issue did contain evidence, however, that Lewis and his system were fully supported by the highest levels of Boston's intellectual community. John D. Philbrick, superintendent of the Boston public schools, contributed an article on "The Want of Physical Training"; and Mary Mann, Horace's widow, wrote to congratulate Lewis for fulfilling her husband's dream that physical training be introduced into the public schools. Other people also contributed. Mrs. M. L. Taylor wrote from Lasell Seminary for women to report on the success of her students. Helen Lewis contributed to the journal, as she did to most of her husband's affairs, beginning what became a regular column in the journal on dress reform and women's health. Dio's contributions to the first issue included an article entitled "Gymnastics for the Insane," detailing his work at the McLean Asylum; a lengthy report of his appearance before the American Institute of Instruction; instructions for several beanbag games; and a description of the proper use of the Blowgun, a device used to help expand the chest.

Throughout the remaining months of 1860 and all of 1861, Lewis's journal contained a variety of articles on physical culture matters and continued to feature the opinions of some of the most prominent members of the Boston community. From a press run of sixty for the first issue, the journal's subscription list grew to more than four thousand names by October of the next year.[5] In January 1862, however, Lewis changed the journal's title to *Lewis's Gymnastic Monthly and Journal of Physical Culture*, reduced the size of the pages, and began including lengthy, illustrated articles describing how to perform a variety of exercises both with and without implements. Lewis advertised that volume two "will present a complete guide in Gymnastics, for the Gymnasium, the School and the Family."[6] It appears from an examination of several issues of the *Gymnastic Monthly* that as he finished them, Lewis began printing, in the *Monthly*, verbatim, sections of his work in progress, *The New Gymnastics for Men, Women and Children.*[7] In fact, with the exception of the page numbers, he apparently used the same printing plates for both the *Monthly* and his textbook. "The *Gymnastic Monthly* my husband put into book form in 1862," Helen explained in answer to a question of Luther Gulick's on this matter.[8] In another letter she clarified the fact that Dio had not codified his system before the magazine began. "Yes," she wrote, "the Gym. monthly was published while the exercises where [sic] being developed and was then put into book form of which you have a copy 1862."[9] The *Gymnastic Monthly* ended with the final issue of volume two.

### The New Gymnastics for Men, Women and Children

The first edition of Lewis's *The New Gymnastics for Men, Women and Children*, published by Ticknor and Fields, appeared in 1862. In his preface to the work, Lewis made plain his commitment to the physical education of women: "Like air and food," he wrote, these exercises "are adapted to both sexes, and to persons of all ages." Lewis further claimed that the system "has been introduced into female seminaries with complete satisfaction. Its beautiful games, graceful attitudes, and striking tableaux, possess a peculiar fascination for girls." It is the author's "ardent hope," he concluded, that "his humble labors may contribute something to the beauty and vigor of his countrymen."[10]

Unlike most nineteenth-century exercise texts, the first edition of *The New Gymnastics* was remarkably spare of physiological and

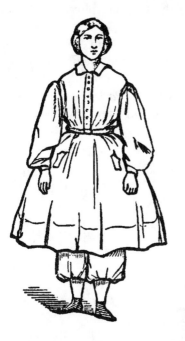

Figure 66: This drawing of appropriate exercise attire for women was modeled, according to Lewis, on an ambrotype taken in 1861 of one of his teachers. [Dio Lewis] "Ladies Gymnastic Dress," *Lewis' New Gymnastics for Ladies, Gentlemen and Children and Boston Journal of Physical Culture 1* (May 1861):106.

pedagogical theory. "I have nothing to say of the importance of Physical Education," Lewis began his first chapter. "Presuming that all who read this work are fully cognizant of the imperative need which it calls forth," he continued, "I shall enter at once upon my task."[11]

Following brief descriptions of proper gymnastic dress—which for women should consist of rubber-soled shoes, flannel pantaloons, shortened skirts, and a loose-fitting blouse allowing "perfect liberty about the waist and shoulders"—Lewis stressed the importance of music as an adjunct to exercise and gave instructions on how to prevent dust by using wax to fill the cracks in the gymnasium floor.[12] Lewis's energetic prose then marched the reader through 115 pages of descriptions of exercises that, taken together, he claimed as *his* system of New Gymnastics. There were thirty beanbag exercises,[13] fifty-four exercises involving the use of a partner and a six-inch wooden ring, sixty-seven "wand" exercises using four-foot-long hollow rods inside which several pounds of lead shot could be placed to increase resistance, thirty-four dumbbell drills, and twenty-two Indian club exercises. The final series of exercises that Lewis claimed as part of his system in 1862 were thirty-eight freehand, calisthenic movements. These were very reminiscent of Beecher's recommended exercises, although Lewis attributed them to the German physical educator Daniel Schreber.[14]

The second half of the 1862 edition consisted of Lewis's translation of two German gymnastics texts that he admitted having substantially rewritten so as to "adapt them to the American mind."[15] Professor Maurice Kloss's *The Dumb Bell Instructor for Parlor Gymnasts* began with a brief history of dumbbell training and a few caveats for older

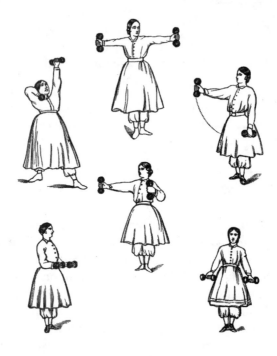

Figure 67: A sampler of dumbell exercises from Dio Lewis's *New Gymnastics for Men, Women and Children* (1862).

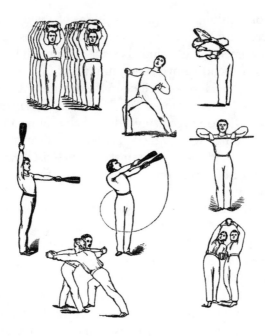

Figure 68: A sampler of wand, club and ring exercises from Dio Lewis's *New Gymnastics for Men, Women and Children* (1862).

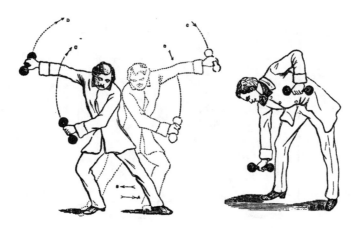

Figure 69: Illustrations from Maurice Kloss's *Dumb Bell Instructor for Parlor Gymnasts* as included in Dio Lewis's *New Gymnastics for Men, Women and Children* (1862).

trainers before settling down to descriptions of a wide variety of relatively difficult dumbbell exercises set to music. Kloss favored large, sweeping movements and included exercises done while standing still, squatting down, bending over, and jumping. Unlike many early exercise books that provide few specifics on the order of the exercises or the correct number of repetitions, *The Dumb Bell Instructor* concluded with specific advice on organizing a dumbbell routine for three different levels of gymnasts: beginners, "somewhat advanced," and "more advanced." In each of these programs, eight exercises were prescribed, with the number of repetitions and the degree of difficulty increasing correspondingly.[16]

Daniel Gottlieb Moritz Schreber's *The Pangymnastikon; or, All Gymnastic Exercises Brought Within the Compass of a Single Piece of Apparatus, as the Simplest Means for the Complete Development of Muscular Strength and Endurance* contained 107 gymnastic movements with a high degree of difficulty.[17] Like the rings of the modern gymnast, the first series of Pangymnastikon exercises included in Schreber's text used only two wooden rings, attached to the ceiling by ropes. However, the ropes of the Pangymnastikon passed over a padded hook allowing the rings to be placed at different heights. In many of the exercises the rings were close enough to the floor that the exercises were reminiscent of Clias's early triangle exercises in which the feet remained on the floor and the gymnast only partially supported the

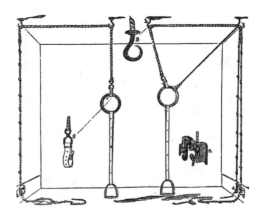

Figure 70: The Pangymnastikon, from Dio Lewis's *Weak Lungs, and How to Make them Strong* (1864).

weight of his body. In many of Schreber's exercises, however, the feet were clear of the floor, and the gymnast performed chins, dips, "summerset forward and backward" rolls, hanging upside down, and exercises in which only one arm supported the weight of the body. To these two suspended rings the gymnast attached a pair of leather straps on the bottom of which were "stirrups." Set up in this way, the Pangymnastikon could be used for a wide variety of swinging exercises, exercises to increase flexibility in the hips and legs, and strengthening exercises in which the Pangymnastikon stirrups were held in place on the floor by the feet while the gymnast executed movements similar to those done with pulleys at gymnasiums. Schreber even included a lengthy section of leaping exercises in which the Pangymnastikon could be used as a high jump standard.[18]

The exercises in Lewis's translation of Schreber's *Pangymnastikon* comprise one of the most difficult and ambitious exercise programs recommended for American women up to that time. Although Lewis no doubt saved money by illustrating the text with Schreber's engravings of a male figure, he closed the book with a special section entitled "Suggestions in Reference to the Use of the Pangymnastikon by Females," in which he categorically stated: "This apparatus will be much used by females of all ages. Of the 107 exercises, there is not one which they may not execute with propriety and profit."[19] What made this particular series of exercises even more difficult than Beaujeu's earlier gymnastics routine was the fact that unlike parallel bars and chinning bars, which are stationary, exercises performed on rings require tremendous upper-body strength simply to keep the apparatus steady. In one exercise, Lewis even recommended that dips be done while swinging through the air. As any modern trainer will attest, performing a dip on stationary bars is relatively easy if one has sufficient triceps and deltoid strength. It is a feat that most men and a few women can do with relatively little training. Performing a dip on hanging rings, however, is an extraordinarily difficult feat, a fact that leaves open to question the number of women who were able to properly perform all of the Pangymnastikon exercises.

But there can be no question that Lewis believed women should use the Pangymnastikon; he considered it of real benefit to women. Cognizant of the social stigma attached to public displays by women, Lewis recommended that women train on their Pangymnastikons at home, in the privacy of their bedrooms. "When a lady is done with her morning cares, and would dress for dinner," he advised, "she slips on

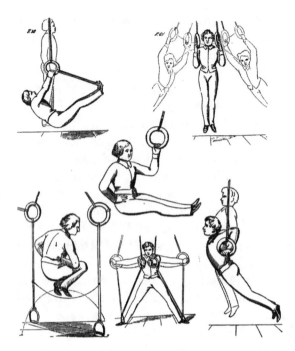

Figure 71: "This apparatus will be much used by females of all ages," Lewis wrote, "There is not one exercise which they many not execute with propriety and profit." Pangymnastikon exercises from Dio Lewis's *New Gymnastics for Men, Women and Children* (1862).

her Zouave, and stepping to the Pangymnastikon, devotes a few minutes to its exercises." The Zouave costume, essential to the proper performance of the exercises, consisted of flannel knickers—with no attached skirt—and a loose-fitting shirt. Lewis argued that it was the only apparel that allowed women the full enjoyment and benefit of the Pangymnastikon.[20]

Lewis advocated that women use their Pangymnastikons on Mondays, Wednesdays, and Fridays. He gave directions for an entire year of training, with the exercises sequenced to gradually strengthen their entire bodies. Women should begin, he advised, with the first ten exercises, performing these ten in the proper order for a full month before tackling the slightly more difficult next ten during the second month, and so on. In addition to the eighty-eight different Pangymnastikon movements, Lewis also described nineteen leaping exercises to be added to the routine at any time after the third month of training.[21]

Although the Pangymnastikon exercises did not appear in the tenth edition of *The New Gymnastics*, released in 1868, Lewis did not abandon his interest in the device or stop recommending it. Sarah Ashley remembered the Pangymnastikon hanging in the basement of Lewis's Beacon Street medical offices when she was his patient in the early 1870s.[22] As late as 1883, *In a Nutshell*, his advice book for college students, carried an advertisement for the device.[23]

Lewis also devoted space in the first edition of *The New Gymnastics* to several gymnastic games. Pin Running was a competitive game, similar to a relay race involving two players, or teams. To begin, Indian clubs were set at distances of fifteen, thirty, and forty-five feet. Standing

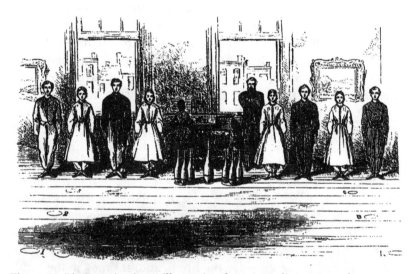

Figure 72: Pin Running in an illustration from J. Madison Watson's *Handbook of Calisthenics and Gymnastics* (1864). Although Watson does not identify the large man in the window on the right as Dio Lewis, the figure certainly resembles him.

in a circle at the starting point, the competitors ran to the first pin and carried it back and placed it in the starting ring. Then off they went for the second, and then the third. The person, or team, able to stand all three clubs in the starting circle first was declared the winner. As a variation, Lewis suggested that a twenty- to fifty-pound bag of beans—or a small boy—be lifted and borne on the shoulder for the final leg of the run.[24] Lewis believed that men and women could compete against each other in this exercise and observed that "the greatest speed I have ever witnessed, has been achieved by women."[25]

The "Birds's Nest Game" helped correct the habit of stooping, Lewis argued. Using beanbags weighing three to four pounds, the students threw the bags onto four wooden nests suspended from the gymnasium ceiling. The largest nest was two feet square and hung overhead thirteen feet from the floor. The smallest was only eight inches square and hung seventeen feet from the floor.[26] Throwing a bag into the largest nest earned one point, into the smallest, four points. Most people needed a number of throws to land a four-pound beanbag on the eight-inch nest seventeen feet in the air and, thus, got plenty of exercise.

The Arm Pull Device was one of several novel exercise implements promoted by Lewis. It consisted of a pair of handles attached to a stout rope. Used both singly and in pairs, Lewis directed his gymnasts to pull against one another, drawing themselves backward and forward without moving their feet.[27] To correct posture, Lewis recommended the regular use of the Gymnastic Crown, an iron diadem decorated with the American eagle and Stars and Stripes. Lewis urged that the crowns, which he sold in graduated weights from three to one hundred pounds, should be worn twice a day for fifteen minutes at a time. With their crowns in place, women were to climb stairs, walk on their tiptoes, walk with their toes turned both inward and outward, walk by placing their heels down first, and perform a series of lunging movements. There were ten different modes of walking, Lewis explained, and, using the crown, they gave the back the most "invigorating" exercise.[28] The final device was the Shoulder Pusher, a rod of two and a half feet, preferably made of ash, to which carved arm pieces were attached. Placed at the shoulder, the elbow, and, at times, in the hand,

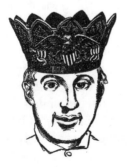

Figure 73: The Gymnastics Crown from Dio Lewis's *New Gymnastics for Men, Women and Children* (1862). The Gymnastics Crown was no doubt inspired by Clias's weighted helmet.

gymnasts pushed against one another, using their partner as resistance.[29]

Several things are striking about Lewis's first edition, the first of which is the strong German influence on his thinking revealed by his inclusion of Schreber's and Kloss's works.[30] The fact that more than half of his book is made up of the translations of other men's ideas not only suggests that Lewis's own technical thinking was not particularly advanced at this point, but that his model of human potential was strongly influenced by these German experts. He did include a number of exercises that appear to be no more fatiguing or difficult than Beecher's light calisthenics; but it is clear that these were merely preparatory and remedial exercises, and that it was expected that women as well as men would gradually find their way to the more difficult dumbbell and Pangymnastikon exercises. Lewis's advocacy of these increasingly difficult moves for women constitutes a major turning point in America's attitude toward appropriate physical education for women. No wonder Beecher felt his system was too vigorous. Flips and chins and somersaults on wooden rings are not the sorts of exercises one normally associates with proper Victorian womanhood.

In August 1862, Lewis discussed his system and the physical potential of women in a twenty-page article in *The Atlantic Monthly*. He attempted a condensation of *The New Gymnastics* in the *Monthly*, but he began his article with a philosophical explanation of his beliefs regarding exercise. He made it plain that his vision of American womanhood was radically different from that of most of his exercise forbearers. Egalitarian to a fault, Lewis argued that every exercise class should be a coeducational class, and he declared that "women need not fall behind men in those exercises which require grace, flexibility and skill," adding that "at the Normal Institute for Physical Education females succeed better than males." In fact, Lewis continued, clearly warming to his subject, "There are in my gymnasium at this time a good many ladies with whom the most ambitious young man need not be ashamed to compete, unless the shame come from being defeated."[31]

Lewis's message fell, it seems, on appreciative ears. The Lewis Scrapbook contains thirty-six different reviews of Lewis's *New Gymnastics*, all of which unfailingly praised Lewis and his ideas on physical training. "We cannot imagine anything more important to the rising generation than the careful study of this volume," observed the *Philadelphia Inquirer*.[32] "This book should reach a sale of hundreds of thousands," wrote another reviewer. "The author is a public benefactor."[33] Although it probably never reached a sales figure that high, the book appears to have outperformed all other nineteenth-century texts. At least four printings were produced in 1862, and six years later a "revised and greatly enlarged" tenth edition appeared. This version remained continuously in print without changes through 1891.[34]

### The 1868 Tenth Edition:
### Breaking European Ties

Lewis's tenth edition of *The New Gymnastics* differed substantially from the 1862 original. Although the tenth edition still contained a long compilation of illustrated exercises using rings, wands, wooden dumbbells, Indian clubs, and so forth, the two long German translations were gone. In their place, Lewis offered a greater number of "his own" exercises and several opening chapters expounding on his system.[35] These opening chapters of the tenth edition are of special interest in understanding Lewis's place in physical education history as he used them to assert his invention of the movements that constitute the New Gymnastics and to denigrate the rival systems of heavy weight lifting and military drill.

In his first chapter, "Origin of the New System of Gymnastics," Lewis detailed, item by item, "what portions of the New System are my own creation."[36] Lewis claimed the invention of the wooden rings and beanbags, the substitution of the wooden for the iron dumbbell, and the use of music as an accompaniment to exercise. He also claimed all but five of the wand exercises and all the club exercises. Half the "free" gymnastics and all the specifics—though not the idea—of the "mutual help exercises," he claimed, were also his.[37]

Lewis's claims to originality are shaky at best. American Movement Cure experts such as George Taylor and Russell Trall had advocated "mutual assistance" exercises since the early 1850s.[38] Donald Walker, author of *British Manly Exercises,* had recommended Indian club exercises in the early 1830s,[39] and Catharine Beecher described cornbag exercises in 1856.[40] Also, beyond Nathaniel Allen's claim that his sister-in-law first suggested Lewis use music, there exist the records of the calisthenics classes at Mount Holyoke from the 1840s and 1850s in which musical accompaniment was part of the regular routine, and of Beecher's advocacy of music for classroom drill in the 1850s.[41] Even more damaging to Lewis's claim is Kloss's statement in his *Dumb Bell Instructor for Parlor Gymnasts*—the German text Lewis translated and incorporated in *The New Gymnastics*—that his exercises "are adapted to music." In fact, Kloss differentiated between those exercises done in 2/2 time, 3/4 time, 4/4 time, and so on, and these instructions were, of course, contained in the first edition of Lewis's book with illustrations showing the rhythmic divisions of each exercise.[42] As for his claim that he developed certain freehand exercises, Lewis would have to get at the end of a very long line of exercise experts that stretched back to the eighteenth century. Just in the decade prior to Lewis's first edition, Mathias Roth (1853), Catharine Beecher (1856), Russell Trall (1857), and P. A. Fitzgerald (1856) had all published works containing similar movements. Trall and Fitzgerald also included dumbbell and Indian club exercises in their texts.[43]

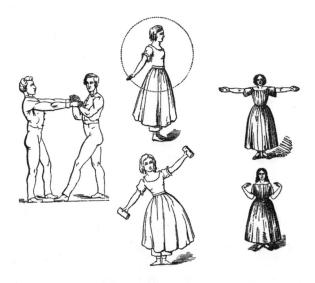

Figure 74: Illustrations from Russell Trall, *Illustrated Family Gymnasium* (1857). Trall borrowed illustrations shamelessly from other authors. His free-hand exercises are direct copies of those in Fitzgerald's *Exhibition Speaker.*

Lewis also used the tenth edition to again attack George Barker Windship, David P. Butler, and the advocates of heavy weightlifting, a print campaign he began in the first issue of his magazine, *Lewis's New Gymnastics.*[44] Situated in Boston as he was, Lewis directly competed with Windship and Butler for both patients and gymnasts, and, in 1868, Butler and Windship were near the height of their popularity.

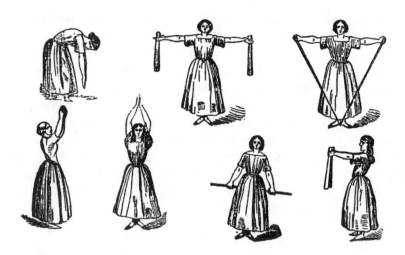

Figure 75: Exercise illustrations from P. A. Fitzgerald's *Exhibition Speaker*. (1856).

Using animal metaphors, Lewis compared the heavy weightlifter to the slow and plodding draft horse, and the New Gymnastics practitioner to the quicker and more agile carriage horse, arguing that "lifting great weights affects him as drawing heavy loads affects the horse. Surely it is only this mania for monstrous arms and shoulders, that could have misled the intelligent gymnast on this point."[45] Besides Windship and the heavyweight club, Lewis's system also had to compete with a resurgence of interest in military drill brought on by the Civil War. In 1864, in fact, a bill that would have required military training for all male students in the state had made it through two readings in the Massachusetts legislature. Although Lewis, Nathaniel Allen, and William Lloyd Garrison were able to get its passage stopped, Lewis felt compelled to use the tenth edition to reiterate his objections to the military system of training.[46]

Lewis also charged that several former students had taken his exercises, reorganized them, and claimed them for their own. He named no names but claimed that an exercise book published in New York "appropriated, without even a mention of my name, all the principle features and much of the detail of the system to which I have devoted so many years."[47] This book was undoubtedly J. Madison Watson's *Handbook of Calisthenics and Gymnastics: A Complete Drill-Book for*

*Schools, Families and Gymnasiums with Music to Accompany the Exercises,* an elegantly illustrated, 388-page textbook adopted for school use by the New York Board of Education in 1864.[48] Although differing from Lewis's work in that it included a lengthy section of vocal exercises, more than two hundred pages of Watson's purposive exercises appear to be direct replications of Lewis's ideas. In the *Handbook* and his greatly abridged *Watson's Manual of Calisthenics: A Systematic Drill-Book Without Apparatus for Schools, Families and*

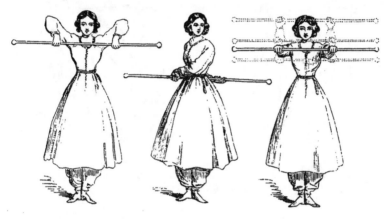

Figure 76: Illustrations from J. Madison Watson's *Handbook of Calisthenics and Gymnastics* (1864).

*Gymnasiums, With Music to Accompany the Exercises,* published that same year, Watson takes his readers through lightweight dumbbell exercises, wand exercises, mutual assistance exercises, Indian club exercises, and partner exercises using wooden rings. Like Lewis, he also urged women to wear shortened skirts and pantaloons or their "bathing dresses" while they exercised.[49] Watson even copied some of Lewis's games. "Pin-running" became the "Indian Club Race."[50]

Despite his overstatements as to the originality of the New Gymnastics, Lewis did leave an exercise legacy of considerable importance. That legacy, however, had less to do with whether his "chest expansion with dumbbells" differed from "chest expansion with dumbbells" by earlier authors than it did with his advocacy of exercise for women and the visual subtext one "reads" in his books. In the tenth edition, for instance, Lewis included a series of "mutual help" exercises in which another person was employed as resistance in a series of pushing and pulling exercises. Although the text speaks of using persons of equal strength for these exercises, the illustrations pair males and females, an explicit example of Lewis's egalitarian stance on the

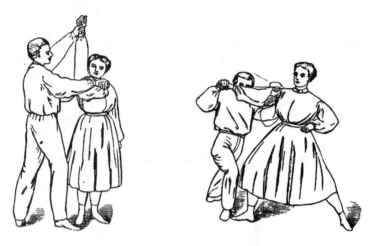

Figure 77: Mutual help exercises from the tenth edition of Dio Lewis's *New Gymnastics for Men, Women and Children* (1868).

question of the physical potential of women. In the first edition as well, there is a boldness in the way women are depicted in the illustrations. Their movements are unhindered by corsets, long skirts, and excessive petticoats. They bend, reach their arms overhead, spread their legs, and lunge as if they were fencers. They appear to use the same dumbbells and clubs, the same wands, and the same beanbags the men use. On page after page, men and women are shown performing the same tasks with the same confident expressions. The females in Lewis's illustrations are not wasp-waisted ingenues but women in their prime who have a look of sturdiness and competence about them. They represent a new type of woman, a woman who understood that the body could be trained and improved and that physical improvement could change the quality of her life.

### Our Girls

Lewis expounded at length on precisely this theme in *Our Girls* (1871), which grew from his experiences with his students at the Family School for Young Ladies in Lexington. *Our Girls* is both an advice book for young women and a philosophical rumination on the doctrine of separate spheres. Opening *Our Girls* with Margaret Fuller's quote, "That her hand must be given with dignity, she must be able to stand alone," Lewis spoke in a stronger voice than ever before about woman's right to dignity, equality, and a life outside the home.[51] In a chapter entitled "Employments for Women," Lewis argued, "There are a great many occupations at present pursued exclusively by men, which offer no considerable difficulties to women."[52] According to Lewis, women could easily be photographers, bank clerks, brokers, secretaries, dentists, lawyers, lecturers, librarians, physicians, preachers, proofreaders, publishers, teachers, gymnastics and dancing instructors, watchmakers, teachers of drawing and painting, architects, engravers, designers, gardeners, merchants, carpenters, sculptors, restaurant owners, and so on.[53] Furthermore, he argued, women should receive the same pay as men did for the same work. Lewis predicted accurately that the public schools soon would be run almost entirely by women teachers, but argued that it was unfair for a male teacher to receive a thousand dollars a year in salary and a female teacher only four hundred. This is "not because of the inferiority of her moral influence in the school, not because the pupils learn less, but because she is a woman."[54]

Historian James Whorton has suggested that Lewis's intent was to set off a "revolution, a winning of physical independence for women."[55] For Lewis, that independence was intimately tied to his new vision of the female body. He attacked the idea that women were somehow inherently frail, arguing that it was ludicrous to adhere to the idea that a pale and sensitive woman was feminine and refined, and one in blooming health was masculine and coarse. What was wrong, he wondered, with women fulfilling their physical potential? After all, he argued, "every acute observer knows that the feminine soul, like the masculine, utters its richest harmonies only through a perfect instrument."[56]

Lewis understood, however, that body ideology was intimately tied to nineteenth-century America's notions of class. "If she looks strong and moves with a will, she will be mistaken for a worker, for a servant," he explained to his readers. "If she looks delicate and moves languidly, it will be seen at once that she does not belong to the working class."[57] "Don't you see now how it is?" he asked rhetorically. "To have a strong and muscular body is to be suspected of work, of service; while a frail, delicate *personnel* is proof of position, of ladyhood." This attitude must stop, Lewis declared. "It is true that many strong, muscular women are coarse and ignorant," he elaborated, but that is because "they have given their lives to hard work and have been denied all opportunities to cultivate their minds and manners." However, he continued, "To compare such with the petted, pampered daughters of social and intellectual opportunity, and then to treat the strong body of one as the source of the coarseness and ignorance within, and, in the other case, to treat the weak, delicate body as the source of the fine culture, is to reason like an idiot."[58]

Lewis believed that woman's role in society was a reflection of the physical size and strength of her body. "Whenever women shall rise to true companionship with men," he argued, "as their equals, and not their toys, then a small woman will no more be preferred than a small man." Lewis devoted an entire chapter to this theme, arguing in "Large vs Small Women" that women of average height should strive to weigh between 140 and 160 pounds. He felt that large women had a more dignified character and greater amiability than did small women. Because of his phrenological leanings, Lewis also subscribed to the belief that large women possessed greater intelligence and were more likely to produce large, intelligent offspring.[59] Small and petite women—by which he meant women between ninety and 110 pounds—were preferred by men because they were like pets or toys, Lewis argued. A man who selects a small wife and dresses her in silks and laces with "little ornaments stuck all over," he wrote, is actually exhibiting the same sort of preference he does when he chooses an exceptionally small lapdog.[60]

Lewis contended that the smallness of many American women could be traced to three sources. "Our girls have no adequate exercise," he wrote, and "exercise is the great law of development." He also maintained that the tight corseting of women reduced their vital capacity by nearly half and particularly affected the reproductive organs, lungs, stomach, and liver. Finally, he asserted that women had no real work. They live "in the shade," as he put it, adding that without a regular occupation, "no person, male or female, can preserve a sound mind in a sound body."[61]

Lewis didn't want women to "live in the shade." He dreamed of majestic, independent women who were equal in all respects to men. Lewis knew that his exercise system could help women achieve that goal. But something more was needed. He needed to prove that women were physically able to stand the rigors of his exercise system and intellectual training at the same time. Only then, he realized, would women have in their possession all the tools they needed to be true participants in the world outside the home.

[1]Lewis, "Physical Culture," *Massachusetts Teacher* (October, November 1860): 377, 404.

[2]Earlier magazines, such as *The Journal of Health* and *The Water Cure Journal and Herald of Reforms,* had also dealt with physical culture issues as part of their advocacy of the Laws of Health. Lewis's was the first magazine, however, to dedicate itself to the cause of exercise.

[3]See "Editorial Notices of my Journal," *Lewis's New Gymnastics for Ladies, Gentlemen and Children and Boston Journal of Physical Culture.* 1 (January 1861): 45, for excerpts from leading New England periodicals following the first issue of Lewis's magazine.

[4][Dio Lewis and Catharine Beecher], "Physiology and Calisthenics," *Lewis's New Gymnastics for Ladies, Gentlemen and Children and Boston Journal of Physical Culture* 1 (November 1860): 1. Lewis ran another excerpt from Beecher entitled "Physical Education" in the February 1861 edition of the journal. See p. 51.

[5]"Important to Subscribers," *Lewis's Gymnastic Monthly and Journal of Physical Culture* 2 (October 1861): 184.

[6]"Lewis's Gymnastic Monthly," *Lewis's Gymnastic Monthly and Journal of Physical Culture* 2 (July 1862): back cover.

[7] Volume two, number one, for instance, devoted eight pages to "Exercises with Rings." The Volume two, number seven, July 1862, issue actually began in the middle of a section of dumbbell exercises—without even a page heading—and then included all of the "Free Gymnastics" exactly as they appeared in his textbook, and finished with twenty-nine pages of Pangymnastikon exercises, again identical in every way to what appears in his book except for the page numbers. By volume two, number five, there were no longer any articles in the magazine other than these exercise descriptions, except for advertisements for the Lewis Normal School, forthcoming publications, and his Essex Street gym. The author is indebted to Dr. Mary Lou LeCompte for her gift of the issues of the *Lewis Gymnastic Monthly* now on deposit at the Todd-McLean Physical Culture Collection at the University of Texas in Austin.

[8]Mrs. Dio Lewis to Doctor Gulick, 21 February 1898, Lewis Scrapbook.

[9]Mrs. Dio Lewis to Dr. Luther Gulick, 8 March 1898, Lewis Scrapbook.

[10]Dio Lewis, *The New Gymnastics for Men, Women and Children,* 3rd ed. (Boston: Ticknor & Fields, 1862), 6-7.

[11]Ibid., 9.

[12]Ibid., 16-19.

[13]The beanbag exercises evolved from several ball games Lewis played in the 1850s. When he noticed the trouble some people experienced catching balls,

he partially deflated them and then switched to the beanbags, which allowed his gymnasts to use greater weight. Catharine Beecher, as noted previously, included exercises using bags of corn in her calisthenic regimens, but Lewis's beanbags were larger in size. In *The Dio Lewis Treasury*, he also recommended using sandbags, made of strong sheepskin of varying weights for the same exercises. Dio Lewis, *The Dio Lewis Treasury* (New York: James R. Barnett, 1886), 606-13.

[14]Russell Trall's *Illustrated Family Gymnasium* (New York: Fowler & Wells, 1857), 78-97, also contained a lengthy condensation of Schreber's exercises with illustrations.

[15]Lewis, *New Gymnastics*, 119.

[16]Ibid., 162-64.

[17]Daniel Schreber, the influential German health and childrearing expert, published a number of books in the mid-nineteenth century. An English translation of his work on the Pangymnastikon appeared as *The Parlour Gymnasium: or, All Gymnastic Exercises Brought Within the Compass of a Single Piece of Apparatus, as the Simplest Means for the Complete Development of Muscular Strength and Endurance* (London: G. W. Bacon & Co., 1866). Schreber's books were influential and bestsellers. His most important work, *Illustrated Medical Indoor Gymnastics*, was in its twenty-sixth edition in 1899 (London: Williams and Norgate). In addition, he published *The Book of Health* (Leipzig: H. Fries, 1839); *The Harmful Body Positions and Habits of Children Including a Statement of Counteracting Measures* (Leipzig: Fleischer, 1853); and *Education Through Beauty by Natural and Balanced Furtherance of Normal Body Growth* (Leipzig: Fleischer, 1858).

Schreber's most famous contribution to medical history, however, came from the psychological trauma he inflicted on his son, Daniel Paul Schreber, a German judge, who became one of Sigmund Freud's most famous patients. According to Morton Schatzman, most modern psychoanalysts base their understanding of paranoia upon Freud's analysis of Schreber. Schatzman argues that the father's radical ideas on health and bodily development contributed to the son's mental problems in adulthood. See Morton Schatzman, M.D., "Paranoia or Persecution: The Case of Schreber," *History of Childhood Quarterly* 1 (Summer 1973): 62-88.

[18]Lewis, *New Gymnastics*, 236-55.

[19]Ibid., 256.

[20]Ibid. Lewis noted that this same costume was worn by the female members of the Zouave Military Clubs.

[21]Ibid., 236-55

[22]Sarah A. Ashley to Luther Gulick, 18 February 1898, Lewis Scrapbook.

[23]In 1862, the Pangymnastikon sold for $9.00 and could be ordered from Lewis's gymnasium. In 1883, it sold for $10.40, including postage. Dio Lewis, *In a Nutshell* (New York: Clarke Brothers, 1883), 209.

[24]Lewis, *New Gymnastics*, 95.

[25] Ibid., 95-96.

[26] Ibid., 96-97.

[27] Ibid., 98-99.

[28] Ibid., 99-100.

[29] Ibid., 100-101.

[30] There are no references to Ling or to Swedish Gymnastics in the first edition.

[31] Dio Lewis, "The New Gymnastics," *The Atlantic Monthly* 10 (August 1862): 132.

[32] Handcopied quotation from the *Philadelphia Inquirer*, Lewis Scrapbook.

[33] Clipping entitled "The New Gymnastics for Men, Women and Children," from *Arthur's Home Life* (n.p., n.d): 258. Lewis Scrapbook.

[34] In 1891, Helen Lewis purchased the copyright from Ticknor and Fields and issued the final edition with the Fowler & Wells Publishing Company. Dio Lewis, *The New Gymnastics for Men, Women and Children*, 25th ed. (New York: Fowler & Wells, 1891).

[35] He concluded the new edition with a lecture by British-based disciple Moses Coit Tyler entitled, "The New System of Musical Gymnastics as an Instrument in Education."

[36] Dio Lewis, *The New Gymnastics for Men, Women and Children*. 10th ed. (New York: Ticknor & Fields, 1868), 9.

[37] Ibid., 6-11.

[38] See Trall, *The Illustrated Family Gymnasium*; 150-58.

[39] See chapter 4.

[40] Catharine E. Beecher, *Calisthenic Exercises for Schools, Families and Health Establishments* (New York: Harper & Brothers, 1856), 44-47.

[41] See chapter 5.

[42] Kloss, *Dumb Bell Instructor and Parlor Gymnast*, included in Lewis's *New Gymnastics*, 129.

[43] Trall, *The Illustrated Family Gymnasium*; and P. A. Fitzgerald, *The Exhibition Speaker: Containing Farces, Dialogues, and Tableaux With Exercises for Declamation in Prose and Verse. Also, a Treatise on Oratory and Elocution, Hints on Dramatic Characters, Costumes, Position of the Stage, Making Up, Etc. Etc. To Which is Added a Complete System of Calisthenics and Gymnastics, With Instructions for Teachers and Pupils, Illustrated with Fifty Engravings* (New York: Sheldon, Lamport & Blakeman, 1856), 219-68.

[44] [Dio Lewis], "Heavy and Light Gymnastics," *Lewis's New Gymnastics for Ladies, Gentlemen and Children and Boston Journal of Physical Culture* 1 (November 1860):16. Lewis suggested a public debate between himself and Windship in the December 1860 issue in an article also entitled "Heavy and Light Gymnastics," on page 29.

[45] Lewis, *New Gymnastics*, 10th ed., 79.

[46] Ibid., 5. See Peter J. Wosh, "Sound Minds and Unsound Bodies: Massachusetts Schools and Mandatory Physical Training," *New England*

*Quarterly* 55 (March-December 1982): 52-59, for a discussion of the military drill movement that arose as a consequence of the Civil War. See Eastman, *The Biography of Dio Lewis,* for the story of Lewis's appearance before the Massachusetts legislature on this issue.

[47]Lewis, *New Gymnastics,* 10th ed., 11.

[48]J. Madison Watson, *Handbook of Calisthenics and Gymnastics: A Complete Drill-Book for Schools, Families and Gymnasiums with Music to Accompany the Exercises* (New York: Schermerhorn, Bancroft & Co., 1864).

[49]J. Madison Watson, *Watson's Manual of Calisthenics: A Systematic Drill-Book Without Apparatus for Schools, Families and Gymnasiums, With Music to Accompany the Exercises* (New York: Schermerhorn, Bancroft & Co., 1864), 23. A second edition appeared in 1882 published by E. Steiger & Co. of New York.

[50]Ibid., 250.

[51]Dio Lewis, M.D., *Our Girls* (New York: Harper & Brothers, 1871), title page.

[52]Ibid., 131. Lewis quoted extensively from Virginia Penny's *Cyclopedia of Woman's Work,* a book that he stated contained more than five hundred employments suitable for women besides housework.

[53]Ibid., 131-72. Harriett Martineau expressed similar sentiments in 1859. Harriett Martineau, "Female Industry," *The Edinburgh Review,* No. 222 (April 1859): 293-336.

[54]Lewis, *Our Girls,* 159.

[55] Whorton, *Crusaders for Fitness,* 278.

[56]Lewis, *Our Girls,* 67.

[57]Ibid., 70.

[58]Ibid., 71.

[59]Lewis, like Orson Fowler, argued that the Founding Fathers—Washington, Jefferson, Franklin, and others—were all large men, most of them weighing more than two hundred pounds. Ibid., 89.

[60]Ibid., 86-87.

[61]Ibid., 92, 103.

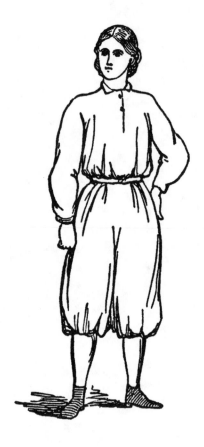

Figure 78: The Zouave costume for use on the Pangymnastikon. From Dio
Lewis's *New Gymnastics for Men, Women and Children* (1862).

# Chapter 10
## The Influence of Dio Lewis:
### "Courage and Strength to Take Up the Battle"

In 1864, Lewis decided to test his radical ideas on American womanhood by founding, under one roof, Dio Lewis's Family School for Young Ladies and a movement cure sanitarium. The sanitarium was a natural outgrowth of his medical practice in Boston. Dr. Dio Lewis's Family School for Young Ladies, on the other hand, was, from the beginning, an experiment. Lewis viewed the school as a means to validate his belief that women were capable of greater physical and intellectual vigor than nineteenth-century medical and social propriety sanctioned. As the 1867 school catalogue explained it, the plan was to "secure a symmetrical development of body, mind and heart; to give due attention to physical, social and moral culture, while providing thorough instruction in Literature, Science, and Art."[1] Several years into the experiment, Lewis wrote, "We are well satisfied, that the common opinion concerning excessive brainwork in our schools is an error; that our girls, even, may double their intellectual acquisitions, provided their exercise, bathing, diet, sleep, and other hygienic conditions be rightly managed."[2]

The closing of the Family School would mark the end of Lewis's active involvement as an exercise entrepreneur. The present chapter explores this period in his life and attempts to assess the impact that he and his system of purposive training had on the lives of American women.

### The Family School for Young Ladies

Lewis chose the Lexington House Hotel for his new combination sanitarium-girls school and purchased it in 1864. The village of Lexington proved to be a good choice. The hotel was only eleven miles from Boston and was connected by a rail line so Dio could commute into the city on the nine o'clock train and return each evening in time to have supper with the students.[3] Patients and students alike viewed Lexington's proximity to Boston favorably. One patient wrote, "One advantage in coming here is the fact that [the] place is near Boston, the centre of the Universe."[4]

Lexington was remarkable both for its healthfulness and good morals, Lewis boasted in his catalogue.[5] Lacking any major industry,

Lexington's air was fresh and clean, and the scenic countryside provided numerous opportunities for walks, picnics, and horseback rides. The old hotel had 110 rooms, including a large ballroom that Dio

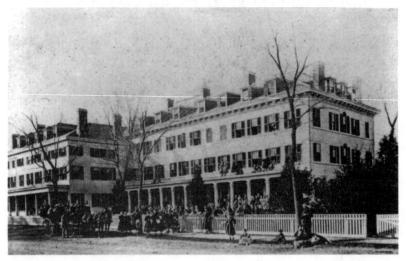

Figure 79: Photograph of Dio Lewis' The Family School for Young Ladies, Lexington, Massachusetts. Courtesy Babson Library, Springfield College, Springfield, Massachusetts.

converted into the gymnastics and assembly hall. In the basement he installed a variety of hydropathic facilities, and upstairs he fitted out special apartments for himself and Helen.[6] Resolving to establish a family atmosphere for the girls at the school, Mrs. Lewis took the role of the "School-mother."[7] More than thirty servants assisted with meal preparations, housekeeping, the sanitarium patients, and the building's maintenance.[8]

The school formally opened in October 1864. The first year only thirty students attended, ranging in age from twelve to twenty-three. The pupils comprising the first class came from the "most intelligent families in New England," Lewis boasted. Intellectually and morally, they "were all we could ask; physically, they were much below the average."[9]

Despite the poor physical condition in which the first students started the year, the thirty young women made remarkable physical progress. Used to teaching gymnastics to people who lived at home and indulged in "fashionable errors" of dress, diet, sleep, and bathing, Lewis confessed that even he was unprepared for the dramatic changes his new lifestyle produced in the students. By having his charges retire early, sleep in well-ventilated rooms, eat plain but nutritious foods, wear gymnastic dress at all times, practice the New Gymnastics for an hour and a half each day, and take five- to ten-mile hikes on the weekends, his students transformed themselves during the first academic year.[10] As it was with Orson Fowler, the standard of improvement used by Lewis in that first year, and ever after, was an increase in size and muscularity. "The general development may be inferred, when it is stated, that, about the upper part of the chest, the average enlargement was two and three-quarter inches," he boasted. Every pupil, he claimed, not withstanding their hard study, "had grown muscular and healthy."[11]

In the second year of the school's operation, and with all the building improvements completed, more than one hundred girls and several boys showed up for the fall term. By this time, Lewis had assembled a thirty-member faculty, headed by former manual-labor advocate Theodore Weld.[12] Abolitionist Angelina Grimke Weld, his wife, taught history. Catharine Beecher joined the faculty in 1867 to lecture on domestic economy and the Laws of Health. Sarah Grimke taught composition and mythology.[13]

The physical improvement of the female students was also marked in the second year of the school's operation. Girls who previously could not climb stairs, Lewis crowed, now walked ten miles with ease. The size of their chests increased an average of two and a half inches and, more importantly, "there was a corresponding change in the size of the arms, and the general muscular system, while the carriage of the body so changed as to excite general remark."[14] Lewis's reference to larger arms and greater overall muscularity suggests that Love Brown's assessment of the Lewis system was correct. Not only was it far more vigorous than the calisthenics of Mount Holyoke, it was a "real" training system designed to produce physical changes in the appearance of the body. In a later article from the North American Review, discussing his Lexington experiment, Lewis claimed that during an eight-month period students made the following measurement increases: chest—2 1/2 inches, waist—5 inches, upper arm—1 1/2 inches, forearm—1 inch.[15]

In its third year of operation, enrollment at the Family School for Young Ladies reached 144 students with an average age of seventeen years.[16] Students came from as far away as California, Central America, and the West Indies that year. The Lewis regimen altered little: loose and comfortable dress, rigorous intellectual study, systematic exercise for at least an hour to an hour and a half each day, simple food, dancing three evenings a week, and bed at 8:30 P.M. A newspaper report from 1866 reported, "Girls who came in feeble health have grown robust, while the strong have grown almost insensible to fatigue. The average expansion of the chest has been 2 1/3 inches."[17]

Although gymnastics played the largest role in effecting the physical transformation of his students, Lewis understood that they also needed recreation. During the extensive remodeling of the Lexington House Hotel, he installed a bowling alley for the use of both students and patients. In the evenings, he organized parlor games in the gymnastic hall, and he designated the hour before bedtime as Recreation Hour, requiring everyone to take part in some sort of amusing activity. According to Eastman, the students' great favorite was "competitive" gymnastics.[18]

### End of an Era

That a fire should effectively end Lewis's great educational experiment was indeed ironic, as both the 1866 and the 1867 catalogues for the Family School contained detailed descriptions of the safety precautions taken during the hotel's renovation to prevent just such a calamity. Lewis boasted that he had installed fire hoses and fire escapes, and had hired an "intelligent" night watchman to patrol the building.[19] Despite these precautions, the old Lexington House Hotel burned to the floor joists on 7 September 1867. A lover of modern conveniences, Lewis had installed gaslights and steam heat in the school just the year before, and the gaslights, along with the $1,700 worth of coal stored in the basement, resulted in the school's total destruction. Some members of the local community had joked about the novel lighting system when Lewis had it installed. One local citizen reportedly said, "What do they need of it? There is gas enough in the house already."[20]

Lewis could at least be grateful that the fire occurred between sessions. The Normal College students had just departed, the fall semester Family School students were not scheduled to arrive for at least twenty days, and so no one was injured in the blaze. The Lewises, however, faced serious financial problems. Not only did they lose their household goods, their personal papers, and the sanitarium and school records, they soon discovered that their fire insurance would cover only about two-thirds of the estimated cost of rebuilding.[21] To get through the next year, Lewis rented a smaller hotel in nearby Arlington on Spy Pond. There they continued the Family School as best they could during the 1867–1868 term, but, because of the cramped facilities, Lewis had to send home all the movement cure patients. In the spring of 1868, dissatisfied with the small facility, Lewis had a decision to make. He only recognized two choices: closing the school or rebuilding on a much larger scale in Lexington. Writing to Luther Gulick, Helen Lewis remembered, "The Doctor had not the means sufficient to rebuild on the large scale necessary to compete with other large schools." So, rather than do a second-class job, Lewis decided officially to close the school in the spring of 1868.[22]

Because of the insurance settlement, Dio and Helen had sufficient funds to purchase a large home across from the Boston Athenaeum on Beacon Street in Boston, and the following year Helen inherited enough money from her family to enlarge their home into an eight-story, brick hotel they called Bellevue. The Lewises lived on the top floor, considered the most healthful, in an apartment that overlooked Boston Harbor. In the basement Dio set up his medical offices, installed Turkish baths, and maintained an exercise space where the Pangymnastikon could be used.[23] He also installed an elevator—the second in the city of Boston. With the renovations finally completed, he leased the hotel to a temperance man for $12,000 a year, a figure that amply covered his living expenses and freed him to pursue writing and lecturing. Under the terms of the lease, he and Helen maintained their right to live on the top floor and have his office in the basement. Financially secure, Dio returned to the lecture circuit, resuming his former pattern of alternating talks on physical education and temperance for the next several years.[24]

## The Normal School Continues

The closing of the Family School for Young Ladies also impacted the Normal College. One of Gulick's correspondents suggested that Lewis "kept up a training school on Essex Street" for a few years following the fire, but whether she meant the normal college or simply Lewis's movement cure/gymnasium is not clear.[25] Articles in the monthly *Herald of Health,* however, suggest that Lewis turned the normal college over to his former student and self-described "right hand man," Folansbee Goodrich Welch, in the summer of 1868. A homeopathic physician, Welch had spent seven years teaching gymnastics for Lewis in Boston and Lexington and had "assisted to some extent in the preparation of his books."[26] Welch had also earned a national

reputation in the field of physical education as a result of his appoint-
ment in 1867 as the head of the physical culture department of Yale
University.[27] According to the *Herald of Health*, Welch had directed an
eight-week normal school at Glenwood Ladies Seminary in West
Brattleboro, Vermont, during the summers of 1868, 1869, and 1870.
Called the Normal Institute for the Training of Teachers in Dio Lewis's
New Gymnastics, Welch's school received a visit from Dio Lewis in
1870 during which Lewis told the students, "When my own classes
were discontinued, I looked about to find someone to take up this
work; and it is a source of no little gratification to me that he was, in
the providence of God, placed at the head of the gymnastics movement
as a teacher of teachers."[28]

Another normal school based on Lewis's system also appears to
have opened during this era. Mary T. Orcutt, who taught gymnastics at
Tilden Ladies Seminary, claimed in her *Manual of Gymnastics* to be the
"Principal of a Normal Institute for Physical Culture" and to have personally taught "thousands of persons of both sexes" the proper
techniques of the New Gymnastics. Orcutt's book, published in 1874,
attributed its ideas to F. G. Welch and his *Moral, Intellectual and
Physical Culture*, which suggests that she may have taught at Welch's
normal school before moving to Tilden Ladies Seminary.[29]

It also appears that late in his life, Lewis briefly returned to teacher
training. He participated in the "Summer Institutes" at Martha's
Vineyard organized by Louis Agassiz,[30] conducting a normal school at
the Institute in both 1883 and 1884. A resolution passed by the class of
1884 thanked Lewis for his "skill and enthusiasm as an instructor, his
genial and admirable qualities as a man, and his unexpected liberality
in the presentation to them of valuable books and apparatus." One of
the seven female names signed to the resolution was that of Delphine
Hanna, who helped establish physical education as a profession for
women.[31] Other evidence that Lewis had not totally abandoned
teacher training can be found in an 1881 letter to Abigail May.
Answering her query about taking on her son as a student, Lewis
wrote: "We have no classes during August and September. I would
teach the young man for a few weeks . . . and I think in that time, I can
help him to teach fifty exercises well."[32]

Although the fate of his Normal School is difficult to trace, Lewis,
the man, continued to cut a wide swath in the world of reform in the
two decades following his closing of the Lexington school. In fact, the
last two decades of Lewis's life appear to have been a typical whirlwind

of activity. He spent most of the 1870s on the road, lecturing about temperance and the rights of women, yet he managed to turn out several important books that continued to keep his ideas about health, exercise, and the equality of women before the public. *Our Girls, Chastity, Chats With Young Women, Prohibition a Failure* and *Our Digestion* all appeared in the early 1870s.[33] In the 1880s, he turned out *Gypsies: Or Three Years's Camp Life in the Mountains of California, Curious Fashions, In a Nutshell,* and, posthumously, *The Dio Lewis Treasury.*[34] He also tried twice, unsuccessfully, to establish new magazines with *Dio Lewis's Monthly* in 1883 and *Nuggets* in 1885.[35] Lewis died in Yonkers, New York, on 21 May 1886.[36]

### Assessing the Influence of the New Gymnastics

With the establishment of his normal school, interest in Lewis's new purposive exercise system had spread rapidly as his teacher-converts left Boston and traveled to many parts of the world. Moses Coit Tyler, for instance, an early trainee of Lewis's, arrived in London in May 1863 with letters of introduction from Lewis and William Lloyd Garrison.[37] Tyler quickly established a school in London for physical culture, placed articles in several British magazines and newspapers, gave lectures before various scientific bodies, and even instructed the royal family.[38] During his stay, Tyler established satellite schools in other parts of England, and penned *The Brawnville Papers,* a satirical novel about the need for exercise that appeared both as a book and as installments in the *Herald of Health,* a leading American physical culture magazine.[39]

Another former student, Adele Parot, introduced Lewis's New Gymnastics to San Francisco in late 1862 and lobbied for the passage of California's mandatory physical education legislation in 1866, the first legislation requiring physical training in the public schools in the United States.[40] During the same period, Dr. Sarah Emerson, who trained at Lewis's gymnasium in Boston, took the system to Honolulu.[41] According to Eastman, schools teaching the Lewis system were also reported in Russia, Germany, Scotland, Africa, India, and "wherever the English language was spoken."[42]

In some American cities, it appears that gymnastics clubs based on Lewis's system formed even though no instructors were available. During the Civil War, for instance, Lewis reported that he sent magazines to the South where groups of women met regularly in some of the larger towns to practice gymnastics.[43]

Undeniably, Lewis's system had its greatest impact on the physical education programs in America's female colleges and seminaries. Miss Evans, the calisthenics teacher at Mount Holyoke, was sent by the trustees to enroll in the Lewis Normal Institute for Physical Education in the summer of 1862. The senior Edward Hitchcock was behind this decision, as he believed that the New Gymnastics were superior to the calisthenics drills the Mount Holyoke girls normally performed. Accompanying Evans to Lewis's school was a Miss Blanchard, and the two women returned to Boston the next winter for another three weeks of instruction.[44] The following year, a Lewis normal school graduate, Miss Trine, traveled out from Boston to give lessons to the entire Mount Holyoke faculty.[45] Vassar also adopted the New Gymnastics as part of their required curriculum.[46] Michigan offered Lewis's system to its few women students early in 1863, although it continued to promote military drill for male students.[47] Lucy B. Hunt, a first-year student at Lewis's Family School for Young Ladies in 1866, introduced the system to newly formed Smith College in 1875. Six years later, she published her own interpretation of the Lewis system entitled *Hand-Book of Light Gymnastics*.[48]

An examination of other exercise books and popular magazines from the next several decades of the nineteenth century also gives solid evidence of Lewis's influence. Dr. M. L. Holbrook, for instance, publisher and editor of the *Journal of Hygiene and Herald of Health*, spent two years studying with Dio Lewis and thought so much of the doctor and his system that he named his son Dio Lewis Holbrook.[49] Also,

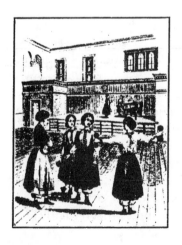

Figure 80: Vassar College Gymnasium in 1866. Note the New Gymnastics implements and the piano for musical accompaniment. From: Fred Eugene Leonard, *A Guide to the History of Physical Education* (1923).

Edward Hitchcock, Jr.'s *A Manual of the Gymnastic Exercises as Practiced by the Junior Class in Amherst College* was essentially a lengthy section of lightweight dumbbell exercises, set to music, to be performed in a large gymnastics hall with a painted floor. Although Hitchcock claimed the exercises as his own, they were clearly derived from Lewis's system.[50] In a letter to Gulick written more than a decade after the publication of his book, Hitchcock admitted that Lewis "was the only *teacher* in gymnastics I ever had." Hitchcock first visited Lewis's gym, he wrote, after having read Lewis's book on *The New Gymnastics*. Hitchcock did not enroll in the Normal School, but he stayed for a period of time as an "honorary pupil." Through the years, Hitchcock reported, he corresponded and visited with Lewis. "I did not regard him as a great master, but now I consider him as the leader in class or aggregate gymnastics . . . give him a due mead of praise," he told Gulick, "for he was a pioneer in our line of work & was by no means a crank."[51]

Cornelia Clapp learned gymnastics from Miss Evans at Mount Holyoke and later assumed the post of gymnastic instructor at her alma mater. In 1883, "at the request of her pupils who were called upon to teach gymnastics in various schools to which they went," Clapp produced a small teaching manual based on Lewis's *New Gymnastics*.[52] Clapp's book, *Manual of Gymnastics Prepared for the Use of the Students of Mt. Holyoke Seminary*, probably did not circulate widely. As an instructional manual for teachers, however, it helped spread the Lewis system throughout the country and kept it viable as a system into the 1890s.[53]

## Courage and Strength to Take Up the Battle

Did Dio Lewis make a difference in the lives of American women? As a physical educator, the answer surely is an unqualified "yes." Lewis's promotional and entrepreneurial skills raised physical education for women to a new level. Lewis did it all. He lectured brilliantly and organized gymnastic clubs; he was a master teacher[54]; he founded the first exercise magazine published in the United States; he established the first normal school for the training of teachers in America; he published a bestselling textbook that stayed in print for thirty years; he insisted on the coeducation and physical equality of the sexes; and he conducted for four years an ambitious experimental school that generated an enormous amount of positive publicity in support of physical training for women.

Lewis's most significant contribution to the history of women's exercise, however, was broadly philosophical and difficult to quantify. It was an attitudinal contribution and resulted in both an emerging physicality and a growing independence among American women. Mrs. W. O. Lincoln reported, "I admired him much. He appeared to me a thoroughly honest man who had the full courage of his convictions and who by his frank and noble personality had the affection of all about him." Continuing, Lincoln wrote, "He was in earnest if any man ever was, and I believe him to have been, though much in advance of his day, a pioneer in the cause of women's advancement."[55]

"I entered his school," Lincoln, recalled, "worn out in body and mind, and a mere bundle of damaged nerves." Yet, following an eight-month stay, and daily doses of Lewis's systematic exercise, "[I] gained there, courage and strength to take up the battle and begin anew." Although deaf, Lincoln experienced so successful a transformation that Lewis offered her a job as a gymnastics teacher for 1867. When the school burned, however, there was no room for Lincoln. Lewis helped her find another position, and for a number of years she made her living as a gymnastics teacher.[56]

Finally, in responding to Gulick's request for information about other Lewis students, Lincoln's pride in the achievements of her classmates is apparent. "They were from all parts of the country and quite a number of them became prominent in various professions," she wrote.[57] Supported by Lewis, Lincoln and her classmates broke with the old pattern of separate sphere domesticity. Following their time with Lewis, the idea that they should have health, independence, and a profession seemed neither preposterous nor a social disadvantage. Eastman commented,

> As the years went on Dr. and Mrs. Lewis had abundant cause to feel satisfaction and pride in the large number of their pupils who not only filled with success the usual sphere of woman in the home, but who, in less accustomed ways became the world's helpers. The names of many of them are widely known as teachers, as physicians, and as artists, while others have been permanently identified with the organization of charities and the noble reform movements of the time.[58]

By 1870, American attitudes toward women's exercise in general and gymnastics in particular had changed to such an extent that female gymnastic teachers could be held up as heroines and role models. This is apparent in many aspects of Mary Alice Seymour's short story "Fern

Grove Gymnasium," in which Marion Berkely, the town's new gymnastics teacher, is painted as a nonpareil among women.[59]

According to Seymour, Berkely was a daredevil horsewoman capable of jumping stone fences. But her femininity was not compromised by this adventuresome behavior, nor by her regular exercise program. Instead, Berkely is described as intelligent, fluent in three languages, and possessed of a figure to rival that of the Venus de Milo. Nor were her attractiveness and femininity at odds with her intelligence or independence. Trained in the New Gymnastics of Dio Lewis, Berkely ran her own gymnastic school in which "the refining influences of Music, Art, Languages and Belles Lettres were adapted to the mind, as the Dio Lewis System was used to develop the body."[60]

It was clearly Seymour's intention to deliver several messages along with her short story. The first, and most obvious, was her championing of Dio Lewis and his system of gymnastic exercises for women. Her second, and equally important, message can be found in her flattering descriptions of Berkely's appearance, bravery, intelligence, and manners. "What fashionable woman of the world can endure as a rival a frank, truthful woman, thoroughly educated, mentally and physically?" Seymour asked in her own voice, suggesting that "young girls who excel in physical culture are the favorites and pets of every social circle in which they move."[61]

Undoubtedly, Dio Lewis would have approved of Marion Berkely. Berkely's physical beauty, fitness, intelligence, and independence exemplified the type of new woman he hoped would populate America. As women trained on his system and read his manifestos for female independence, their newfound physicality and confidence manifested itself in a number of ways. Here, again, Lewis's voice was not the first to deliver this message, but at mid-century his was undoubtedly the loudest and most persuasive. That women ascribed to his theories there can be no doubt. Consider, for instance, the language of "The Dumb Bells," a song dedicated to Dio Lewis:

> Go mount the platform, bells in hand ...
> Let music float from well-strung band ...
> Each heart takes up the gladsome strain ...
> And echo back its tones again ...
> Each fair round muscle leaps the measure ...
> Each eye responsive dances pleasure ...
> The bosom heaves, but not with sighs ...
> Care from the glad heart quickly flies ...
> New life is in the bounding step ...

A sweeter voice upon the lip . . .
The heart this pleasant story tells
We owe it to the "merrie belles."[62]

In a number of ways, Lewis changed forever the basic dialogue concerning women's bodies. Rather than encouraging women to view their physical ideal as small, frail, slightly ill, and painfully weak, Lewis championed health, vigor, and substance. He preached that there was beauty in muscularity and that women should view their bodies as "trainable"—subject to their personal will. These were new, important concepts for American women, concepts that freed women to realize that, within limits, they were actually in charge of their physical destiny.

Lewis must have smiled when he read J. H. Fletcher's comments about women and exercise in an 1871 article in *Good Words* magazine. "What we ought to admire is a form unconfined, well knit, 'supple as that of a panther,' with an arm rounded white and hard as marble, from the well-strung muscles under the polished skin."[63] And surely he must have nodded his head in approval when Prentice Mumford wrote in *Lippincott's* of the "coming woman" saying that she "will not be deficient in nerve or weak in muscle . . . The idea of woman as the weaker sex will become old-fashioned and finally obsolete. Physical strength is not for men alone . . . Male muscle may lift more pounds, but put that of the female in training, and it runs, leaps, and climbs as the female mind jumps at conclusions, as quickly as, if not quicker than, that of the male."[64]

Though it would be decades before American women achieved the full physical emancipation Lewis imagined—and many would argue that this emancipation has not been achieved even in the 1990s—Lewis encouraged American women to take their first faltering steps out of physical bondage. We should do Lewis the justice that Helen Lewis claimed for him more than one hundred years ago; we should realize that his contribution was a major contribution to the history of American womanhood.

[1][Dio Lewis], *Catalogue and Circular of Dr. Dio Lewis's Family School for Young Ladies, Lexington, Mass. 1867* (Cambridge: Welch, Bigelow and Company, 1867), 12.
[2]Ibid., 15.

[3]Lizzie Morley to "Dear Brother," [Edward Morley], 29 April 1866. Folder 5.18. The Edward Williams Morley Collection, California Institute of Technology Archives, Pasadena, CA.

[4]Lizzie Morley to "Dear Brother," [Edward Morley], 29 May 1866. Folder 5.18. The Edward Williams Morley Collection, California Institute of Technology Archives, Pasadena, CA.

[5][Lewis], *Cataogue and Circular for 1867*, 14.

[6]"We have two complete series of hot-air bath-rooms, and every variety of water-bath, with the various forms of spray," Lewis wrote in [Dio Lewis], *Catalogue and Circular* [1866], 5.

[7]On page 4 of both the 1866 and 1867 catalogs, Mrs. Lewis is described as responsible for "Dress, and the Duties of School-mother."

[8]Eastman, *Biography*, 112.

[9][Lewis], *Catalogue*, 1866, 14-15.

[10]Lewis had signs erected every quarter mile on all the roads leaving Lexington to mark the distance the girls walked.

[11]Ibid., 15.

[12]Following his brief career as the secretary of the manual labor society, Weld spent several decades as an itinerant abolitionist. In 1854, having lost his voice from excessive lecturing, he decided to open a school for boys at Eaglewood, New Jersey. Lewis visited Weld's school several times and considered it in some ways a model for his own Family School for Young Ladies. Lewis observed, "The happiest day during the months of preparation for the Lexington School was that on which Mr. Weld consented to join me in its management." Quoted in Eastman, Biography, 96-97. See also Robert H. Abzug, *Passionate Liberator: Theodore Dwight Weld and the Dilemma of Reform* (New York: Oxford University Press, 1980): 286-87.

[13]The subjects covered by the thirty-member faculty included Physical Culture, Anatomy, Physiology, Hygiene, Chemistry, Mental and Moral Science, Logic, Rhetoric, English Classics, Ancient Classics, Natural Science, English Philology, History, French, Zoology, Geometry, Natural Sciences, Mathematics, German, Italian, Spanish, English Literature, Elocution, Piano, Voice, Painting in Water Colors, Natural Theology, Local History, Ethics, Domestic Economy and Laws of Health, and Gymnastics.

[14][Lewis], *Catalogue* [1866], 16.

[15]Dio Lewis, Elizabeth Cady Stanton, and James Read Chadwick, "The Health of American Women," *The North American Review*, No. 313 (December 1882): 506.

[16]Charles Hudson, *History of the Town of Lexington, Middlesex County, Massachusetts, From its First Settlement to 1868, With a Genealogical Register of Lexington Families* (Boston: Wiggin & Lunt, 1868), 376.

[17]"Letter from Lexington, Mass.," 9 June 1866, newspaper clipping, Lewis Scrapbook.

[18]Eastman, *Biography*, 101.

[19]Lewis not only bragged about the intelligence of his night watchman, but he installed a time clock and required the security guard to punch in on an hourly basis to make sure he didn't sleep. [Lewis], *Catalogue, 1867*, 29.

[20]Lizzie Morley to "My dear Brother," [Edward Morley], 9 November 1866. Folder 5.20. The Edward Williams Morley Collection, California Institute of Technology Archives, Pasadena, CA.

[21]Throughout her correspondence with Luther Gulick, Mrs. Lewis refers to the fact that the Lexington fire destroyed most of their papers and records. In 1898, she did not have a full set of school catalogues, a school diploma, or a full set of Lewis's *Gymnastic Monthly*. See, for instance, Mrs. Dio Lewis to Luther Gulick, 25 March 1898, Lewis Scrapbook.

[22]Ibid.

[23]Sarah A. Ashley to Luther Gulick, 18 February, 1898, Lewis Scrapbook.

[24]See Eastman, *Biography*, 117-25, for details on the fire and return to Boston.

[25]Mrs. W. O. Lincoln to Luther Gulick, 17 August 1898, Lewis Scrapbook. Eastman's biography of Lewis made no mention of the normal school following the fire.

[26]F. G. Welch to Luther Gulick, 19 February, 1898, Lewis Scrapbook.

[27]Leonard, *A Guide to the History of Physical Education*, 271. Welch also directed physical education at Dartmouth College in 1867–1868, and at Wesleyan University in 1868–1869.

[28]T. J. Ellinwood, "Prof. Welch's School of Physical Culture," *The Herald of Health and Journal of Physical Culture* 16 (November 1870): 227. Welch also promoted the Lewis system through the publication of *Moral, Intellectual, and Physical Culture; or, The Philosophy of True Living*, (New York: Wood & Holbrook, 1869), a textbook on gymnastics and healthy living that contained a lengthy section on Lewis's theories. According to Welch, his condensation of the Lewis system occurred with the "full consent and best wishes of my friend Dr. Dio Lewis" (p. viii).

[29]F. G. Welch, M.D., *Manual of Gymnastics, Published in this Form (By Permission of the Author) for her own Class, By Mary T. Orcutt, Teacher of Gymnastics in Tilden Ladies' Seminary* (Rutland: Tuttle & Co., 1874) 1.

[30]Eastman, *Biography*, 364.

[31]Resolution passed by the Martha Vineyeard Summer Institute class, 1 August, 1884, Lewis Scrapbook.

[32]Dio Lewis to Abigail May, Boston, Massachusetts, 18 July, 1881. A-134, Folder 37, May-Goddard Family Collection, Schlesinger Library, Vassar College, Cambridge MA.

[33]He also published an anti-smoking pamphlet: *Dio Lewis, Tobacco* (Boston: W. L. Green & Co, 1870). Dio Lewis, M.D., *Our Girls* (New York: Harper & Brothers, 1871); Dio Lewis, *Curious Fashions* (New York: Clarke Brothers, 1883); *Chats With Young Women* (New York: Fowler & Wells, 1874); *Chastity*

(New York: Fowler & Wells, 1874); *Our Digestion* (New York: Fowler & Wells, 1873), *Prohibition a Failure* (New York: Fowler & Wells, 1875).

[34]*Gypsies: Or Three Years' Camp Life in the Mountains of Califiornia* (Boston: Eastern Book Company, 1881); *In a Nutshell* (New York: Clarke Brothers, 1883); *Curious Fashions* (New York: Clarke Brothers, 1883); *The Dio Lewis Treasury* (New York: James R. Barnett, 1886).

According to Mrs. Lewis, Dio wrote three other books that were never published. *Longevity* was not issued, she reported to Gulick, because "the plates for a book cost so much," and she was uncertain she could regain her investment. Lewis also wrote two novels: *My Two Husbands* and *The Medfields*. According to Mrs. Lewis, "The first tells of the gradual decline of the first husband by consumption under the usual practise, and the recovery of the second husband of the same disease by a life in the open air and Hygienic treatment." *The Medfields* attempted to examine the laws of heredity in a large family. It focused, according to Helen Lewis, on the physical condition of the mother. "My husband did not publish these," she wrote, "fearing novels might detract from the interest in his other works on physical culture, which was his life work." Mrs. Lewis possessed the manuscripts for these novels and the book on longevity at the time of this letter. Mrs. Dio Lewis to Luther Gulick, 25 March 1898, Lewis Scrapbook.

Edward Hitchcock also reported that Lewis sent him a manuscript to review that dealt with female reproductive problems. Like *Longevity*, this book was never published. Hitchcock to Gulick, 24 March, 1898. Lewis Scrapbook.

[35]Both magazines ran for less than a year.

[36]According to his obituary in *The Auburn Bulletin*, Dio contracted "erysypilas," suffered for two or three days, and died. It was unexpected. He left the following written request regarding his body: "Although I am averse to the somewhat unpleasant notoriety which as yet cremation involves, my very strong conviction is that it is the right disposition of the dead. I leave directions that my body be cremated and that the ashes shall not be put into an urn, but in the earth, over which my wife may lovingly plant forget-me-nots. I direct also with my dear wife's assent, that all funeral parade and expense shall be avoided and that my remains be placed in a pine casket for removal to the crematory. I desire also that no flowers may be sent by my friends." The cremation took place on 24 May 1886. "Dr. Dio Lewis Cremated," *The Auburn Bulletin*, 24 May 1886.

[37]William Lloyd Garrison to William and Mary Howitt, 15 March, 1863, Massachusetts Historical Society, Boston, MA.

[38] See Moses Coit Tyler, *The New System of Musical Gymnastics as an Instrument in Education: A Lecture Delivered Before the College of Preceptors* (London: William Tweedie, 1864); and Eastman, *Biography*, 82-83.

[39]Moses Coit Tyler, *The Brawnville Papers: Being Memorials of the Brawnville Athletic Club* (Boston: Osgood and Company, 1869). The *Herald of Health*

series began with "Minutes of the Brawnville Athletic Club," *The Herald of Health and Journal of Physical Culture* 10 (August 1867): 50-54.

Upon returning to the United States, Tyler taught literature at Dio Lewis's Family School in 1867, and subsequently joined the faculty at the University of Michigan. At Michigan, Tyler remained dedicated to the cause of physical education and chaired the committee to examine the need for a department of physical education. See Moses Coit Tyler, chairman, *Report on a Department of Hygiene and Physical Culture in The University of Michigan, by a Committee of the University Senate* (Ann Arbor, MI: 1870).

[40]Robert Knight Barney, "Adele Parot: Beacon of the Dioclesian Lewis School of Gymnastic Expression in the American West," *Canadian Journal of Sport History* 5 (December 1974): 72-75.

[41]Helen Castle to Luther Gulick, 12 February 1898, Lewis Scrapbook.

[42]Eastman, *Biography*, 86-87.

[43]"Southern Subscribers," Lewis's *New Gymnastics for Ladies, Gentlemen and Children and Boston Journal of Physical Culture* 1 (May 1861): 112.

[44]Persis Harlow McCurdy, "The History of Physical Training at Mount Holyoke College," *American Physical Education Review* 14 (1909): 145-46.

[45]Mount Holyoke Journal Notebook VII, Box 10, 1 February 1863. Mount Holyoke College Archives, South Hadley MA.

[46]Leonard, *History of Physical Education*, 275.

[47]Nancy Struna and Mary L. Remley, "Physical Education for Women at the University of Wisconsin, 1863–1913: A Half Century of Progress," *Canadian Journal of History of Sport and Physical Education* 4 (May 1973): 8-9.

[48]Lucy B. Hunt, *Hand-Book of Light Gymnastics* (Boston: Lee and Shepard, 1881). See Thomas Woody, *A History of Women's Education in the United States* (New York: The Science Press, 1929) 120-22, for a discussion of the early physical education program at Smith. Hunt is listed as a first-year student in the 1866 catalogue of the Lewis Family School for Young Ladies.

[49]M. L. Holbrook to Luther Gulick, c. February 1898, Lewis Scrapbook.

[50]Edward Hitchcock, *A Manual of the Gymnastic Exercises as Practiced by the Junior Class in Amherst College* (Boston: Ginn, Heath & Co., 1884), 7. See also Edward Hitchcock, M.D., "A Report of Twenty Years Experience in the Department of Physical Education and Hygiene in Amherst College, to the Board of Trustees, 27 June 1881" (Amherst: C. A. Bangs & Co., 1881); and Edward Mussey Hartwell, M.D., *Physical Training in American Colleges and Universities: A Report to the Bureau of Education* (n.p., 1885), 31-32.

[51]Edward Hitchcock to Luther Gulick, 24 March 1898, Lewis Scrapbook. "I got a great many rudimentary ideas from him, which helped me to start & work class gymnastics at Amherst." From Lewis, Hitchcock learned to "systematically and conjointly handle dumbbells, wands, rings, bean bags & marches."

[52]McCurdy, *Physical Training at Mount Holyoke College*, 146-47.

[53]Mildred S. Howard, "History of Physical Education at Mount Holyoke College: 1837–1955," ts., Mount Holyoke Archives, Mount Holyoke College, South Hadley, MA.

[54]Besides teaching Edward Hitchcock, Lewis also taught Robert J. Roberts, who would go on to direct the physical training programs of the YMCA. Alfred Albert Smith, "Dio Lewis, Pioneer Physical Educator" (master's thesis, Springfield College, 1914), 20-21.

[55]Mrs. W. O. Lincoln to Luther Gulick, 17 August 1898, Lewis Scrapbook.

[56]Ibid.

[57]Ibid.

[58]Eastman, *Biography*, 119.

[59]Mary Alice Seymour, "Fern Grove Gymnasium," The *Herald of Health* 15 (March 1870): 110-12.

[60]Ibid.

[61]Ibid. 110.

[62]"The Dumb Bells," Lewis Scrapbook. This song was sung to the tune of "Kremo Kramo." Elipses in the song indicate the placement of a repeating line, "Ring-turn limber up the joints and toes," and the chorus:
Dumb-bell, rings, and amazing little clubs,
Me-nigh, Me-low, Me-arms
Twist 'em round, and turn 'em over
Ring-turn limber up the joints and toes."

[63]J. H. Fletcher, "Feminine Athletics," *Good Words* 20 (December 1871): 534.

[64]Prentice Mumford, "The Coming Woman," *Lippincott's Monthly Magazine* 9 (January 1872): 107.

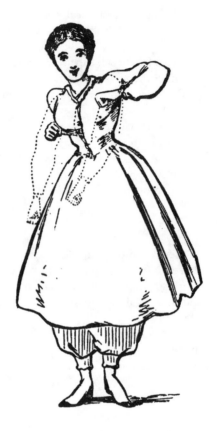

Figure 81: Healthy young womanhood as portrayed in *Watson's Manual of Calisthenics* (1864).

# Chapter 11
## "Reaping the Reward":
## The Quest for Health by
## Lizzie Morley and Her Sisters

A s a case study of the influence purposive exercise had on the lives of many antebellum women, "Lizzie" Morley's letters to her brother, the chemist Edward William Morley, provide solid evidence that such exercise often had a life-changing effect. Twenty-three-year-old Anna Elizabeth Morley became a patient of Dr. Dio Lewis in 1866. Prior to her arrival at Lewis's Family School for Young Ladies in Lexington, she had endured five years of gradually diminishing vitality. Under Lewis's supportive egalitarian care, however, this trend was soon reversed. Delighted by the newfound health and vigor she acquired at the Family School, Lizzie wrote in 1866, "I am improving very rapidly indeed. It took me a long time to get accustomed to the strain of gymnastics and the different modes of treatment," but now, she continued, "I am reaping the reward of my patience."[1]

Morley was born into an upper-class New England family. Her father was the Yale-educated minister Sardis Brewster Morley. Her mother was Anna Clarissa Treat, whose surviving letters suggest a woman of education and intellect. Lizzie and her brother, Edward, a student at Andover Theological Seminary when the correspondence opened, hoped to become teachers and make a contribution to the world.[2] Lizzie began this quest by entering Mount Holyoke Female Seminary in 1861. Almost at once, however, she began to chafe at the way the school's strict regulations and demanding timetable eroded her intellectual ambitions and her physical health.

Although clearly striving to maintain a note of optimism in other parts of her letters, eighteen-year-old Lizzie complained frequently about the school's unrealistic academic standards. "We are required to spend 2¼ hours on every lesson," Lizzie explained to Edward. "I . . . cannot learn the lessons in that time," she continued. For instance, I cannot read from 50 to 100 pages in Goldsmith's Greece, study five or six pages in Classical Dictionary, and learn the history lesson in 2¼ hours." Lizzie reported that she spent at least three hours on every lesson. She told Edward that the Mount Holyoke schedule and academic demands were so rigorous that "perhaps you have heard the remark that if any one lost a minute at Mt. Holyoke Seminary they could not make it up in a year. Now this remark is not strictly true but much truer than I ever supposed till I came here and learned something of its truth by experience, certainly the half hours and hours never flew so rapidly. 'Tempus doesn't fugit,' is not true here."[3]

Returning after the Christmas break to begin another semester at Mount Holyoke, Lizzie again complained of the school's heavy demands. "Our time is occupied somewhat as follows," she wrote to Edward in January 1862. "School exercises and domestic work, 3 3/4 hours, half an hour singing, half an hour gymnastics, half an hour writing, half an hour walking . . . about an hour and a half at table, including evening devotions, then allow for all necessary interruptions, and I have the whole care of our coal fire, and how much time is left for a lesson? . . . I think a body has enough to do."[4] Realizing that she had not yet bothered to ask about her brother's health, Lizzie slowed her diatribe to inquire, "Oh! dear how do you feel?" before finally commenting on her own state, "I am as ugly and cross as ever I can be, provoked and discouraged in the bargain. If we could sit up as late as we want, or else rise as early, there would be some common sense in it. But the idea that you can't stir without breaking some of the 70 rules is provoking."[5]

A major factor in Lizzie's frustration with Mount Holyoke's repressive timetable was that it allowed her so little time for exercise. Although she, like all Mount Holyoke students, practiced calisthenics every day and felt lucky that her manual labor assignment was ironing tablecloths—"pretty good work," Lizzie told Edward—she clearly did not view either of these activities as particularly recreative.[6] Apparently, neither did Edward, for on 5 December 1861, he sent her money to buy a pair of ice skates. Lizzie wrote in thanks, "Some skates are exactly what I needed to draw me away from my studies, in order to take more exercise."[7]

Although the letters never reveal a diagnosis of the health problems that began to affect Lizzie in 1863, it is possible that emotional factors—particularly in response to the overly protective attitudes of some members of Mount Holyoke's faculty—contributed to her physical decline. Trying to explain to Edward her growing feelings of depression, ill health, and weakness, Lizzie wrote,

> You remember when I was at home, almost everyone said that I was looking very strong and healthy, better than at any time since I've lived at W[illiamstown]. Here, everyone says that I look sick, and knows I am not well. Now exactly what to think I don't know . . . I

am rather amused sometimes when Miss Ward begins to ask me how
I do. I always insist that I am perfectly well and she ends off with
some good advice to be very careful.[8]

Another instructor, Miss Homer, also contributed to Lizzie's con-
fusion. "I went down to see Miss Homer about my health last night,"
Lizzie wrote to Edward in May 1863. "I believe she is going to doctor
me the rest of the term. She advises me to stay out of any kind [of]
school next year, remain at home without studying, and try to rest."
Lizzie was unable to accept Miss Homer's suggestion and told her, "I
did not know which corner of creation she intended putting me in if
she expected to stop my studying [for] a whole year."[9]

Morley's ambition and intellectual competitiveness may well have
contributed to her health problems. "I have easy studies and get along
nicely in both of them," Lizzie reported to Edward in June 1863. "Still I
am too ambitious to be contented. I want to do something that will
count: something worth speaking of." But Lizzie wondered how to
achieve those goals,

> when I seem everywhere to get the reputation of undertaking more
> than I ought. Last Thanksgiving, Miss Ward told me quite seriously
> one day that there was one lesson she wished I could learn, but she
> was afraid I never should. At any rate she was sure if I did it would be
> one of the hardest I ever mastered. I inquired with considerable
> interest what it was, thinking if it was so difficult it would be best to
> commence it immediately. My ardor cooled very much when she
> said it was only 'to learn to never go beyond my strength and do
> more than I am able, whatever the inducements may be.' I tried to
> laugh it off, but she was so solemn and earnest that I have not forgot-
> ten it, especially as she gives me a good many cautions.[10]

Although the only tangible physical ailments Lizzie ever discussed
in her letters to Edward were an occasional headache and a pain in her
side, her time at Mount Holyoke clearly eroded her confidence in her
health and vigor. In January 1863, Lizzie told her brother, "I am *tired*
but don't want to rest, can't rest."[11] Less than a week later, Lizzie wrote,
"I hardly know what is the matter with me, but think it may be because
I am tired. I have been suffering a good bit this week from depression
of spirits."[12] In May, she wrote, "I cannot tell you how glad I was to
receive your letter, I was feeling very blue and low spirited . . . I have
been feeling so for some time and cannot succeed in throwing it off
entirely, but account for it on the ground that I am not very well. Not

that I would have you think that I acknowledge that I am sick, not so by any means." Lizzie tried to believe there was little wrong with her that a good rest wouldn't cure. "But bah! what the use?" she asked Edward. "I am not sick, only of medicine. My side has not troubled me half as much since I grumbled a little about it. I was tired and worn out, so it took it upon itself to complain, that's all." Just the same, she concluded, "I am going to be careful."[13]

Despite her vow to be careful, Lizzie continued to have physical problems. Over the objections of her teachers, Morley decided to take a year's leave and study during 1863—1864 at the Abbott Academy in Andover, Massachusetts. She took a lighter academic load at Abbott, but because of her proximity to Edward did not write any letters. In the summer of 1864, Lizzie moved home where she attempted the rest cure recommended by her Mount Holyoke instructors. When, after approximately eighteen months, that approach also failed to produce vitality and vigor, Lizzie and her family decided that she should try more radical measures to restore her health. Thus it was that in late March or early April of 1866, Lizzie arrived at the Family School for Young Ladies in Lexington, Massachusetts, to become a patient of Dr. Dio Lewis.[14]

Although Lizzie always identified herself as a patient while in Lexington, she also participated in academic classes at the Family School for Young Ladies, and she prepared a piece to be read at the Spring Graduation Exhibition.[15] She commented favorably on Lewis's educational philosophy. "The Institution is not only a literary institution but is also designed for physical education . . . My own conviction of the matter is, that whereas in other schools the pupils are pushed unmercifully at times, here they have adopted a happy medium. The classes certainly accomplish a great deal of work as seen in their rapid improvement."[16]

Morley also spoke well of the teachers she met at the school. Lewis has recruited a "very fine corps of teachers," she wrote, adding that "in every department, Dr. Lewis [has hired] . . . the most capable persons that he possibly can [find]."[17] The patients and students "come from all parts of the United States and even from England, " Morley explained. "This school is gaining a wide reputation . . . It is an aristocratic school—as much so as any in the country . . . the society is most select. Certainly there is a very nice set of girls here this year."[18]

Although Mount Holyoke had sent two instructors to receive training in Lewis's methods in 1862, it does not appear that Lizzie participated at Mount Holyoke to any great extent in their version of Lewis's gymnastics. Whether that was through a conscious decision on her part or because of the school's concern with her health is not clear. In January 1863, while on vacation, Lizzie made herself a red flannel gymnastics dress. When she returned to Mount Holyoke, she wrote to Edward, "I have not yet begun to practice gymnastics, at least not since I finished my dress. I should rather like to try it but presume I shall [get] enough chances by and by."[19] If Morley did get her chance before leaving school in June, she did not mention it in her letters to Edward.

Once she arrived in Lexington, however, Lizzie spent almost all of her time involved in either the practice of the New Gymnastics, recreational games, or horseback riding. "After leaving you at the depot," she wrote to Edward on 29 April 1866, "I hurried back to the Doctor's parlor and found another game of Jack Straws just commenced. I joined the company and we played for a while when Doctor Lewis proposed a game of Squails . . . We were no sooner started than it was time for a general exercise in school . . . Soon came our dancing lesson."[20] Lewis's movement cure prescription for Lizzie included horseback rides twice a day—prior to breakfast and at six o'clock each evening. The evening rides often lasted two hours. "We ride just in time to see the *gorgeous sunsets* which we have here," she told Edward, "some of the most beautiful I ever saw."[21] Lizzie also reported that Lewis insisted on her riding even when she was not feeling particularly well. Forced to ride on a Saturday evening when she had asked to be excused, Lizzie later admitted to Edward that she felt Lewis had been right to encourage her. "I was very tired when I returned," she noted, "but rested from it in a few hours."[22]

Lizzie found much to admire in Dio Lewis. She described him as "frank and openhearted,"[23] "very kind and considerate," and she told her brother that she believed he would like Lewis "as a *man*."[24] Lizzie certainly did. " I like Dr. Lewis very much," she wrote, "and also his wife." Furthermore, she wrote to Edward in another letter, praising the doctor and his system of gymnastics, Dr. Lewis is a "very generous man, and is constantly making outlays for the benefit of teachers, scholars and patients."[25] However, what clearly pleased Lizzie most about her stay in Lexington was the fact that Lewis treated his patients and students as adults. "Dr. Lewis does not make a strict code of rules, and then set spies to watch the scholars," Morley wrote. "He controls the pupils by love and they would consider it dishonorable to deceive him or to try to evade his wishes."[26]

Lizzie's only dissatisfaction with Lexington was that her health did not improve as rapidly as she had hoped. She made gradual progress throughout April, but in May 1866, she burdened Edward with the tale of roommate troubles, a situation that had left her emotionally depressed and "completely exhausted." Describing her frustrations to Edward, Lizzie wrote, "I fear I have not gained as I ought to since being here . . . It makes me feel very much discouraged . . . I'd like to be a caterpillar for the privilege of resting in a little sanctuary of my own with none to molest or make [me] afraid."[27] One week later, however, having moved into a more favorable room and away from her troublesome roommate, Lizzie reported a noticeable change in her health. "I am now improving rapidly and am in good spirits," Lizzie wrote to Edward, adding, "I feel better today than I have for months."[28]

The move to a private room was a turning point in Lizzie's physical and emotional transformation. Writing to Edward in June, she claimed to be gaining "very rapidly indeed. I don't know of but one patient," she wrote, "that is gaining faster than I am and hers is a different case entirely. Within the last two or three days as I have come to realize how very fast I am improving, I have hardly been able to think or talk of anything else."[29] Furthermore, Lizzie told Edward, "I am not writing this today merely because it is one of my very brightest days, but because I know what I write is true. Dr. Lewis . . . the nurse . . . and all that knew me when I first came here speak of the change in me. Are you not glad for me?"[30]

"Last night," Lizzie reported in the same letter, "I saw Dr. Lewis professionally. He thinks I am gaining very rapidly and says I shall make a *strong* woman [Morley's emphasis]. I am now put on a diet, a thing that I am very glad of. For dinner I have beef and graham bread, for breakfast, graham bread and butter and stewed fruit with cracked wheat and butter. I am to have nothing else for the present, not even sugar, milk, gravy or anything of the kind." Delighted by her progress and the imminent prospect of a total cure, Lizzie vowed to Edward, "I am glad for it is best for me and I am willing to deny myself anything for the sake of health." Continuing, Lizzie added, "It seems . . . as if I was waking up from a long, terrible dream, as if a dark cloud were passing away that had clouded my whole life. It makes me very happy to live once more."[31]

In July, with the opening of Dio Lewis's normal school, Lizzie's enhanced strength and fitness allowed her to participate in the school as an unenrolled student. Writing on 13 July 1866, she reported that she practiced with the normal school students every day and "so far have enjoyed it very much." There were forty students in the class, and she told her brother that "some of them will make very fine gymnasts and do credit to their teachers and to the Institution."[32] "I have become very ambitious in regard to gymnastics," she confided to Edward. "To tell the truth I have been perfectly fascinated with gymnastics."[33]

Even Lizzie's mother got involved in exercise, with Lewis's blessing. In September, Anna Morley went to Lexington for a six-week visit during which she also took part in the exercise program. In a letter to Edward, accompanying one of Lizzie's letters, Mrs. Morley encouraged him to visit Lexington as well and participate in the exercise sessions. "For awhile it is hard," she wrote, "bringing out aches and pains unknown before," but once past that time, she claimed, "one often gains rapidly."[34]

Perhaps the most remarkable thing about Lizzie's letters from Lexington is the sense of her growing independence. Although she still suffered from occasional spells of weakness, she seemed more resolute in her decision to exercise and remain healthy. Morley also grew in political understanding, becoming increasingly critical of the traditional roles assigned to women by Catharine Beecher, the ardent proponent of separate spheres, who had joined Lewis's faculty in the fall of 1866.[35] Despite the fact that Lewis described Beecher as vital to the life of the school, Lizzie found her lectures silly. "Miss Catherine Beecher is here now lecturing to the girls," she wrote to Edward. "Her lectures consist of a good deal of twaddle about young ladies of position learning to do housework and to take care of children. She has a *few* very good ideas," Lizzie wrote, "but they are mingled with so much nonsense that one becomes completely disgusted."[36]

Beecher could also be rude, according to Lizzie, who told Edward that upon entering the school's sitting room one evening, she found Beecher reading a newspaper. Beecher invited Lizzie to join her for a visit, but throughout their conversation continued to look at the paper, even reading aloud small sections from time to time. "She was so rude that I [was] almost offended," Lizzie told Edward. "I treated her as politely as I could while I remained, but I can assure [you] I felt determined not to be caught so again and made a hasty retreat."[37]

Although Lizzie Morley was only one woman, her experiences with the New Gymnastics and the Lexington school suggest that Lewis helped to bring about the emergence of a new type of nineteenth-century woman. Not only did Lewis point Morley in the direction of strength, vigor, and physical endurance, he also opened her eyes to the possibility of a different kind of life. Although she did not become a gymnastics teacher, her exposure to Lewis's exercise regimen and to his social philosophy changed the course of her life. Lizzie understood that her battle for health was as real as the war that had just riven the country. "Had I been less courageous," she wrote on one occasion, "I should have despaired of being benefitted."[38]

The record is not clear as to when, or how, Lizzie left Lexington. Her collection of letters to Edward end in November 1866, and the surviving letters from other family members provide no information on her relationship to exercise. What *is* known about the remaining years of Morley's life is that she finally found a job that allowed her to fulfill her earlier dream and "to do something that will count, something worth speaking of."[39] In the mid-1870s, she traveled to China as an independent missionary, taught school there for approximately fifteen years, and then married, at age fifty, the Reverend Howard Stanley Nichols. They were "very, very happy" together and adopted a Chinese daughter in 1906.[40] Lizzie and her husband stayed in China until 1915, and then retired to Wilton, New Hampshire, where she died in 1918, at age seventy-five.[41]

*****

Lizzie Morley was not the only nineteenth-century woman whose life improved through an involvement with purposive exercise. In 1842, Julia Stillman, a former Mount Holyoke student, wrote from her home to tell Mary Lyon that, "I have been perfectly well, following the adoption of a plan of exercise."[42] In 1864, a woman described at one time as "emaciated almost to a skeleton" reported to hydropathic exercise advocate Russell Trall that "I have lately had plenty of outdoor exercise, and have grown so strong and robust you would hardly know me."[43] And Fanny Johnson, who adopted the shortened skirts of the "American costume," as well as a program of regular exercise, reported to physician and *Letter Box* editor Harriet Austin in April 1858, "I am pretty well and keep most of the flesh I gained. I spend much of my leisure time riding or romping out of doors with the children or the dog."[44] In that same issue of *The Letter Box*, Lizzie Lawrence reported from Boston that she took at least a mile walk each morning.[45] From physician Eliza Rodgers came news that there were twenty-five women in Pleasant Valley, Wisconsin, and its two neighboring communities who adopted the "masculine mode of riding" as a regular form of exercise in 1864.[46]

Hattie Smith reported in the *Laws of Life* on her twenty-year experiment with hygienic living in 1872. A former water cure patient, Smith maintained that "in all my efforts to regain lost health, I regard exercise as one of the most important agencies." Smith walked every day and on several occasions traveled as far as twenty miles in a day without any noticeable distress. "I *like* to walk," she confided. "No one knows how much I enjoy my excursions."[47] Mary Raymond of Melrose, Wisconsin, claimed that her health and strength dramatically improved after she decided to follow the laws of health and partake of regular, vigorous, outdoor exercise.[48] Emeline Dodge reported a similar transformation in 1868. To cure her weak back, Dodge adopted the American costume, changed her diet, and began doing regular exercise. "At the end of six months, I had gained ten pounds in flesh," she reported. At the end of eighteen months, "[I] walked five miles at one time."[49] Women even recognized that their matrimonial chances might improve if they increased their physical development. Twenty-three-year-old "Constance" wrote in her personal ad in the *Water Cure Journal* that she had a "tolerably well developed body" but hoped to improve it even further with appropriate exercise.[50]

Some women during the period of this study turned their physical conversions into business ventures. The female students who trained at Dio Lewis's normal school, for instance, found that the stronger muscles and improved health they achieved from their use of dumbbells and Indian clubs were good preparation for the new profession of physical education. Other women explored other ways to turn exercise advocacy into a living. After practicing the movement cure for a few months, Mrs. Z. R. Plumb became a "full-chested and rosy-cheeked woman" and opened her own school of physical training on West Fourteenth Street in New York City. According to *Herald of Health* editor Russell Trall, Mrs. Plumb's gym, called the Academy of Physical Culture, had a large patronage and "is doing a good work in teaching the young muscles to grow, and the old ones how to stir."[51] Another woman, Mary Hall, opened the Brooklyn Ladies Gymnasium at 176 Atlantic Street in October 1859. The *American Phrenological Journal* reported that the opening of Hall's gym was attended by a distinguished group of educators, politicians, and theologians and that the group had nothing but praise for the competence of Miss Hall and the idea of a woman's gym.[52] Far more significant to the growth of the idea of exercise for women in the United States, however, was the syndicate of female lecturers, organized by health reformer Harriet Austin. The syndicate traveled throughout the Western states in the late 1860s and 1870s delivering the health reform and exercise message and serving as agents for Austin's *Laws of Life* journal.[53]

During the period between 1880 and 1900, several new systems of purposive training challenged the preeminence of Lewis's New Gymnastics in the field of physical education for women. The Sargent System—named after Harvard professor Dudley Allen Sargent—was eclectic, borrowing movements from a variety of sources. Also competing for recognition was a new version of Swedish Gymnastics introduced by Dr. Hartwig Nissen in Washington, D.C., and subsequently promoted by wealthy Boston socialite Mary Hemenway.[54] Both systems produced normal schools—Sargent's School of Physical Education and the Boston Normal School of Gymnastics—and trained women teachers. So successful were these newer systems that, by the early 1890s, Lewis's New Gymnastics had been largely supplanted as the most popular method of exercise for women.[55] What was never replaced in the hearts and minds of some American women, however, was Lewis's implicit promise that purposive training was important to their struggle for identity and equality. Feminist author Charlotte Perkins Gilman, for instance, the grandniece of Catharine Beecher, claimed to have been fundamentally changed by her love of gymnastics. According to historian Patricia Vertinsky, "Gilman's dedication to physical fitness derived partly from her ongoing feeling, intensified at adolescence, that she needed strength to cope with what she was beginning to perceive as the female burden of economic dependence and a confining domestic role."[56] Gilman's desire for strength and independence compelled her to learn to "vault and jump . . . go up a knotted rope, walk on my hands under a ladder, kick as high as my head and revel in the flying rings." "But best of all," Gilman reported, "were the traveling rings, those widespaced, single ones, stirrup-handled, that dangled in a line the length of the hall."[57] Gilman described her strength as "glorious" and reported that she could run a mile in seven minutes. In 1881, at age twenty-one, she even convinced Providence, Rhode Island, gymnasium owner, Dr. John Brooks, to open his gym to women so that she could continue to improve.[58]

Elizabeth Cady Stanton was another staunch proponent of women's exercise.[59] Although Stanton's age and increasing girth kept her from enjoying the bicycle fad of the 1880s and 1890s, she understood the movement's political importance. "Many a woman," she reported, "is riding to suffrage on a bicycle."[60] Frances Willard and the leadership of the Women's Christian Temperance Union also recognized the importance of physical training to the cause of women's rights. At the W.C.T.U.'s national convention for 1891, the group voted to establish a "Department of Physical Culture" to be headed by Frances W. Leiter. In her annual report for 1892, Leiter forcefully defended the temperance group's interest in physical training: "Physical education materially concerns the future success of women . . . the girl who can enter womanhood with a liberal education and good health can command the world." According to Leiter, "The success of all our plans for the advancement of women will largely be determined by her prevailing physical condition."[61]

By the end of the century, the physical condition of American women had considerably improved thanks to the efforts of Lewis and the other early exercise reformers. Their advocacy of exercise and a more robust physical model for womanhood offered an ideal healthier than that of the slender, ethereal, "steel-engraving" type of woman associated with the Jacksonian era. This larger, stronger, and more intelligent model of womanhood was epitomized by the glowing tribute paid to lecturer Frances D. Gage of St. Louis, Missouri. In a biographical study for *The Laws of Life*, Gage, yet another proponent and practitioner of purposive training for women, was described as a "large-hearted, large-headed, large-bodied, and in every way extraordinary woman . . . whose voice is melodious, her language . . . excellent, [and] her appearance majestic."[62] Health reformer and women's rights advocate James C. Jackson also picked up the banner for the ideal of Majestic Womanhood in the 1860s, and continued to wave it into the 1880s. Jackson argued that the women who have contributed most to America "have been of more than ordinary physical size—not always in their height, but in their muscular structure and the robustness of their physical frames."[63]

Through the end of the century, body size and proportion remained a critical issue in physical education and facilitated the growth of the new discipline of physical anthropometry. Phrenology's linking of exercise, body size, and intelligence also continued. As late as 1903, Dr. Wlliam T. Porter argued that a study of the children of St. Louis had proven that "those who had succeeded in getting into the highest grades were the tallest, and weighed the most, and that those who were in the lowest grades were the shortest, and weighed the least." A study in England supposedly corroborated this, causing American *Mind and Body* magazine to argue, "In other words, it has been found that, at corresponding ages, the more intelligent classes are taller and heavier than the less intelligent." Proper physical training, the article reasoned, would help improve intelligence.[64]

But it was not just the size of American women that had improved by the turn of the century; they were less often ill and less troubled by their monthly menstruation. As Martha Carey Thomas, president of Bryn Mawr College, argued in 1908, several generations of college-educated women tended to prove that "college women were not only not invalids, but that they were better physically than other women in their own class of life."[65] Furthermore, several turn-of-the-century statistical studies proved to the satisfaction of most members of the physical education community that there was no evidence, as conservative physician Edward H. Clarke suggested in 1873, that women impaired their future childbearing capacities through pursuing purposive exercise *and* intellectual education.

Although Dio Lewis no doubt had hoped that the widespread success of his system would forever silence Rousseau's eugenic apostles, Clarke's troublesome *Sex in Education* attempted to reopen the debate.[66] Clarke claimed that women could not stand the rigors of physical and intellectual education and must take to their beds with the onset of their menses each month. This time around, however, and largely because of the example of Lewis's Family School for Young Ladies, fewer physical educators were willing to accept Clarke's Rousseauian message regarding the need for gender-specific exercise. Women's colleges and private schools got around the Clarke problem by hiring physicians to help oversee their physical training programs. As numerous women's colleges opened throughout the United States in the closing decades of the century, provisions were made at nearly all of them for purposive exercise.[67] Harvard's head of physical education, the physician Dudley Allen Sargent, used his prestigious professional credentials to further the cause of women's training by establishing a women's gymnasium, opening the Sargent School for Physical Education, and evangelizing for women's exercise in mainstream newspapers and magazines.[68] Senda Berenson, director of women's physical training at Smith College from 1892—1911, knew from personal experience that involvement with purposive training could be a life-changing experience that would strengthen, rather than weaken, women. Born in Russia in 1868, Berenson immigrated to

Boston's crowded West End in 1875. According to historian Betty Spears, Berenson's adolescent dream was to find some way to escape the tenement where she lived with her extended family. Ill throughout childhood, Berenson entered the Boston Conservatory of Music at age twenty-one, hoping for a career as a music teacher. When health problems forced her to drop out of the conservatory, she applied for admission to the Boston Normal School of Gymnastics where she planned to train only long enough to regain her health and resume her musical education. Berenson became fascinated with exercise, however, and found the strength and good health she had never enjoyed during girlhood. Two years later, she took over as the director of physical training at Smith College.[69] Although Berenson's historical canonization was assured when she introduced basketball to her women students—an event that forever changed the course of women's physical education—school records and her surviving papers reveal that she continued to have a deep commitment to Swedish gymnastics and other forms of purposive training. Like Fowler and Lewis, Berenson believed, "All things being equal—the physically strong are the most intellectual of moral people."[70] In lecture and letter notes from the early 1890s, Berenson told of two young women, previously excused from exercise because of ill health, who, after performing supervised gymnastics, had gained "more vitality [and] strength." One of the young women even claimed, "Gymnastics is just what I needed." In her notes, Berenson wrote, "I could tell of many more students who have been put on the right road to larger usefulness, but what I have written is perhaps sufficient to show that this sort of work is much needed and very much worthwhile."[71]

In the closing decades of the nineteenth century, physical educators, along with other academic groups, struggled to establish a professional identity. At the Adelphi Academy in Brooklyn, New York, Dio Lewis met with forty-eight other American physical educators on 27 November 1885 to discuss by-laws for the first professional physical education society—the American Association for the Advancement of Physical Education.[72] Over the next century, as this professional group evolved into the approximately thirty thousand- member American Alliance for Health, Physical Education, Recreation, and Dance, advocacy of purposive training has remained an important focus of the physical education community's mission.

Reliance on purposive exercise as a major focus of the collegiate physical education curriculum for women, however, did considerably diminish following Senda Berenson's introduction of basketball to her students at Smith in the early winter of 1892. By 1910, sports and games had become common to the collegiate physical education curriculum, a change that led to the birth of intercollegiate sport for women and, ultimately, professional and Olympic competition for women.[73] Physical educators never totally abandoned purposive exercise, however. Freehand calisthenics remained a staple of physical education throughout the twentieth century, and the late 1970s saw the reemergence of resistance exercise and cardiovascular training as important components of a new curricular emphasis on physical fitness and "wellness." Thus it is no surprise that the basic tenets of late twentieth-century fitness and "wellness" mimic almost exactly the nineteenth-century's paean to moderation called the Laws of Health.

Even though professional physical educators of both sexes embraced sports such as basketball, field hockey, tennis, and rowing as replacements for most purposive exercise in early twentieth-century schools, many private physical culture entrepreneurs continued to promote purposive training outside the ivied walls of America's universities and academies. Following the Civil War, physical culture entrepreneurship escalated dramatically. Rubber chest expanders, dumbbells, Indian clubs, and a wide variety of home gymnasium appliances came on the market, while books such as William Blaikie's popular *How to Get Strong and How to Stay So* (1879) delivered the exercise-purposive training message to the middle and lower classes.[74] Bernarr Macfadden was the most successful of the many *fin de seicle* entrepreneurs, but he learned the tricks of this trade from men such as David L. Dowd and Eugen Sandow, who preceded him. Stirred by the same grand vision of the physical potential of women that inspired Lewis, Macfadden launched his own campaign to promote strength and exercise for women. This campaign resulted, in October 1900, in the first women's exercise magazine, *Woman's Physical Development*. Three years later, Macfadden held a woman's physique show in Madison Square Garden.[75]

Throughout the twentieth century, private entrepreneurs have continued advocating the benefits of various forms of purposive training for women. Women were taught to emulate swimming star Annette Kellerman in the Teens, to do Walter Camp's Daily Dozen in the Twenties, to "Streamline Your Figure" in the Thirties,[76] to lift weights with the Muscle Beach Girls in the Forties, to attend figure "salons" in the Fifties, to work out with Jack LaLanne and Bonnie Prudden on TV in the Sixties; to jazzercise in the Seventies, and to aerobicize or body-build in the Eighties and Nineties. But woven throughout the multitude of exercise prescriptions for twentieth-century women can be found most of the basic principles of early nineteenth-century purposive training.

One apt summation of the sea-change in the lives of American women brought about by the work of Lewis and other pioneers comes from one of Bernarr Macfadden's columnists, Helen Rowland, a regular contributor to *Physical Culture* magazine. Writing in 1900, Rowland asked,

> Where are the delicate creatures of yesteryear? Gone ... Walk down the main street of your city any fine morning, and note the army of bright-eyed, broad shouldered, straight-limbed young business women on their way to the shops and offices ... These are embryo women deluxe, and they know that in order to do their work they must keep themselves in perfect physical condition ... They are as proud of their Gibson shoulders, high chests and muscular arms as the old-fashioned woman was of her white hands and soft cheeks.[77]

The words of physician J. H. Hanaford are perhaps equally apropos. "Woman has muscles and she has a right to use them in a proper manner ... there is no reason why she should ignore them or be ashamed to develop them ... What if her limbs become a little rotund, her hands enlarged, her brow somewhat bronzed ... She need not be ashamed of it, since such efforts will impart just the vivacity, suppleness, stamina, and endurance that she will need."[78] Even more to the point is this message from *The Herald of Health,* as true for modern women as it was for Lizzie Morley and all the other women at whom it was aimed in 1870: "If we may presume to offer a word of advice to the 'weaker sex' it would be this: 'The country is ready to let you have your rights just as fast as you can take them. The true way to convince mankind that you have strength enough to qualify you for the privileges of human beings, is to get up and show the strength ... Fewer words and more deeds! Stop not to complain, but act!' "[79]

[1]Lizzie A. Morley to "My Dear Brother" [Edward Morley], 10 June 1866. File 5.19. Edward Williams Morley Collection, California Institute of Technology Archives, Pasadena, CA. Unless noted, all subsequent citations to correspondence between Lizzie and her family shall be from the Morley Collection at Cal Tech.

[2]Information on the Morley family can be found in Howard R. Williams, *Edward William Morley* (Easton PA: Chemical Education Publishing

Company, 1957), 3-13. Edward Morley's investigation of the effect of ether on the propagation of light—known as the Michelson-Morley experiment—supported Einstein's relativity theory.

[3]Lizzie Morley to "My dear Brother" [Edward Morley], 24 October 1861. Folder 5.1.

[4]Lizzie Morley to "My dear Brother" [Edward Morley], 28 January 1862. Folder 5.2.

[5]Lizzie Morley to Edward Morley, 28 January 1862.

[6]Lizzie Morley to Edward Morley, 24 October 1861.

[7]Lizzie Morley to "My dear Brother" [Edward Morley], 7 December 1861. Folder 5.1.

[8]Lizzie Morley to "My dear Brother" [Edward Morley], 20 May 1863. Folder 5.12.

[9]Ibid.

[10]Ibid.

[11]Lizzie Morley to "My dear Brother" [Edward Morley], 16 January 1863. Folder 5.12.

[12]Lizzie Morley to Edward Morley, 22 January 1863.

[13]Lizzie Morley to Edward Morley, 20 May 1863.

[14]The exact date of her arrival is not known. The first letter from Lexington is dated 10 April 1866. Folder 5.18.

[15]In a letter dated 10 April 1866, Folder 5.18, Lizzie asked her brother to bring her a copy of *Gray's Botany* so she could use it in the class she was to join. Lizzie referred to her piece for the exhibition in a letter dated 25 May 1866. Folder 5.18.

[16]Lizzie Morley to "My dear Brother" [Edward Morley], 29 May 1866. Folder 5.18.

[17]Lizzie Morley to "Dear Brother" [Edward Morley], 24 May 1866. Folder 5.18.

[18]Lizzie Morley to Edward Morley, 29 May 1866.

[19]Lizzie Morley to Edward Morley, 16 January 1863.

[20]Lizzie Morley to "Dear Eddie" [Edward Morley], 29 April 1866. Folder 5.18.

[21]Ibid.

[22]Lizzie Morley to "Dear Eddie" [Edward Morley], 3 September 1866. Folder 5.20.

[23]Lizzie Morley to "Dear Brother" [Edward Morley], 8 May 1866. Folder 5.18.

[24]Lizzie Morley to "Dear Brother" [Edward Morley], 17 May 1866. Folder 5.18.

[25]Lizzie Morley to "Dear Brother" [Edward Morley], 19 May 1866. Folder 5.18.

[26]Ibid.

[27]Lizzie Morley to Edward Morley, 29 May 1866.

[28]Lizzie Morley to Edward Morley, 25 May 1866.

[29]Ibid.

[30]Lizzie Morley to "Dear Brother" [Edward Morley], 10 June 1866. Folder 5.19.

[31]Ibid.

[32]Lizzie Morley to "Dear Eddie" [Edward Morley], 30 July 1866. Folder 5.19.

[33]Ibid.

[34][Anna Clarissa Treat Morley] to Dear Son [Edward Morley], 19 September 1866. Folder 5.20.

[35]Mae Haverson, "Catharine Beecher: Pioneer Educator" (Ph.D. diss., University of Pennsylvania, 1932) 227; and [Lewis], Catalogue and Circular of Dr. Dio Lewis's Family School for Young Ladies, 1866, 6. Beecher stayed in Lewis's employ for two years. She apparently left when a fire destroyed the Lexington facility, although it is remarkable how little Beecher had to say about her time in Lexington or about Dio Lewis in her autobiography. See Beecher, Educational Reminiscences and Suggestions, 85.

[36]Lizzie Morley to "My Dear Brother" [Edward Morley], 23 October 1866. Folder 5.20.

[37]Ibid.

[38]Lizzie Morley to Edward Morley, 10 June 1866.

[39]Lizzie Morley to "Dear Brother" [Edward Morley], 3 June 1863. Folder 5. 12.

[40]Elizabeth Morley Nichols to "Susie" [identity unknown], February 1908, Mount Holyoke College Archives, South Hadley, MA.

[41]Biographical File: Anna Elizabeth Morley Nichols, Mount Holyoke College Archives, South Hadley, MA.

[42]Julia Stillman to Mary Lyon, 29 August 1842. Sr. B. Writings, LD 7082.25 1837. Mount Holyoke College Archives.

[43] Quoted in [Russell Trall], "Rambling Reminiscences-No 30," The Herald of Health 3 (1864): 45.

[44]"Correspondence," The Letter Box 1 (15 April 1858): 23.

[45]Ibid.

[46]Eliza S. Rodgers, M.D., "The Riding Suit," The Herald of Health 4 (December 1864): 185.

[47]Hattie Smith, "My Experience in Health Reform," Laws of Life and Journal of Health 15 (July 1872): 203.

[48]"Extracts from Letters," The Letter Box 2 (February 1859): 11.

[49]Emeline Dodge, "How I Was Cured of a Weak Back," The Laws of Life 11 (October 1868): 151.

[50]"Matrimony," Water Cure Journal and Herald of Reforms 20 (October 1855): 95.

[51][Russell Trall], "Mrs. Plumb's Academy," The Herald of Health 2 (December 1863): 226.

[52]"Ladies Gymnasium," *American Phrenological Journal* 30 (November 1859): 76-77. Hall had run a women's gym at another address in Brooklyn the previous year.

[53]"Women Lecturing in the West," *The Laws of Life* 11 (July 1868): 109.

[54]Arthur Weston, *The Making of American Physical Education* (New York: Appleton-Century-Crofts, 1962), 34-39.

[55]Ibid. and Betty Spears and Richard Swanson, *History of Sport and Physical Activity in the United States* (Dubuque IA: William C. Brown, 1978), 177.

[56]Patricia Vertinsky, *The Eternally Wounded Woman: Women, Exercise, and Doctors in the Late Nineteenth Century* (New York: Manchester University Press, 1990), 206.

[57]Charlotte Perkins Gilman, *The Living of Charlotte Perkins Gilman: An Autobiography* (New York: D. Applegate and Co., 1935), 66-67.

[58]Charlotte Perkins Gilman, "The Providence Ladies Gymnasium," *Providence Journal* 8 (23 May 1883): 2.

[59]See, for instance, Dio Lewis, Elizabeth Cady Stanton, and James Read Chadwick, "The Health of American Women," *North American Review*, No. 313 (December 1882): 510-17.

[60]Quoted in Ann Koedt, Ellen Levine, and Anita Rapone, *Radical Feminism* (New York: Quadrangle Books, 1973), 32.

[61]Frances W. Leiter, *National Woman's Christian Temperance Union Department of Physical Culture* (n.p, 1892). Included in Scrapbook I, Health and Gymnastics in America, Department of Hygiene and Physical Education, Wellesley College Archives, Wellesley, MA.

[62]"Mrs. Frances D. Gage, of St. Louis, Mo.," *The Laws of Life* 3 (January 1860): 3.

[63]James C. Jackson, "Marriage and its Correlations," *The Laws of Life* 3 (November 1860): 159.

[64]"Physical Culture Underlies Success," *Mind and Body* 9 (January 1903): 249.

[65]Martha Carey Thomas, *Present Tendencies in Women's College and University Education* (n.p., February 1908), quoted in William O'Neill, ed., *The Woman Movement: Feminism in the United States and England* (Chicago: Quadrangle Books, 1969), 168.

[66]Edward H. Clarke, M.D., *Sex in Education: Or a Fair Chance for Girls* (Boston: James R. Osgood, 1873).

[67]Betty Spears, "The Emergence of Women in Sport," in *Women's Athletics: Coping with Controversy*," Barbara J. Hoepner, ed. (Oakland, CA: DGWS Publications, 1974), 26-31.

[68]W. Scott, *Physical Training in New England Schools* (Cambridge, MA: The People Publishing Company, 1899). See also Debbie Cottrell, "Women's Minds, Women's Bodies: The Influence of the Sargent School for Physical Education," (Ph.D. diss., University of Texas at Austin, 1993).

[69]Betty Spears, "Senda Berenson Abbott—New Woman: New Sport," in *A Century of Women's Basketball: From Frailty to Final Four,* Joan Hult and Marianna Trekell, eds. (Reston, VA: American Alliance for Health, Physical Education, Recreation, and Dance, 1991): 19-22.

[70]Senda Berenson, speech notes, typed copy, p. 29, from Box 42, "Publication-Speeches-Notes," Senda Berenson Collection, Smith College Archives, Northampton, MA.

[71]Draft of Senda Berenson's report to the Honorable Trustees of Smith College, Box 42, 44-45, "Publication-Speeches-Notes," Senda Berenson Collection, Smith College Archives, Northampton, MA. Ibid., 29. See also Senda Berenson, Speech notes, typed copy, 39-40, from Box 42, "Publication-Speeches-Notes," Senda Berenson Collection, Smith College Archives, Northampton, MA.

[72]Roberta Park, "Physiologists, Physicians, and Physical Educators: Nineteenth-Century Biology and Exercise, Hygienic and Educative," *Journal of Sport History* 14 (Spring 1987): 43.

[73]Ibid., 39. See also Roberta Braden Powell, "Women and Sport in Victorian America" (Ph.D. diss., University of Utah, 1981).

[74]William Blaikie, *How To Get Strong and How To Stay So* (New York: Harper & Brothers, 1879).

[75]See Jan Todd, "Bernarr Macfadden: Reformer of Feminine Form," in Jack Berryman and Roberta J. Park, eds., *Sport and Exercise Science: Essays in the History of Sports Medicine* (Urbana, IL: University of Illinois Press, 1992), 213-32.

[76]See, for instance, Charles M. Postl, *How To Streamline Your Figure* (Chicago: W. J. Fitzpatrick Co., 1939).

[77]Helen Rowland, "The Passing of the Helpless Woman," *Physical Culture,* undated clipping in D. A. Sargent Papers, Harvard University Archives, Cambridge, MA.

[78]J. H. Hanaford, M.D., "More Muscle for Women, *The Laws of Life* 16 (October 1870): 168.

[79]"The Weaker Sex," *Herald of Health* 15 (May 1870): 228.

# Methodology

The story of American women's involvement with purposive exercise began in New England. It was in New England that the first European exercise books reached American shores, it was there that the first school physical education programs began, it was there that the first public lectures on the need for physical training were delivered, and it was there that most of America's publishing houses first opened for business. For these reasons, this volume deals more completely with the growth of physical training in this region of the United States than it does with that of any other geographic area. It is my hope that future research on this topic will enable me to explore in greater detail the spread of these various exercise systems to other regions of the United States.

As a methodological imperative, I tried to balance this writing between a descriptive history of the books, magazines, and major historical figures that promoted physical training for women in the nineteenth century and a sociocultural analysis of the explicit and implicit promises such experts and their books made to American women. As I researched the antebellum era, it became clear that a significant body of didactic literature existed that remained largely unexamined. Because this research is one of the first attempts to examine systematically these early texts, content analysis has played a significant role in this treatise. As other sport scholars have done when looking at the nineteenth century, I include references in my analysis to some European texts, especially British texts.[1] However, I limited my use of non-American books to those that were reviewed in the United States or that had American editions—books to which I had reason to believe antebellum Americans had had access.

One of my primary research goals was to find first person evidence of women's participation in purposive exercise. To this end, I examined letters, manuscripts, and diaries in the university archives of Mount Holyoke College, Smith College, Wellesley College, Springfield College, and Harvard University. I spent time at the Arthur M. and Elizabeth Schlesinger Library on the History of Women in America at Radcliffe College, I examined the manuscript collections of the Boston Public Library, and I did research at the Massachusetts Historical Society. In these New England archives I was pleased to find scattered references by women to their pursuit of purposive exercise in the antebellum period. Unquestionably, the archives of Mount Holyoke College, which introduced purposive exercise in 1837, proved most useful in this quest.[2] I did not, however, find in my two research trips to New England a significant collection of letters (or a diary) kept by one person over a period of years that discussed issues related to health and exercise. This missing link turned up several thousand miles away, in the archives of the California Institute of Technology. At Cal Tech, in the family papers of scientist Edward Morley, reside a series of letters related to his sister, Anna Elizabeth Morley Nichols. Lizzie Morley's lively letters finally gave me the consistent voice I needed to corroborate my theories about the importance of exercise to American women.

My search for women's voices led me away from the conventional medical literature that has formed the basis of most studies on women's health and exercise and into the less well-known world of radical health reform literature. Here I found women frequently speaking about their own experiences and accommodations to health reform, just as twentieth-century historians might look in the letters' columns of *Shape, Muscle & Fitness*, and *Women's Sports and Fitness* rather than in the *Journal of the American Medical Association* or the *New England Journal of Medicine* for an understanding of how women actually incorporate exercise into their daily lives. I found the *Water-Cure Journal & Herald of Reforms*, the *American Phrenological Journal*, and the *Herald of Health & Journal of Physical Culture* to be rich in material related to the body and exercise. In *The Letter Box* and its successor, *The Laws of Life*, I discovered the liberating opinions of physician-publisher Harriett Austin, a hydropathic rebel, who began publishing so that her patients might stay in touch and continue to share their feelings about health, diet, and exercise. *Lewis's New Gymnastics for Ladies, Gentlemen and Children and Boston Journal of Physical Culture*, in its brief run in the early 1860s, gave me another view, especially in the monthly column purportedly written by Helen Lewis, the doctor's wife and most celebrated patient.

In addition to looking at every available issue of the above journals for the period of my study, I also combed the entire run of Sarah Hale's *The Ladies Magazine* and its successor, *Godey's Ladies Book*. For insight into feminist attitudes I examined all of Amelia Bloomer's *The Lily*. I also examined all issues of the *Journal of Health*, all of Horace Mann's *Common School Journal*, the entire run of the *American Journal of*

*Education*, all of William Brown's *The Mother's Assistant and Young Lady's Friend*, and *Dr. Buchanan's Journal of Man* between 1849 and 1853. Using *Poole's Index to Periodical Literature* and *The Wellesley Index to Victorian Periodicals*, I also traced references to women's purposive exercise in popular magazines such as the *Atlantic Monthly*.[3] Finally, I examined *Mind and Body*, published by the North American Gymnastic Union, for secondary source information on German-style gymnastics; *The Posse Gymnasium Journal*, for information on Swedish gymnastics; and *Dr. Hall's Journal of Health* and Bernarr Macfadden's *Physical Culture*, in an attempt to assess the course of women's purposive exercise after 1875.

Besides the letters of Lizzie Morley, the most significant archival discovery I made was that of a large scrapbook, compiled by physical educator Luther Gulick, on the life and contributions of Dio Lewis.[4] Gulick planned to write a biography of Lewis's life and set out, in the late 1890s, to contact Mrs. Lewis and as many of Lewis's former students and teachers as he could find. The resulting correspondence, clippings, and memorabilia provide an important personal dimension of a man I regard as one of the most important figures in the history of women's purposive exercise. Although Catharine Beecher's life has produced several scholarly biographies, Lewis's has not produced even one because of the lack of primary source material. Now, however, with the discovery of Gulick's scrapbook, we at last have some first person material on Lewis's life—through letters from Mrs. Lewis to Dr. Gulick; letters of reminiscence from Lewis's associates Moses Coit Tyler, Nathaniel T. Allen, and F. G. Welch; and letters from Lewis's students who, thirty years later, still remembered favorably their participation in the New Gymnastics. In part because of this discovery, I devote greater space in the present study to the life and contributions of Lewis than I do to any other exercise advocate. While I realize that this may skew the balance of my research findings, I feel strongly that these personal anecdotes and reflections provide a previously unexamined dimension to our understanding of Dio Lewis and his radical ideas about women that scholars of women's sport and exercise have not had previously.

---

[1]Both Patricia Vertinsky and Nancy Struna argue that nineteenth-century America and England shared similar sets of concerns about women's involvement with sport and exercise. See Patricia Vertinsky, *The Eternally Wounded Woman: Women, Exercise and Doctors in the Late Nineteenth Century* (New York: Manchester University Press, 1990), 17; and Nancy

Struna "Puritans and Sport: The Irretrievable Tide of Change," in Steven Riess, ed., *The American Sporting Experience: A Historical Anthology of Sport in America* (Champaign, IL: Leisure Press, 1984) 17.

[2]Smith and Wellesley also have impressive student archives, but the items they house primarily fell outside my time frame.

[3]William Frederick Poole, *Poole's Index to Periodical Literature, Vol. 1, 1802–1881*, rev. ed. (New York: P. Smith, 1938 [1882]) and *The Wellesley Index to Victorian Periodicals: 1824–1900* (Toronto: Toronto University Press, 1966).

[4]Gulick had a fervent interest in physical training and also collected books, pamphlets, and magazines on the subject, amassing an extensive collection that is now part of the Springfield College Library. There are numerous treasures in the Gulick Collection—a 1672 edition of *De Arte Gymnastica*, several scrapbooks put together by Edward Hitchcock, an unpublished speech by Dudley Allen Sargent and so on.

# Bibliography

## Archives and Manuscript Sources

Babson Library, Springfield College, Springfield, Massachusetts. Rare Books and Manuscripts Collection; Dio Lewis Scrapbook; Luther Halsey Gulick Thesis Collection; Luther Halsey Gulick Papers; Edward Hitchcock, Jr. Scrapbooks.

Boston Public Library, Boston, Massachusetts. Rare Books and Manuscripts. William B. Fowle Papers; Catharine Beecher Papers; and Boston School Board Records: 1850-1870.

California Institute of Technology, Pasadena, California. Institute Archives. Morley Family Papers, Edward William Morley Collection.

Harvard University, Cambridge, Massachusetts. Pusey Library, Harvard University Archives. George Barker Windship: Biography Files; *Record of the College Faculty*, vol. 14: 1845-1850; vol. 15: 1850-1855; Papers of Dudley Allen Sargent; Papers of the Physical Education Department.

Massachusetts Historical Society, Boston, Massachusetts. George Barker Windship Collection. Windship-May Family Papers.

Mount Holyoke College Library/Archives, South Hadley, Massachusetts. Mary Lyon Papers; Physical Education Department Collection; Mildred S. Howard Papers.

Radcliffe College, Cambridge, Massachusetts. Arthur M. and Elizabeth Schlesinger Library on the History of Women in America. Elizabeth Blackwell Papers; Phrenology File.

Smith College Library, Northampton, Massachusetts. Sophia Smith Collection and College Archives. Senda Berenson Collection; Physical Education Department Records; General Biographical Files.

University of Texas at Austin. The Todd-McLean Physical Culture Collection. Cursio-Herbst Naturopathy Collection; The Ottley Coulter Collection; The David P. Willoughby Collection; Amelia Bloomer Collection; James C. Jackson and Harriett Austin Collection; Sylvester Graham Collection.

Wellesley College, Wellesley, Massachusetts. Margaret Clapp Library, Wellesley College Archives. Papers of the Department of Hygiene and Physical Education, Including the Papers of the Boston Normal School of Gymnastics.

## Additional Unpublished Materials

Albertson, Roxanne. "Physical Education in New England Schools and Academies from 1780-1860: Concepts and Practices." Ph.D. diss., University of Oregon, 1974.

Borish, Linda J. "'The Lass of the Farm": Health, Domestic Roles, and the Culture of Farm Women in Hartford County, Connecticut, 1820-1870." Ph.D. diss., University of Maryland, 1990.

Bregman, Sydell. "William A. Alcott: A Teacher for Today." Master's thesis, Farleigh Dickinson University, 1972.

Bruland, Esther Byle. "Great Debates: Ethical Reasoning and Social Change in Antebellum America—The Exchange Between Angelina Grimke and Catharine Beecher." Ph.D. diss., Drew University, 1990.

"Mrs. Chapman"s Phrenology." [London] n.d. Mss. Boston Public Library.

Cole, Edith Walters. "Sylvester Graham, Lecturer on the Science of Human Life: The Rhetoric of a Dietary Reformer." Ph.D. diss., Indiana University, 1975.

Conklin, William D., comp. *The Jackson Health Resort: Pioneer In Its Field; As Seen By those who Knew It Well; Being an Account of the Institution"s Fiftieth Anniversary With Records of the Seventieth and the One Hundreth.* Dansville NY: 1971. Typescript. Todd-McLean Collection.

Cross, A. L. "GutsMuths: His Life and Ideas, In Relation to the Physical Training Movement." Master's thesis, Springfield College, n.d. Luther Gulick Thesis Collection. Babson Library, Springfield College.

Federle, James C. "Bodies, Gardens and Pedagogies in Late Eighteenth-Century Germany." Ph.D. diss., University of California at Berkeley, 1991.

Fish, Alanson Lester. "Life, Work, and Influence of Dio Lewis, A.M., M.D." Master's thesis, Springfield College, 1898. Gulick Thesis Collection. Babson Library, Springfield College.

Haddad, Gladys Marilyn. "Social Roles and Advanced Education for Women in Nineteenth-Century America: A Study of Three Western Reserve Institutions." Ph.D. diss., Case Western Reserve University, 1980.

"'Harriett Austin,' A lecture written at the request of Susan B. Anthony. Delivered at the Annual Suffrage Meeting of 16 January 1893, Metzerott"s Hall, Washington D.C." Herbst-Cursio Files, The Todd-McLean Collection, University of Texas at Austin.

Harveson, Mae Elizabeth. "Catharine Esther Beecher: Pioneer Educator." Ph.D. diss., University of Pennsylvania, 1932.

Kennard, June. "Women, Sport, and Society in Victorian England," Ph.D. diss., University of North Carolina at Greensboro, 1974.

Kent, Stanley Gregory. "Redefining Health: The Rise and Fall of the Sportswoman, A Survey of Health and Fitness Advice for Women, 1860-1940." Ph.D. diss., University of Kentucky, 1991.

Kreamer, Kate. "The Impact of Women"s Movements on the Emergence of Women"s Athletics and Sports in the United States." Masters thesis, University of Kansas, 1986.

Leiter, Frances W. *National Woman's Christian Temperance Union: Department of Physical Culture, 1892.* Pamphlet contained in Scrapbook I, *Health and Gymnastics in America.* Department of Hygiene and Physical Education, Wellesley College Archives.

Lindley, Susan Hill. "Woman's Profession in the Life and Thought of Catharine Beecher." Ph.D. diss., Duke University, 1974.

May, Samuel J. "The Rights and Conditions of Women: A Sermon, Preached in Syracuse, November 1845." Ts. Photocopy. Todd-McLean Collection, University of Texas at Austin.

McAllister, Marie Maguire. "The Educational Experiences of Margaret Fuller." Ph.D. diss., Boston College, 1984.

Natterson, Paul David. "Dio Lewis and Physical Fitness: A Social Innovator in a Scientific Sphere." Senior honors thesis, Harvard University, 1985. Harvard Archives.

Noever, Janet Hubley. "Passionate Rebel: The Life of Mary Gove Nichols, 1810-1884." Ph.D. diss., University of Oklahoma, 1983.

Parsons, Ellen. "A Plea for a Gymnasium: Oration Given at 1863 Mount Holyoke Seminary Graduation," Ts. College History Collection, Mount Holyoke College Library/Archives.

"Phrenological Character of Miss Ellen Goddard." 2 May 1852. Reading given by S. P. Butler at 142 Washington Street, Boston. Mss. May-Goddard Collection. Schlessinger Library, Radcliffe College.

Powell, Roberta Braden. "Women and Sport in Victorian America." Ph.D. diss., University of Utah, 1981.

Reekie, Shirley M. "A History of Sport and Recreation for Women in Great Britain, 1700-1850." Ph.D. diss., Ohio State University, 1982.

Sargent, D. A. "The Achievements of the Century in Gymnastics and Athletics Together with Notes and Questions: An Address Delivered to the Students of Springfield College, 1903." Typescript. Babson Library, Springfield College.

Sawyer, J. H. "Henry Ward and Catherine [sic] E. Beecher and Their Influence on the Physical Work of the Young Men"s Christian Association." Masters thesis, Luther Gulick Thesis Collection. Babson Library, Springfield College.

Smith, Alfred Albert. "Dio Lewis: Pioneer Physical Educator." Master"s thesis, Springfield College, 1914. Gulick Thesis Collection. Babson Library, Springfield College.

Todd, Jan. "Beyond The Ivy-Clad Walls: New Directions for Women"s Sport History." Paper presented at the North American Society for Sport History, Halifax, Nova Scotia, 1992.

Todd, Jan. "A Legacy of Strength: The Cultural Phenomenon of the Professional Strongwomen." Paper presented at the North American Society for Sport History, Columbus, Ohio, 1987.

Todd, Jan. "The Strong Lady in America: Professional Athletes and the *Police Gazette*." Paper presented at the North American Society for Sport History, Clemson, South Carolina, 1989.

Todd, Terence. "A History of Resistance Exercise and Its Role in United States Education." Ph.D. diss., University of Texas at Austin, 1966.

Vincenti: Virginia Bramble. "A History of the Philosophy of Home Economics." Ph.D. diss., Pennsylvania State University, 1981.

Walker, William B. "The Health Reform Movement in the United States: 1830-1870." Ph.D. diss., Johns Hopkins University, 1955.

Warner, Patricia Campbell. "Clothing the American Woman for Sport and Physical Education, 1860-1940: Public and Private." Ph.D. diss., University of Minnesota, 1986.

Welch, J. Edmund. "Edward Hitchcock, M.D.: Founder of Physical Education in the College Curriculum." Ph.D. diss., East Carolina College, 1962.

Ziegler, Earle F. "A History of Professional Preparation for Physical Education in the United States, 1861-1948." Ph.D. diss., Yale University, 1950.

## Primary Sources

### Books, Sermons, Catalogs, and Reports

Adams, Charles Francis, ed. *Letters of Mrs. Adams, The Wife of John Adams. With an Introductory Memoir.* 4th ed. Boston: Wilkins, Carter and Company, 1848.

Alcott, William A. *An Address Delivered Before the American Physiological Society: March 7, 1837.* Boston: Light & Stearns, 1837.

_____. *Forty Years in the Wilderness of Pills and Powders; or, the Cogitations and Confessions of an Aged Physician.* Boston: John P. Jewett, 1859.

_____. *Gift Book for Young Ladies; or Familiar Letters on Their Acquaintainces, Male and Female Employments, Friendships, etc.* New York: Miller, Orton and Mulligan, 1855.

_____. *The Laws of Health: Or, Sequel to the "House I Live In."* Boston: John P. Jewett, 1857.

_____. *Lectures on Life and Health; Or, The Laws and Means of Physical Culture.* Boston: Phillips, Sampson and Company, 1853.

_____. *Letters to a Sister; or Woman"s Mission.* Buffalo: George H. Derby and Co., 1850.

_____, ed. *The Library of Health and Teacher on the Human Constitution.* 4 vols. Boston: George W. Light, 1837.

_____, ed. *The Moral Reformer and Teacher on the Human Constitution.* 2 vols. Boston: Light & Horton, 1835.

_____. *The Young Wife, Or Duties of Woman in the Marriage Relation.* Boston: Charles H. Pierce, 1848.

_____. *The Young Woman's Book of Health.* New York: Miller, Orton and Mulligan, 1855.

_____. *The Young Woman's Guide.* Boston: Charles H. Pierce, 1847.

*The American Boys Book of Sports and Games: A Repository of In-and Out-Door Amusements for Boys and Youth.* New York: Dick & Fitzgerald, Publishers, 1864.

Andry, Nicolas. *Orthopaedia: Or, The Art of Correcting and Preventing Deformities in Children: By Such Means as May Easily be Put in Practice by Parents Themselves, and All Such as Are Employed in Educating Children: To Which is Added, A Defence [sic] of the Orthopaedia, by way of Supplement, by the Author.* 2 vols. London: A. Millar, 1743.

Armstrong, John, M.D. *Miscellanies; The Art of Preserving Health in Four Books.* London: T. Cadell, 1744.

Austin, Harriett N. *The American Costume: Or, Woman's Right to Good Health*. Dansville, NY: Austin, Jackson & Co., 1876.

Austin, Harriet N. *Hygienic Tract #4: Health Dress*. Dansville, NY: Hygienic Tract Society, n.d.

Barnett, S. M. *Barnett's Patent Parlor Gymnasium*. New York: J. Becker and Co., 1871.

Beach, Wooster, M.D. *Beach's Family Physician and Home Guide for the Treatment of the Diseases of Men, Women and Children, on Reform Principles With an Appendix, From Eminent Writers, Giving The Laws of Health, and Important Suggestions for the Attainment of Comfort, Prosperity and Happiness*. Forty-fifth thousand, revised and enlarged. Cincinatti: Moore, Wilstach, Keys & Co., 1862.

Beaujeu, J. A. *A Treating [sic] on Gymnastic Exercise, or Calisthenics, For the Use of Young Ladies Introduced at the Royal Hibernian Military School, Also at the Seminary for the Education of Young Ladies, Under the Direction of Miss Hinks in 1824*. Dublin: R. Milliken and Son, 1828.

Beck, Charles, trans. *Treatise on Gymnasticks Taken Chiefly from the German of F. L. Jahn*. Northampton: Simeon Butler, 1828.

[Beecher, Catharine E]. *The Annual Catalogue of the Hartford Female Seminary Together With an Account of the Internal Arrangements, Course of Study, and Mode of Instructing the Same*. Hartford: 1831.

_____. *Calisthenic Exercises for Schools, Families and Health Establishments*. New York: Harper & Brothers, 1856.

_____. *Catalogue and Circular of the Hartford Female Seminary*. Hartford, by the author, 1827.

_____. *Educational Reminiscences and Suggestions*. New York: J. B. Ford and Co., 1874.

_____. *An Essay on the Education of Female Teachers*. Lyceum address, 1835.

_____. *Letters to the People on Health and Happiness*. New York: Harper & Brothers, [1855] 1856.

_____ *Physiology and Calisthenics for Schools and Families*. New York: Harper & Brothers, 1856.

_____. *Suggestions Respecting Improvements in Education*. Hartford: Packard and Butler, 1829.

_____. *A Treatise on Domestic Economy for the Use of Young Ladies at Home, and at School*. New York: Thomas H. Webb & Co., 1841.

_____. *A Treatise on Domestic Economy for the Use of Young Ladies at Home, and at School*. rev. ed. New York: Harper & Brothers, 1850.

_____. *Woman Suffrage and Women's Profession*. Hartford: Brown & Gross, 1871.

Bell, Sir Charles. *Expression: Its Anatomy and Philosophy*. New York: Fowler & Wells, 1883.

*The Bijou Book of Manly Exercises*. London: Frederick Warne and Co., 1868.

Blackwell, Elizabeth, M.D. *Counsel to Parents on the Moral Education of Their Children*. New York: Fowler & Wells, 1879.

_____. *The Laws of Life with Special Reference to the Physical Education of Girls*. New York: George P. Putnam, 1852.

_____. *Pioneer Work in Opening the Medical Profession to Women*. London: Longmans Green and Company, 1895. Reprint edition. New York: Source Book Press, 1970.

Blundell, J. W. F. *The Muscles and Their Story from the Earliest Times; Including the Whole Text of Mercurialis, and the Opinions of Other Writers, Ancient and Modern on Mental and Bodily Development*. London: Chapman and Hall, 1864.

Board of Censors. *Lectures Delivered Before the American Institute of Instruction, Boston, Massachusetts, August 21, 1860*. Boston: Ticknor & Fields, 1861.

Brennar, Madame. *Gymnastics for Ladies, A Treatise on the Science and Art of Calisthenic and Gymnastic Exercises*. London: by the author, 1870.

Brigham, Amariah, M.D. *Remarks on the Influence of Mental Cultivation and Mental Excitement Upon Health*. 2nd ed. Boston: Marsh, Capen & Lyon, 1833.

Brinton, D. G., M.D., and George H. Napheys, M.D. *Personal Beauty: How to Cultivate and Preserve It in Accordance with the Laws of Health*. Springfield, MA: W. J. Holland, 1870.

_____. *The Laws of Health in Relation to the Human Form*. Springfield, MA: W. J. Holland, 1871.

Buchan, William, M.D. *Domestic Medicine: or, a Treatise on the Prevention and Cure of Diseases by Regimen and Simple Medicines*. Boston: Joseph Bumstead, 1813.

Butler, D. P. *Butler's System of Physical Training—The Lifting Cure: An Original Scientific Application of the Laws of Motion or Mechanical Action to Physical Culture and the Cure of Disease. With a Discussion of True and False Methods of Physical Training*. Boston: by the author, 1868.

Caldwell, Charles. *Thoughts on Physical Education: Being a Discourse Delivered to a Convention of Teachers in Lexington, Kentucky on the 6th and 7th of November, 1833*. Boston: Marsh & Co. 1834.

*Calisthénie ou Gymnastique des Jeunes Filles, Traité Élémentaire Des Differéns Exercises, Propres A Fortifier Le Corp, A Entretnir La Sante, Et A Preparer Un Bon Tempérament*. Paris: [1828] 1830.

*Calisthénie, ou Somascétique Naturelle, Appropriée A L'Education Phyisique Des Jeunes Filles*. Besançon, France: Charles Deis, 1843.

Capen, Nahum. *Reminiscences of Dr. Spurzheim and George Combe and a Review of the Science of Phrenology From the Period of Its Discovery by Dr. Gall to the Time of the Visit of George Combe to the United States, 1838, 1840*. New York: Fowler & Wells, 1881.

Capron, George, M.D., and David B. Slack, M.D. *New England Popular Medicine*. Providence: J. F. Moore, 1846.

Chavasse, P. H. *The Physical Training of Children With a Preliminary Dissertation By F. H. Getchell, M.D.* Chicago: New World Publishing, 1875.

Chiosso, James. *The Gymnastic Polymachinon*. New York: H. Balliere, 1855.

_____. *Gymnastics an Essential Branch of National Education, Both Public and Private; The Only Remedy to Improve the Present Physical Condition of Man*. New York: H. Balliere, 1854.

Chreiman, Miss. *The Scientific Physical Training of Girls: A Lecture Delivered in the Lecture Room of the Exhibition, July 25th, 1884*. Printed and published for the Executive Council of the International Health Exhibition, and for the Council of the Society of Arts. London: William Clowes and Sons, 1884.

Clapp, Cornelia. *Manual of Gymnastics Prepared for the Use of the Students of Mt. Holyoke Seminary*. Boston: Beacon Press, 1883.

Clias, Peter Henry. *Anfangsgrunde der Gymnastik oder Turnkunst*. Bern: 1816.

_____. *An Elementary Course of Gymnastic Exercises; Intended to Develope and Improve the Physical Powers of Man*. London: Sherwood, Jones and Co., 1823.

_____. *An Elementary Course of Gymnastic Exercises; Intended to Develope and Improve the Physical Powers of Man; With the Report to the Medical Faculty of Paris on the Subject and a New and Complete Treatise on the Art of Swimming*. 4th ed. London: Sherwood, Gilbert and Piper, 1825.

_____. *Kalisthenie oder Uebungen zur Schoenheit und Kraft fuer Maedchen*. Bern: 1829.

_____. *Principes de Gymnastique*, Paris: 1819.

Coates, Reynell, M.D. *Popular Medicine: or, Family Adviser; Consisting of Outlines of Anatomy, Physiology, and Hygiene, With Such Hints on the Practice of Physic, Surgery, and the Diseases of Women and Children, As May Prove Useful in Families When Regular Physicians Cannot Be Procured: Being a Companion and Guide for Intelligent Principals of Manufactories, Plantations, and Boarding Schools, Heads of Families, Masters of Vessels, Missionaries, or Travellers; and a Useful Sketch for Young Men about Commencing the Study of Medicine*. Philadelphia: Carey, Lea and Blanchard, 1838.

Cogswell, Joseph C. and George Bancroft. *Prospectus for a School to be Established at Round Hill, Northampton, Massachusetts*. Cambridge: by the authors, 1823.

Coles, L. B., M.D. *The Philosophy of Health; or Health Without Medicine: A Treatise on the Laws of the Human System*. Boston: William D. Ticknor & Co., 1848.

Colthrup, Samuel Robert. *A Lecture on Physical Development and its Relation to Mental and Spiritual Development*. Boston: Ticknor & Fields, 1859.

Combe, Andrew, M.D. *The Principles of Physiology Applied to the Preservation of Health and to the Improvement of Physical and Mental Education*. Edinburgh: 1835.

_____. *The Principles of Physiology Applied to the Preservation of Health and to the Improvement of Physical and Mental Education*. Reprinted with notes and observations by Orson S. Fowler, based on the 7th Edinburgh ed. New York: Fowler & Wells, [1838] n.d.

Combe, George. *The Constitution of Man Considered in Relation to External Objects*. Edinburgh: MacLachlan and Stewart, [1828] 1844.

_____. *The Constitution of Man Considered in Relation to External Objects*. 9th ed. Edinburgh: MacLachlan and Stewart, 1860.

_____. *Lectures on Phrenology: Including its Application to the Present and Prospective Condition of the United States*. 3rd ed. New York: Fowler & Wells, 1882.

_____. *Notes on the United States of North America During a Phrenological Visit in 1838-39-40*. 3 vols. Edinburgh: Maclachlan, Stewart and Company, 1841.

Cooper, Alfred B. *Paul Preston's Book of Gymnastics: Instructions for Sports and Exercises To Promote the Health and Long Life of His Youthful Friends.* Rev. ed. New York: James Miller, 1866.

*A Course of Calisthenics for Young Ladies in Schools and Families With Some Remarks on Physical Education.* Hartford: H and F. J. Huntington, 1831. [Published simultaneously in Boston, New York, and Philadelphia.]

Curtis, A., M.D. *Lectures on Midwifery and the Forms of Disease Peculiar to Women and Children, Delivered to the Members of the Botanico-Medical College of Ohio.* 2nd ed. Columbus, OH: by the author, 1841.

Curtis, John Harrison, M.D. *Observations on the Preservation of Health, in Infancy, Youth, Manhood and Age; With the Best Means of Improving the Moral and Physical Condition of Man, Prolonging Life, and Promoting Human Happiness.* 2nd ed. London: Henry Renshaw, 1838.

*A Defence of the Graham System of Living: Or, Remarks on Diet and Regimen.* New York: W. Applegate, 1835.

De Laspee, Henry. *Calisthenics; or, The Elements of Bodily Culture, On Pestalozzian Principles: A Contribution to Physical Education.* London: Darton and Co., n.d.

*DeWitt's Athletic Exercises For Health and Strength: Training, Walking, Running, Dumb Bells, Indian Clubs, Etc.* New York: De Witt, n.d.

Dubois, J. B. *Plan and Proposals for Building by Subscription an Academy for Riding, Fencing and Dancing: With a View to Facilitate the Acquirement of those Elegant and Useful Exercises, Upon a System of General Accommodation.* London: 1793.

Duffin, E. W., M.D. *Influence of Modern Physical Education of Females, in Producing and Confirming Deformity of the Spine.* London: 1830.

Eastman, H. E. *Eastman's System of Calisthenic Culture and Manual.* Milwaukee: Riverside Printing House, 1872.

Eastman, Mary F. *The Biography of Dio Lewis, A.M., M.D.* New York: Fowler & Wells, 1891.

Fairchild, James H. *Oberlin: The Colony and the College: 1833-1883.* Oberlin OH: E. J. Goodrich, 1883.

Farnham, Eliza W. *Woman and Her Era.* 2 vols. New York: A. J. Davis & Co., 1864.

Ferrero, Edward. *The Art of Dancing, and Ball Room Instructor. To Which is Added A Few Hints on Etiquette; Also, The Figures, Music and Necessary Instruction For the Performance of the Most Modern and Approved Dances, as Executed at the Private Academies of the Author, Together With a Complete Description of the Various Figures of the Celebrated German or Cotillion.* New York: Dick & Fitzgerald, 1859.

Fish, Alanson Lester. *Calisthenic Dictionary.* Springfield MA: Seminar Publishing Company, 1902.

Fitzgerald, P. A. *The Exhibition Speaker: Containing Farces, Dialogues, and Tableaux With Exercises for Declamation in Prose and Verse. Also, a Treatise on Oratory and Elocution, Hints on Dramatic Characters, Costumes, Position of the Stage, Making Up, Etc. Etc. To Which is Added a Complete System of Calisthenics and Gymnastics, With Instructions for Teachers and Pupils, Illustrated with Fifty Engravings.* New York: Sheldon, Lamport & Blakeman, 1856.

Follen, E. L. *The Life of Charles Follen.* Boston: Thomas H. Webb & Co., 1844.

Fowler, Orson S. *Creative and Sexual Science or: Manhood, Womanhood and Their Mutual Inter-Relations: Love, Its Laws, Power, Etc.* New York: by the author, 1870.

_____. *Education and Self Improvement: Comprising Physiology—Animal and Mental, Self Culture and Perfection of Character, Memory and Intellectual Development.* 26th ed. New York: Fowler & Wells, 1847.

_____. *Hereditary Descent: Its Laws and Facts Applied to Human Improvements.* New York: Fowler & Wells, 1848.

_____. *Human Science: or Phrenology; its Principles, Proofs, Faculties, Organs, Temperaments, Combinations, Conditions, Teachings, Philosophies, etc. etc. as Applied to Health, its Value, Laws, Functions, Organs, Means, Preservation, Restoration, etc., Mental Philosophy, Human and Self Improvement, Civilization, Home, Country, Commerce, Rights, Duties, Ethics, etc., God, His Existence, Attributes, Laws, Worship, Natural Theology, etc., Immorality, its Evidences, Conditions, Relations to Time, Rewards, Punishments, Sin, Faith, Prayer, etc., Intellect, Memory, Juvenile and Self Education, Literature, Mental Discipline, the Senses, Sciences, Arts, Avocations, A perfect Life, etc. etc. etc.* Philadelphia: National Publishing Company, 1868.

_____. *Love and Parentage Applied to the Improvement of Offspring; Including Important Directions and Suggestions to Lovers and the Married Concerning the Strongest Ties and the Most Sacred and Momentous Relations of Life.* 7th ed. New York: Fowler & Wells, 1846.

_____. *Maternity or the Bearing and Nursing of Children Including Female Education and Beauty.* 2nd ed. New York: Fowler & Wells, 1850 [1848].

_____. *Matrimony as Taught by Phrenology and Physiology.* Boston: O. S. Fowler, 1859.

_____. *Memory and Intellectual Improvement Applied to Self-Education and Juvenile Instruction. New York: Fowler & Wells, 1847.* Included in Fowler, Orson S. *Education and Self-Improvement.* New York: Fowler & Wells, n.d.

_____. *On Matrimony: Or, Phrenology and Physiology Applied to the Selection of Congenial Companions for Life; Including Directions to the Married for Living Together Affectionately and Happily.* New York: O. S. and L. N. Fowler, 1842.

_____. *Phrenology and Physiology Explained and Applied to Education, and Self-Improvement; Including the Intellectual and Moral Education and Government of Children: Mental Discipline & The Cultivation of Memory; and the Means of Regaining and Preserving the Health By Pointing Out the Methods of Increasing and Decreasing the Phrenological Organs in Children and One's Self.* New York: O. S. & L. N. Fowler, 1842.

_____. *Physiology, Animal and Mental: Applied to the Preservation and Restoration of Health of Body and Power of Mind.* 6th ed. New York: Fowler & Wells, 1851.

_____. *Private Lectures on Perfect Men, Women and Children, In Happy Families; Including Gender, Love, Mating, Married Life, and Reproduction, Paternity, Maternity, Infancy and Puberty; Together with Male Vigor and Female Health Restored, and their Ailments Self-Cured, etc.; as Taught by Phrenology and Natural Science.* Sharon Station, NY: Mrs. O. S. Fowler, 1883.

_____. *Religion; Natural and Revealed; or the Natural Theology and Moral Bearings of Phrenology and Physiology.* New York: Fowler & Wells, 1844.

_____. *Self-Culture and Perfection of Character: Including the Management of Youth.* New York: Fowler & Wells, 1847. Included in Fowler, Orson S. *Education and Self-Improvement.* New York: Fowler & Wells, n.d.

_____. *The Illustrated Self-Instructor in Phrenology and Physiology.* New York: Fowler & Wells, 1854.

_____. *Sexual Science; Including Manhood, Womanhood, and Their Mutual Interrelations; Love Its Laws, Power, etc., Selection or*

*Mutual Adaptations, Married Life Made Happy, Reproduction, and Progenal Endowment, or Paternity, Maternity, Bearing, Nursing, and Rearing Children, Puberty, Girlhood, etc., Sexual Ailments Restored, Female Beauty Perpetuated, etc. etc. as Taught by Phrenology.* Philadelphia: National Publishing Company, 1870.

_____. *Temperance and Tight Lacing: Founded on the Laws of Life as Developed by the Sciences of Phrenology and Physiology.* New York: Fowler & Wells, 1845.

Fuller, Francis. *Medicina Gymnastica: Or a Treatise Concerning the Power of Exercise with Respect to the Animal Economy and the Great Necessity of it in the Cure of Several Distempers.* London: printed by John Matthews, 1705.

Fuller, S. Margaret. *Woman in the Nineteenth Century.* Facsimile of the 1845 edition. Columbia: University of South Carolina Press, 1980.

Gove, Mary S. *Lectures to Women on Anatomy and Physiology with an Appendix on Water-cure.* New York: Harper & Brothers, 1846.

Graham, Sylvester. *The Aesculapian Tablets of the Nineteenth Century.* Providence: Weeden and Cory, 1834.

_____. *Lectures on the Science of Human Life.* 2 vols. Boston: March, Capen, Lyon and Webb. 1839.

Griscom, John H., M.D. *Animal Mechanism and Physiology; Being a Plain and Familiar Exposition of the Structure and Functions of the Human System.* New York: Harper & Brothers, 1839.

Guilford, L.T. *The Use of a Life: Memorials of Mrs. Z. P. Bannister.* New York: American Tract Society, 1885.

Gunn, John C. *Gunn's New Family Physician: Or, Home Book of Health; Forming a Complete Household Guide . . . With Supplementary Treatises on Anatomy, Physiology and Hygiene or Domestic and Sanitary Economy.* 100th ed. New York: Moore, Wilstach & Baldwin, 1866 [1830].

GutsMuths, Johann Christoph Friedrich. *Gymnastics for Youth: Or a Practical Guide to Healthful and Amusing Exercises for the Use of Schools. An Essay Toward the Necessary Improvement of Education, Chiefly as it Relates to the Body; Freely Translated from the German of C.G. Salzmann, Master of the Academy at Schnepfenthal and Author of Elements of Morality.* Philadelphia: William Duane, 1802.

GutsMuths, Johann Christoph Friedrich [Attributed to C. G. Salzmann]. *Gymnastics for Youth: Or a Practical Guide to Delightful and Amusing Exercises for the Use of Schools, An Essay Toward the Necessary Improvement of Education, Chiefly as it Relates to the Body.* London: Printed for J. Johnston, 1800.

_____. *Gymnastik fur die Jugen. Enthaltend eine Praktische Anwisung zu Leibesubungen. Ein Beytraq zur Nothigsten Verbesserung der Korperlichen Erziehung.* Schnepfenthal: Buchhandlung der Erziehunganstalt, 1793.

_____. *Turnbuch für dir Sohne des Baterlandes.* Frankfurt: 1817.

Hale, Sarah Josepha. *Biography of Distinguished Women: or, Woman's Record, From the Creation to 1869. Arranged in Four Eras with Selections from Authoresses of Each Era.* New York: Harper & Brothers, 1876.

Hamilton, Gustavus. *The Elements of Gymnastics for Boys and Calisthenics for Young Ladies.* London: 1827.

Hanaford, Phebe, A. *Daughters of America; or, Women of the Century.* Augusta, ME: True and Company, 1882.

Harrison, Professor. *Indian Clubs, Dumb-Bells, and Sword Exercises.* London: Dean and Son, n.d.

Hartwell, E. M., M.D. *Physical Training in American Colleges and Universities: A Report to the Bureau of Education.* N.p.: 1885.

_____. *School Document No. 22-1891. Report of the Director of Physical Training, December 1891.* Boston: Rockwell and Churchill, 1891.

Higginson, Thomas Wentworth. *Common Sense About Women.* New York: Longmans, Green and Co. 1894.

_____. *Women and the Alphabet: A Series of Essays.* Boston: Houghton Mifflin Co., 1881.

Hitchcock, Edward Jr., M.D. *A Report of Twenty Years Experience in the Department of Physical Education and Hygiene in Amherst College, to the Board of Trustees, June 27, 1881.* Amherst, MA: C. A. Bangs & Co., 1881.

_____. *A Manual of the Gymnastic Exercises As Practiced by the Junior Class in Amherst College.* Boston: Ginn, Heath & Co., 1884.

_____. *The Power of Christian Benevolence Illustrated in the Life and Labor of Mary Lyon.* Northampton: Hopkins, Bridgman & Co., 1852.

Hoffman, Friedrich. *On Motion, the Best Medicine for the Body.* Halle, Germany: 1701.

_____. *The Incomparable Advantages of Motion and of Bodily Exercises, and How They are to be Employed for the Preservation of Health.* Halle: 1819.

Hunt, Lucy B. *Handbook of Light Gymnastics.* Boston: Lee and Shepard, 1881.

Hutchison, Joseph C. *A Treatise on Physiology and Hygiene for Educational Institutions and General Readers.* New York: Clark and Maynard, 1870.

*Influence of Modern Physical Education of Females in Producing and Confirming Deformity of the Spine.* New York: Charles G. Francis, 1830.

Jackson, James C. *American Womanhood: Its Peculiarities and Necessities.* Dansville NY: Austin, Jackson and Co., 1870.

_____. *How To Treat The Sick Without Medicine.* 10<sup>th</sup> ed. Dansville, NY: Austin, Jackson and Co., 1868.

_____. *Shall Our Girls Live or Die?* Dansville, NY: Austin, Jackson & Co., n.d.

_____. *Student Life: Or, How to Work With The Brain Without Overworking the Body.* Dansville, NY: Austin, Jackson & Co., 1868.

_____. and Harriet N. Austin. *Our Home on the Hillside: What We Are Trying to Do and How We are Trying to Do It.* Dansville, NY: n.d.

Jacques, D[aniel] H. *Hints Toward Physical Perfection; or, the Philosophy of Human Beauty; Showing How to Acquire and Retain, Bodily Symmetry, Health and Vigor, Secure Long Life, and Avoid The Infirmities and Deformities of Age.* New York: Fowler & Wells, 1859.

Jahn, Friedrich Ludwig. *Deutsches Volksthum.* Lübeck, Germany: 1810.

_____ and Ernst Eiselen. *Die Deutsche Turnkunst zur Einrichtung der Turnplatze Dargestellt von Friedrich Ludwig Jahn und Ernst Eiselen.* Berlin: Kosten der Herausgeber, 1816.

James, Ed., comp. *How to Acquire Health, Strength and Muscle; Including Treatment for Free Livers and Sedentary People, About Air, Clothing, Food and Stimulants; also Best Modes of Exercise for All Ages, Cures and Preventives for Various Diseases, Proportions of a Perfect Human Figure; Sketches of Dr. G. B. Winship's [sic] and R. A. Pennell's Methods, Remarkable Feats of Strength, Measurements of Noted Athletes, The Muscular System, Tables of Nutrition and Digestion.* 12<sup>th</sup> ed. New York: Ed James, 1878.

James, Ed. *Practical Training for Running, Walking, Rowing, Wrestling, Boxing, Jumping and all Kinds of Athletic Feats; Together With Tables of Proportional Measurements for Height and Weight of Men In and Out of Condition; Including Hints on Exercise, Diet, Clothing, and Advice to Trainers; Also Banting's System of Reducing Corpulency, and Record of Fast Athletic Performances.* New York: Ed James, 1877.

Janes, Lewis G. *Health-Exercise: The Rationale and Practice of the Lifting-Cure or Health Lift.* New York: Lewis G. Janes, 1871.

Kehoe, Sim D. *The Indian Club Exercise With Explanatory Figures and Positions. Photographed from Life; and General Remarks on Physical Culture.* New York: American News Company, 1866.

Kellogg, J. H., M.D. *Ladies Guide in Health and Disease, Girlhood, Maidenhood, Wifehood, Motherhood.* Des Moines, IA: W. D. Condit & Co., 1888.

Knox, Samuel. *An Essay on the Best System of Liberal Education, Adapted to the Genius of the Government of the United States.* Baltimore, 1799.

*The Ladies Library.* 3 vols. London: Sir Richard Steele, 1739.

Lamarck, J. B. *Zoological Philosophy: An Exposition with Regard to the Natural History of Animals.* London: MacMillan, 1809.

Leavitt, John W. *Exercise a Medicine; or, Muscular Action as Related to Organic Life.* New York: J. W. Leavitt, 1870.

[Lewis, Dio]. *Catalogue and Circular of Dr. Dio Lewis's Family School for Young Ladies, Lexington, Massachusetts, 1866.* Cambridge: John Wilson and Son, 1866.

[_____]. *Catalogue and Circular of Dr. Dio Lewis's Family School for Young Ladies, Lexington, Massachusetts, 1867.* Cambridge: Welch, Bigelow and Company, 1867.

_____. *Chastity; or, Our Secret Sins.* Philadelphia: G. MacLean, 1874.

_____. *Curious Fashions.* New York: Clarke Brothers, 1883.

[_____]. Dr. Dio Lewis's Training School for Teachers of the New Gymnastics. [Circular] Cambridge: John Wilson and Son, 1866.

_____. *The Dio Lewis Treasury.* New York: James R. Barnett, 1886.

_____. *Five Minute Chats With Young Women.* New York: Harper & Brothers, 1874.

_____. *Gypsies, or Why We Went Gypsying in the Sierras.* Boston: Eastern Book Company, 1881.

_____. *Lewis's Normal Institute for Physical Education.* Boston: published by the Normal Institute for Physical Education, 1863.

_____. *The New Gymnastics for Men, Women and Children.* 3rd ed. Boston: Ticknor & Fields, 1862.

_____. *The New Gymnastics for Men, Women and Children.* 10th ed. Boston: Ticknor & Fields, 1868.

_____. *The New Gymnastics for Men, Women and Children*. 25th ed. New York: Fowler & Wells, 1891.

_____. *Our Girls*. New York: Harper & Brothers, 1871.

_____. *Weak Lungs and How to Make Them Strong. Or Diseases of the Organs of the Chest, With Their Home Treatment by the Movement Cure*. Boston: Ticknor & Fields, 1864.

Lieber, Franz. *The Stranger in America; or, Letters to a Gentleman in Germany, Comprising Sketches of the Manners, Society and National Peculiarities of the United States*. Philadelphia: Carey, Lea and Blanchard, 1835.

Lion, J. C. *Why is the German System of Gymnastics Entitled to Recognition?* [Pamphlet] Milwaukee: Freidenker Publishing, n.d.

Livermore, Mary A. *What Shall We Do With Our Daughters? Superflous Women and Other Lectures*. Boston: Lee & Shepard Publishing, 1883.

Locke, John. *Some Thoughts Concerning Education*. Cambridge: University Press, [1693] 1913.

McRae, David. *The Americans at Home*. rev. ed. Glascow, 1860.

Mann, Horace. *Lectures on Education*. Boston: Wm. B. Fowle, 1848.

Martineau, Harriet. *Society in America*. Reprint ed. Seymour Martin Lipset, ed. Garden City, NY: Doubleday, 1962.

Mason, Samuel W. *Manual of Gymnastic Exercises for Schools and Families*. Boston: Crosby and Nichols, 1863.

Mavor, William F. *The Catechism of Health, Containing Simple and Easy Rules and Directions for the Management of Children, and Observations on the Conduct of Health in General. For the Use of Schools and Families*. New York: Samuel Wood & Sons, 1819.

Mendell, Miss and Miss Hosmer. *Notes of Travel and Life*. New York: Mendell and Hosmer, 1835.

Milo, William with Additions, Alterations, Notes, and Illustrations by Handsome Charles, the Magnet. *Notes on Beauty, Vigor and Development; or How to Acquire Plumpness of Form, Strength of Limb, and Beauty of Complexion: With Rules for Diet and Bathing and a Series of Improved Physical Exercises*. New York: Samuel R. Wells, n.d.

Neal, John. Wandering Recollections of a Somewhat Busy Life: An Autobiography. Boston: Roberts Brothers, 1869.

Nichols, Mary Gove. *Experience in Water-cure: A Familiar Exposition of the Principles and Results of Water Treatment in the Cure of Acute and Chronic Diseases*. New York: Fowler & Wells, 1849.

[Pardon, George Frederick]. *Captain Crawley's Gymnastics Containing Dumb Bell Exercises, Indian Clubs, Parallel Bars, The Horizontal Bar, and the Trapeze*. London: Ward, Lock and Co., n.d.

[Payne, J. A.]. *Philadelphia Natatorium and Physical Institute*. [Brochure] (N.p.) The Todd-McLean Collection, University of Texas at Austin.

*Peck & Snyder Price List of Out and Indoor Sports and Pastimes*. New York, 1886.

*The Phrenological Miscellany; or, The Annuals of Phrenology and Physiognomy From 1865 to 1873*. New York: Fowler & Wells, 1882.

Power, John, M.D. *Essays on the Female Economy. 1. On the Periodical Discharge of the Human Female; with New Views on its Nature, Causes and Influence on Disease; to Which are Added, Directions for its Management in the Different Stages of Life. 2. On a Species of Abortion Not Heretofore Described, to Which Delicate Females in High Life are Peculiarly Liable; With a Mode of Treatment Which Has Secured a Happy Termination of the Preganancy Where Previously Repeated Disappointment Had Been Experienced*. London: Burgess and Hill, 1821.

Ricketson, Shadrach, M.D. *Means of Preserving Health, and Preventing Diseases: Founded Principally on an Attention to Air and Climate, Drink, Food, Sleep, Exercise, Clothing, Passions of the Mind, and Retentions and Excretions*. New York: Collins, Perkins and Company, 1806.

Riofrey, Bureaud, M.D. *Physical Education; Specially Adapted to Young Ladies*. 2nd ed. London: Orme, Brown, Green and Longmans, [1838].

Ross, Joel H., M.D. *Hints and Helps to Health and Happiness: Long Life and Little Physic*. 3rd ed. Auburn, NY: Derby and Miller, 1852.

Roth, M[athius]. *The Free Gymnastic Exercises of P. H. Ling, Arranged by H. Rothstein*. London & Boston: Groombridge & Sons, 1853.

Rousseau, Jean Jacques. *Emile*. Included in Linda A. Bell, ed. *Visions of Women*. Clifton, NJ: Humana Press, 1983.

Rush, Benjamin. *Sermons to Gentlemen Upon Temperance and Exercise*. Philadelphia: 1772.

Sargent, Dudley Allen. *Dudley Allen Sargent: An Autobiography*. Philadelphia: Lea and Febiger, 1927.

Schaible, Charles Henry. *An Essay on the Systematic Training of the Body: A Memorial Essay Published on the Occassion of the First Centenary Festival of Friedrich Ludwig Jahn*. London, Trubner & Co. 1878.

Schreber, D[aniel]. G. M. *The Book of Health.* Liepzig: H. Fries, 1839.
_____. *Education Through Beauty by Natural and Balanced Furtherance of Normal Body Growth.* Liepzig: Fleischer, 1858.
_____. *The Harmful Body Positions and Habits of Children Including a Statement of Counteracting Measures.* Liepzig: Fleischer, 1853.
_____. *The Parlour Gymnasium: or, All Gymnastic Exercises Brought Within the Compass of a Single Piece of Apparatus, as the Simplest Means for the Complete Development of Musuclar Strength and Endurance.* London: G. W. Bacon & Co., 1866.
_____. *Illustrated Medical In-Door Gymnastics or a System of Medico-Hygienic Exercises Requiring No Mechanical or Other Aid, and Adapted to Both Sexes and All Ages, and for Special Cases.* Translated from the 3rd German ed. by Henry Skelton. London: Williams and Norgate, 1856.
Scott, W. *Physical Training in New England Schools.* Cambridge: The People Publishing Company, 1899.
Seelye, L. Clark. "The Need of A Collegiate Education for Woman: A Paper Read Before the American Institute of Instruction at North Adams, July 28, 1874." Published by vote of the convention, 1874.
Shew, Joel, M.D. *Consumption: Its Prevention and Cure by the Water Treatment.* New York: Fowler & Wells, 1855.
_____. *The Water-Cure Manual: A Popular Work Embracing Prescriptions of the Various Modes of Bathing, The Hygienic and Curative Effects of Air, Exercise, Clothing, Occupation, Diet, Water-Drinking, & C. Together With Descriptions of Diseases and the Hydropathic Means to be Employed Therein. Illustrated With Cases of Treatment and Cure.* New York: Fowler & Wells, n.d.
_____. *Consumption: Its Prevention and Cure by the Water Treatment.* New York: Fowler & Wells, 1855.
Shew, M. L. *Water-Cure for Ladies: A Popular Work on the Health Diet, and Regimen of Females and Children and the Prevention and Cure of Diseases; With A Full Account of the Processes of Water-Cure; Illustrated with Various Cases.* Revised by Joel Shew, M.D. New York: Wiley and Putnam, 1844.
Sinclair, John. *A Collection of Papers on the Subject of Athletic Exercises.* London, 1806.
Sinclair, John. *Result of the Inquiries Regarding Athletic Exercises.* London, 1807.

_____. *The Code of Health and Longevity; or, a Concise View of the Principles Calculated for the Preservation of Health, and the Attainment of Long Life. Being an Attempt to Prove the Practability of Condensing, Within a Narrow Compass, The Most Material Information Hitherto Accumulated, Regarding the Most Useful Arts and Sciences, Or Any Particular Branch Thereof.* 4 vol. 2nd ed. Edinburgh: Arch Constable & Co., 1807.

Sizer, Nelson. *Forty Years in Phrenology; Embracing Recollections of History, Anecdote and Experience.* New York: Fowler & Wells, 1892.

*Songs for Calisthenics.* Springfield: Horace S. Taylor, 1849.

*Songs for Calisthenics.* Northampton: Hopkins, Bridgman & Co, 1857.

Speir, Robert F. *Going South for the Winter; With Hints to Consumptives.* New York: by the author, 1873.

Spurzheim, G., M.D. *Outlines of Phrenology . . . Being Also a Manual of Reference for the Marked Bust.* Boston: Marsh, Capen and Lyon, 1834.

_____. *Phrenology In Connection With the Study of Physiognomy to Which is Prefixed a Biography of the Author by Nahum Capen.* Boston: Marsh, Capen and Lyon, 1833.

*Sure Methods of Improving Health and Prolonging Life; or, A Treatise on the Art of Living Long and Comfortably, By Regulating Diet and Regimen. Embracing all the Most Approved Principles of Health and Longevity and Exhibiting the Remarkable Power of Proper Food, Wine, Air, Exercise, Sleep, & c. In the Cure of Chronic Diseases, as well as in the Preservation of Health, and Prolongation of Life. To Which is Added, The Art of Training for Health, Rules for Reducing Corpulence, and Maxims of Health, For the Bilious and Nervous, The Consumptive, Men of Letters, and People of Fashion.* London: by the author, 1827.

[Taylor, George H]. *A Brief Sketch of Principles Involved in Dr. George H. Taylor's Remedial Methods.* New York: Drs. Taylor and Patchen, 1887.

_____. *Diseases of Women: Their Causes, Prevention, and Radical Cure.* New York: George Maclean, 1871.

_____. *An Exposition of the Swedish Movement-Cure, Embracing the History and Philosophy of this System of Medical Treatment, with Examples of Single Movements, and Directions for Their Use in Various Forms of Chronic Disease, Forming a Complete Manual of Exercises; Together with a Summary of the Principles of General Hygiene.* New York: Samuel R. Wells, 1868.

_____. *Health by Exericise Showing What Exercises to Take and How to Take Them to Remove Physical Weakness, Embracing the History and Philosophy of Medical Treatment by this System, Including the Process of Massage.* New York: Fowler & Wells, 1883.

_____. *Health for Women. Showing the Causes of Feebleness and the Local Diseases Arising Therefrom; With Full Directions for Self-Treatment by Special Exercises.* New York: American Book Exchange, 1880.

_____. *Health for Women. Showing the Causes of Feebleness and the Local Diseases Arising Therefrom; With Full Directions for Self-Treatment by Special Exercises.* 12$^{th}$ ed. New York: Health Culture Company, 1923.

_____. *An Illustrated Sketch of the Movement Cure: Its Principles, Methods and Effects.* New York: Published at the Institute, 1866.

_____. *Mechanical Aids in the Treatment of Chronic Forms of Disease.* New York: George W. Rodgers, 1893.

Ticknor, George. *Life, Letters and Journals of George Ticknor.* 2 vols. Boston: Harper & Wells, 1876.

Tissot, Clement Joseph. *Gymnastique medicinale et chirurgicale, ou essai sur l'utilite du mouvement, on des differens exercises du corps, et du repos dans la cure de maladies.* Paris: Bastien Libraire, 1780.

Tissot, Simon André, M.D. *An Essay on Diseases Incident to Literary and Sedentary Persons. With Proper Rules for Preventing their Fatal Consequences and Instructions for Their Cure.* Dublin: printed for James Williams, 1772.

Titcomb, Miss. *Calisthenic Exercises.* N.p, [1852]. Pamphlet. Rare Books and Manuscripts, Babson Library, Springfield College.

Tracy, Stephen, M.D. *The Mother and Her Offspring.* New York: Harper & Brothers, 1853.

Trall, Russell, T. *The Illustrated Family Gymnasium; Containing the Most Improved Methods of Applying Gymnastic, Calisthenic, Kinesipathic, and Vocal Exercises to the Development of the Bodily Organs, the Invigoration of Their Functions, The Preservation of Health, and the Cure of Diseases and Deformities.* New York: Samuel R. Wells, 1873.

Tyler, Moses Coit. *The Brawnville Papers: Being Memorials of the Brawnville Athletic Club.* Boston: Osgood and Company, 1869.

_____, chairman. "Report on a Department of Hygiene and Personal Culture in The University of Michigan, By a Committee of the University Senate." Ann Arbor: Published by the University, 1870.

_____. *The New System of Musical Gymnastics as an Instrument in Education. A Lecture Delivered Before the College of Preceptors.* London: William Tweedie, 1864.

Vanderpoel, Emily Noyes. *Chronicles of a Pioneer School from 1792-1833; Being the History of Miss Sarah Pierce and Her Litchfield School.* ed. Elizabeth C. Barney. Cambridge: University Press, 1903.

_____. *More Chronicles of a Pioneer School from 1792-1833; Being Added History On The Litchfield Female Academy Kept By Miss Sarah Pierce and Her Nephew, John Pierce Brace.* New York: Cadmus Book Shop, 1927.

Voarino, Signor G. P. *A Second Course of Calisthenic Exercises: With a Course of Private Gymnastics for Gentlemen: Accompanied with a Few Observations on the Utility of Exercise.* London: published by James Ridgeway, Boosey and Sons, Royal Exchange, and Rolandi Italian Library, 1828.

_____. *A Treatise on Calisthenic Exercises Arranged for the Private Tuition of Ladies.* London: printed for N. Hailes, 1827.

Walker, Alexander. *Intermarriage or the Mode in Which and the Causes Why Beauty, Health and Intellect Result from Some Unions and Deformity, Disease and Insanity from Others.* Philadelphia: Lindsay and Blakiston, 1856 [1839].

_____ *Beauty; Illustrated Chiefly by an Analysis and Classification of Beauty in Woman. Preceded by a Critical View of the General Hypotheses Respecting Beauty, by Hume, Hogarth, Burke, Knight, Alison, etc., and Followed by A Similar View of the Hypotheses of Beauty in Sculpture and Painting, by Leonardo DaVinci, Winckelmann, Mengs, Bossi, etc.* London: Effingham Wilson, 1836.

[Walker, Donald]. *British Manly Exercises; In Which Rowing and Sailing Are Now First Discussed.* London, 1834.

_____. *Exercises for Ladies; Calculated to Preserve and Improve Beauty and to Prevent and Correct Personal Defects, Inseparable from Constrained or Careless Habits: Founded on Physiological Principles.* 2nd ed. London: Thomas Hurst, 1837.

[_____]. *Walker's Manly Exercises: Containing Rowing, Sailing, Riding, Driving, Racing, Hunting, Shooting, and Other Manly Sports. The Whole Carefully Revised or Written, by "Craven."* 11th ed. London: George Bell & Sons, 1888.

*The Water-cure in America: Over Three Hundred Cases of Various Diseases Treated with Water, by Drs. Wesselhoeft, Shew, Bedortha, Schieferdecker, Trall, Nichols, and Others. With Cases of Domestic*

*Practice; Designed for Popular as Well as Professional Reading, Edited by a Water Patient.* New York: Fowler & Wells, 1852.

Watson, J. Madison. *Handbook of Calisthenics and Gymnastics: A Complete Drill-Book for Schools, Families and Gymnasiums With Music to Accompany the Exercises.* New York: Schermerhorn, Bancroft & Co., 1864.

_____. *Watson's Manual of Calisthenics: A Systematic Drill-Book Without Apparatus, for Schools, Families and Gymnasiums With Music to Accompany the Exercises.* New York: Schermerhorn, Bancroft & Co., 1864.

_____. *Watson's Manual of Calisthenics: A Systematic Drill-Book Without Apparatus, for Schools, Families and Gymnasiums With Music to Accompany the Exercises.* New York: E. Steiger & Co. 1882.

Welch, F. G., M.D. *Manual of Gymnastics, Published in this Form (By Permission of the Author) for her own Class, By Mary T. Orcutt, Teacher of Gymnastics in Tilden Ladies' Seminary.* Rutland: Tuttle & Co., 1874.

_____. *Moral, Intellectual and Physical Culture; or the Philosophy of True Living.* New York: Wood & Holbrook, 1869.

Weld, Theodore D. *First Annual Report of the Society for Promoting Manual Labor in Literary Institutions Including the Report of Their General Agent: January 28, 1833.* New York: S. W. Benedict & Co., 1833.

Wells, Samuel R. *Wedlock; Or the Right Relations of the Sexes: Disclosing the Laws of Conjugal Selection and Showing Who May and Who May Not Marry.* New York: Samuel R. Wells, 1874.

_____. *New Physiognomy or, Signs of Character, As Manisfested Through Temperament and External Forms, and Especially in the Human Face Divine.* New York: Samuel R. Wells, 1868.

Willard, Frances E. *How to Win: A Book for Girls.* New York: Funk & Wagnall, 1888.

_____. *Glimpses of Fifty Years: The Autobiography of An American Woman.* Chicago: Women's Temperance Publication, 1889.

Willis, A. E. *A Treatise on Human Nature and Physiognomy.* Chicago: Cameron, Amberg & Co., n.d.

Wollstonecraft, Mary. *A Vindication of the Rights of Woman.* Girard KS: Haldeman-Julius Publications, 1944.

*Woman's Worth; or, Hints to Raise The Female Character.* New York: D. Appleton & Co., 1844.

Woolson, Abba Goold. *Woman in American Society*. Boston: Roberts Brothers, 1873.

## Serial Articles

Alcott, William A. "Progress of Physical Education." *American Journal of Education* 1 (1826): 22.

"American Institute of Instruction, Interesting Proceedings, Gymnastics in Schools—Lectures and Discussions—Educational Movements in Different States—Closing Scenes." *New York Times*, 27 August 1860, 2.

"Appropriate Exercise." *The Journal of Health* 1 (23 September 1829): 22.

Austin, Harriett N. "Letter No. 16." *The Water-Cure Journal and Herald of Reform* 27 (May 1859): 69.

_____. "Letter No. 19." *The Water-Cure Journal and Herald of Reform* 28 (August 1859): 20.

_____. "Letter No. 20." *The Water-Cure Journal and Herald of Reform* 28 (September 1859): 34-35.

_____. "Letter No. 22." *The Water-Cure Journal and Herald of Reform* 28 (November 1859): 67-68.

_____. "Thoughts About Health. Extracts from an Address Delivered at a Health Convention in Cooper Institute, New York, Thirty-One Years Ago." *The Laws of Life* 32 (September 1886): 260-61.

_____. "Thoughts About Health." *The Water-Cure Journal and Herald of Reform* 28 (February 1860): 25-29.

_____. "Woman"s Present and Future." *The Water-Cure Journal and Herald of Reform* 16 (September 1853): 57.

Beard, George, M.D. "The Physical Future of the American People." *Atlantic Monthly* 43 (June 1879): 718-28.

Beecher, Catharine E. "Female Education." *The American Journal of Education* 2 (April 1827): 219-23.

_____. "Female Education." *The American Journal of Education* 2 (May 1827): 264-69.

_____. "Health of Teachers and Pupils." *American Journal of Education* 2 (September 1856): 399-408.

_____. "To the Alumni of the West Newton Normal School." *The Common School Journal* 8 (15 January 1846): 21-24.

"Benefits of Exercise." *The Journal of Health* 2 (27 October 1830): 51-53.

Billberg, Harald. "Swedish Gymnastics." *Murray's Magazine* 9 (1863): 825-29.

Bishop, Mrs. Coleman E. "One Law of Life—Exercise." *The Laws of Life* 32 (December 1889): 357.

[Bloomer, Amelia]. "The American Costume." *The Lily* 4 (March 1852): 33.

[_____]. "A Sure Method for the Destruction of Woman"s Health." *The Lily* 3 (December 1851): 178.

[_____]. "Dress Reform." *The Lily* 3 (December 1851): 183.

[_____]. "Dress Reform." *The Lily* 4 (August 1852): 70-71.

[_____]. "Lectures on Anatomy and Physiology." *The Lily* 4 (April 1852): 42.

[_____]. "Loss of Health and Happiness per Consequence of the Follies of Dress." *The Lily* 7 (September 1855): 131.

[_____]. "Woman"s Power of Endurance." *The Lily* 8 (October 1856): 108.

"Bodily Exercise the Best Medicine." *Water-Cure Journal and Herald of Reforms* 25 (August 1857): 46.

Bridge, J. D. "The Moral Power of Women." *The Mother"s Assistant & Young Lady's Friend* 3 (August 1843): 181-186.

Brigham, Charles H. "What Exercises Shall We Take?" *The Herald of Health and Journal of Physical Culture* 14 (October 1869): 162-66.

Bronson, M. A. "Women Need More Courage." *The Lily* 7 (February 1855): 22.

"Buffalo High School." *American Annals of Education and Instruction* 3 (April 1828): 233-35.

Caldwell, Charles, M.D. "Physical Education—With Notes and Illustrations Addressed to Teachers and Others." Six parts. *The Phrenological Journal and Life Illustrated* 51 (July, August, September, October, November, and December 1870): 14-18; 94-100; 167-71; 232-37, 333-39; 392-98.

"Calisthenics." *The Journal of Health* 2 (23 February 1831): 190.

"Calisthenic Exercises." *The Journal of Health* 2 (27 April 1831): 250.

"Cartesian System of Penmanship." *American Journal of Education* [New Series] 1 (August 1830): 378.

Cheever, D. W. "The Gymnasium." *Atlantic Monthly* 3 (May 1859): 529-543.

"Claims of the Lifting Cure." *The Herald of Health and Journal of Physical Culture* 13 (May 1869): 231.

Coffin, J. G. "Intelligence." *American Journal of Education* 1 (November 1826): 699.

"Col. Amoros Gymnastic School, Paris." *American Journal of Education* 1 (November 1826): 689-90.

Coles, George. "Thoughts on Dress." *The Mother's Assistant* 3 (January 1843): 19-21.

"Commencement Exercises at the Normal Institute for Physical Education." *Lewis's New Gymnastics for Ladies, Gentlemen and Children and Boston Journal of Physical Culture* 1 (October 1861): 178.

"A Course of Calisthenics for Young Ladies in Schools and Families With Some Remarks on Physical Education." *The Ladies Magazine* 5 (February 1832): 91-92.

"Course of Education in the New York High School." *The American Journal of Education* 1 (January 1826): 23-29.

"The Darien Seminary for Young Ladies." *The Phrenological Journal and Life Illustrated* 51 (August 1870): 5.

"Dio Lewis: A Noted Son of Auburn Dies Today." *The Auburn Bulletin,* 21 May 1886.

"Dr. Dio Lewis Cremated." *The Auburn Bulletin.,* 24 May 1886.

"Dr. Elizabeth Blackwell." *Litell's Living Age* 58 (1858): 231-34.

"Dr. Grigg's Lecture." *The Ladies Magazine* 4 (November 1831): 517.

Dunton, Delos. "Items from Home of the Free." *The Herald of Health and Journal of Physical Culture* 4 (September 1864): 103.

Edgerton, S. C. "Female Culture." *The Mother's Assistant & Young Lady"s Friend* 3 (April 1843): 94-95.

Ellinwood, T. J. "Professor Welch's School of Physical Culture." *The Herald of Health and Journal of Physical Culture* 16 (November 1870): 225-27.

Fairchild, M. Augusta, M.D. "The Fitness of Things." *Herald of Health and Journal of Physical Culture* 4 (July 1864): 37.

"False Attitudes." *The Journal of Health* 2 (30 November 1830): 91-92.

"Female Teachers." *The Common School Journal* 9 (March 1847): 96.

"The First Boston Gymnasium." *Mind and Body* 6 (January 1900): 251-52.

"Flannels—Dyspepsy—Gymnasium." *The Journal of Health* 2 (8 December 1830): 111.

Flecther, J. H. "Feminine Athletics," *Good Words* 20 (December 1871): 534.

Fowle, William B. "The Animal Mechanism and Economy." *Boston Medical Intelligencer* 5 (24 October 1826): 196-97.

_____. "Boston Monitorial School: Report to the Trustees, 23 December 1825," *American Journal of Education* 1 (January 1826): 29-41.

_____. "Boston Monitorial School: Report to the Trustees, 23 December 1825." *American Journal of Education* 1 (February 1826): 164-65.

_____. "Gymnastic Exercise for Females." *Journal of Education* 1 (November 1826): 698-99.

[_____]. "Health of Teachers." *The Common School Journal* 10 (1 August 1848): 234-37.

[_____] "Physical Exercise." *The Common School Journal* 10 (1 September 1848): 266-68.

[Fowler, Orson]. "Practical Phrenology—No. 1: Directions for Making Examinations with Rules for Finding the Organs." *American Phrenological Journal* 4 (1 January 1842): 14-16.

[_____]. "Health—Its Value and Conditions, Including the Means of Preserving and Regaining It." *American Phrenological Journal* 6 (May 1844): 136-37.

Gleason, R. B. "Hints to Women." *The Water-Cure Journal and Herald of Reforms* 15 (January 1853): 7-8.

Gorton, D. A., M.D. "Practical Hydropathy—No. II." *The Water-Cure Journal and Herald of Reforms* 28 (October 1859): 55-56.

_____. "Theory and Practice—No. VIII: Remedial Agents—Exercise." *The Water-Cure Journal and Herald of Reforms* 28 (August 1853): 17-18.

"Gymnastics." *The Journal of Health* 4 (27 October 1830): 51-53.

"Gymnastics for Girls." *Scientific American Supplement #753* 7 (June 1890).

"Gymnastics in Schools." *The Herald of Health and Journal of Physical Culture* 14 (October 1869): 178.

"Gymnastic Exercises." *The Journal of Health* 1 (13 January 1830): 132.

[Hale, Sarah]. "A Chapter to be Read." *The Ladies Magazine and Literary Gazette* 5 (December 1832): 518.

[_____]. "Female Seminaries." *The Ladies Magazine and Literary Gazette* 6 (March 1833): 142-43.

[_____]. "Hints About Phrenology." *The Ladies Magazine and Literary Gazette* 6 (April 1833): 173-75.

[_____]. "Introduction." *The Ladies Magazine and Literary Gazette* 1 (January 1828): 1.

[_____]. "Literary Notices: A Course of Calisthenics, for Young Ladies in Schools and Families." *The Ladies Magazine and Literary Gazette* 5 (September 1832): 91-92.

[_____]. "On Domestic Industry." *The Ladies Magazine and Literary Gazette* 6 (July 1833): 289-92.

[_____]. "Dr. Grigg"s Lecture." *The Ladies Magazine and Literary Gazette* 4 (November 1831): 514-18.

Hall, Lucy M. "Health and Ill Health of Women—IV." *The Laws of Life* 30 (June 1887): 164-65.

Hanaford, J. H., M.D., "More Muscle for Women." *The Herald of Health and Journal of Physical Culture* 16 (October 1870): 167-69.

"Harriett Martineau on George Combe." *The Phrenological Miscellany; or, the Annuals of Phrenology and Physiognomy from 1865-1873, Revised and Contained in One Volume.* New York: Fowler & Wells, 1882.

"Hartford Female Seminary." *The American Journal of Education* 2 (April 1827): 252-53.

"Hartford Female Seminary." *The American Journal of Education* 3 (August 1828): 461.

"Hartford Female Seminary and Its Founder." *The American Journal of Education* 3 (August 1878): 81-82.

Hawks, Betsy D. "Suggestions to Young Women on Self-Culture." *The Lily* 6 (April 1854): 51.

Higginson, Thomas Wentworth. "The Murder of the Innocents," *Atlantic Monthly* 4 (September 1859): 345-56.

_____. "Gymnastics." *The Atlantic Monthly* 7 (March 1861): 283-302.

_____. "The Health of Our Girls." *The Atlantic Monthly* 9 (June 1862): 722-31.

Holloway, Laura. "The Women of the South." *The Phrenological Journal and Life Illustrated* 51 (September 1870): 208-209.

Hubbard, L. V. "Brookline Gymnasium." *American Journal of Education* 3 (April 1828): 231-33.

"In-Door Exercises." *The Journal of Health* 1 (27 January 1830): 151-52.

"The Influence of Woman on Society." *The Ladies Magazine and Literary Gazette* 4 (June 1831): 261.

Jackson, James C. "A Morning Lecture." *The Laws of Life* 32 (September 1889): 261-63.

_____. "An Open Letter to a Young Mother." 3 parts. *The Laws of Life* 32 (October, November, December 1889): 289-92, 321-24, 353-56.

Jacques, D. H. "Hints Toward Physical Perfection; or, How to Acquire and Retain Beauty, Grace, and Strength, and Secure Long Life and Continued Usefulness." *The Water-Cure Journal and Herald of Reforms* 23 (April, June 1857): 77-78; 123-26 and 24 (July, August, September, October, November, December 1857): 3-5; 29-30; 53-55; 77-79; 100-102; 116-17.

Janes, Lewis G. "George Barker Windship, M.D.—His Relations to Physical Culture." *The Herald of Health* [no volume or date available]. George Barker Windship Papers, Massachusetts Historical Society.

_____. "The Lifting Cure." *The Herald of Health and Journal of Physical Culture* 14 (November 1869): 206-208.

_____. "The Lifting Cure." *The Herald of Health and Journal of Physical Culture* 14 (December 1869): 258-60.

"The Journal of Health." *The Ladies Magazine and Literary Gazette* 6 (March 1833): 46-47.

"Kinesipathic Institute." *The Water-Cure Journal and Herald of Reforms* 28 (August 1859): 29.

Kirk, Eleanor. "Two Women of the Present." *The Phrenological Journal and Life Illustrated* 51 (July 1870): 57-58.

"Letter of the Deputation of the University to the Chairman of the Committee on the Subject of Establishing a Gymnasium in Boston." *American Journal of Education* 1 (July 1826): 444-45.

[Lewis, Dio]. "Boston Gymnasia." *Lewis's New Gymnastics for Ladies, Gentlemen and Children and Boston Journal of Physical Culture* 1 (November 1860): 11.

[_____]. "Commencement Exercises at the Normal Institute for Physical Education. *Lewis's New Gymnastics for Ladies, Gentlemen and Children and Boston Journal of Physical Culture* 1 (October 1861): 178.

[_____]. "Editorial Notices of My Journal." *Lewis's New Gymnastics for Ladies, Gentlemen and Children and Boston Journal of Physical Culture* 1 (January 1861): 45.

_____. "Female Dress." *The Herald of Health and Journal of Physical Culture* 8 (October 1866): 152.

[_____]. "First Graduates of the Normal Institute for Physical Education." *Lewis's New Gymnastics for Ladies, Gentlemen and*

*Children and Boston Journal of Physical Culture* 1 (October 1861): 188.

[_____]. "Gymnastics Before the American Institute of Instruction at Its Recent Meeting in Tremont Temple, Boston, Mass." Lewis's *New Gymnastics for Ladies, Gentlemen and Children and Boston Journal of Physical Culture* 1 (November 1860): 15-16.

[_____]. "Gymnastics in the Atlantic Monthly." *Lewis's New Gymnastics for Ladies, Gentlemen and Children and Boston Journal of Physical Culture* 1 (October 1861): 178.

[_____]. "Heavy and Light Gymnastics." *Lewis's New Gymnastics for Ladies, Gentlemen and Children and Boston Journal of Physical Culture* 1 (November 1860): 16.

[_____]. "Heavy and Light Gymnastics." *Lewis's New Gymnastics for Ladies, Gentlemen and Children and Boston Journal of Physical Culture* 1 (December 1860): 29.

[_____]. "Important to Subscribers." *Lewis's Gymnastic Monthly and Journal of Physical Culture* 2 (October 1861): 184.

[_____]. "Ladies Gymnastic Dress." *Lewis's New Gymnastics for Ladies, Gentlemen and Children and Boston Journal of Physical Culture* 1 (May 1861): 106.

[_____]. "Miss Beecher and her Western College." *Lewis's New Gymnastics for Ladies, Gentlemen and Children and Boston Journal of Physical Culture* 1 (August 1861): 155.

[_____]. "Mistakes in Gymnastics." *Lewis's New Gymnastics for Ladies, Gentlemen and Children and Boston Journal of Physical Culture* 1 (November 1860): 12.

[_____]. "Movement Cure in Boston." *Lewis's New Gymnastics for Ladies, Gentlemen and Children and Boston Journal of Physical Culture* 1 (November 1860): 12.

_____. "The New Gymnastics." *The Herald of Health and Water-Cure Journal* 1 (January 1863): 8-10.

_____. "The New Gymnastics: Exercises With Wands." *The Herald of Health and Water-Cure Journal* 1 (February 1863): 60-62.

_____. "The New Gymnastics: The Pangymnastikon." *The Herald of Health and Water-Cure Journal* 1 (March 1863): 112-15.

_____. "The New Gymnastics: Continued." *The Herald of Health and Water-Cure Journal* 1 (April 1863): 144-46

_____. "The New Gymnastics: Continued." *The Herald of Health and Water-Cure Journal* 1 (May 1863): 189-90.

_____. "The New Gymnastics." *Atlantic Monthly* 10 (August 1862): 129-43.

[_____]. "Normal School for Gymnastics." *Lewis's New Gymnastics for Ladies, Gentlemen and Children and Boston Journal of Physical Culture* 1 (April 1861): 91.

_____. "Physical Culture." Parts I & II. *The Massachusetts Teacher* 13 (October, November 1860): 377, 404.

[_____]. "Physical Training of Girls." *Lewis's Gymnastic Monthly for Ladies, Gentlemen and Children and Boston Journal of Physical Culture* 1 (April 1861): 99.

[_____]. "Second Course of Lewis's Normal Institute for Physical Education." *Lewis's New Gymnastics for Ladies, Gentlemen and Children and Boston Journal of Physical Culture* 1 (October 1861): 190.

[_____]. "Teachers of Gymnastics." *Lewis's New Gymnastics for Ladies, Gentlemen and Children and Boston Journal of Physical Culture* 1 (April 1861): 87.

[_____]. "Southern Subscribers." *Lewis's New Gymnastics for Ladies, Gentlemen and Children and Boston Journal of Physical Culture* 1 (May 1861): 112.

[_____]. "Teachers of Gymnastics." *Lewis's New Gymnastics for Ladies, Gentlemen and Children and Boston Journal of Physical Culture* 1 (April 1861): 87.

[_____]. "Teachers of the New Gymnastics." *Lewis's New Gymnastics for Ladies, Gentlemen and Children and Boston Journal of Physical Culture* 1 (December 1860): 30.

[_____ and Catharine Beecher]. "Physiology and Calisthenics." *Lewis's New Gymnastics for Ladies, Gentlemen and Children and Boston Journal of Physical Culture* 1 (January 1861): 45.

[_____]. "Physical Education." *Lewis's New Gymnastics for Ladies, Gentlemen and Children and Boston Journal of Physical Culture* 1 (November 1860): 1.

_____, Elizabeth Cady Stanton and James Read Chadwick. "The Health of American Women." *The North American Review* 135 (December 1882): 503-24.

[Lieber, Franz.] "A Review: Art. VI.—A Treatise on Gymnastics: Taken Chiefly from the German of F. L. Jahn. 8 vols. Northampton, Massachusetts: 1828." *American Quarterly Review* 3 (March 1828): 126-50.

"The Lift Cure." *The Phrenological Journal and Life Illustrated* 51 (November 1870): 5 in "Journal Miscellany."

"London Gymnastic Institution." *American Journal of Education* 1 (October 1826): 79-80.

M. M. K. "Reform for Women." *Phrenologial Journal and Life Illustrated* 51 (July 1870): 27-28.

"Maine Wesleyan Seminary." *Quarterly Register and Journal of the American Education Society* 2 (November 1829): 63, 110-12.

Mann, Horace. "Gymnasia." *The Common School Journal* 7 (10 June 1845): 12.

[_____]. "Physical Exercise: Dr. Thayer's Gymnastic Apparatus, Boylston Hall, Boston." *The Common School Journal* 7 (16 June 1845): 177-79.

_____. "Prospectus." *The Common School Journal* 1 (November 1838): 10-11.

Martineau, Harriet. "On Female Education." *Monthly Repository* 17 (October 1822): 77-81.

_____. "Female Industry." *The Edinburgh Review* 222 (April 1859): 293-336.

"Measuring Man." 3 parts. *Phrenological Journal and Life Illustrated* 51 (July, September, October 1870): 9-10; 156-58; 304-306.

"Miscellany: The Green Mountain Boys." *The American Phrenological Journal and Miscellany* 6 (February 1844): 46.

"Miss Harriett N. Austin, M.D." *The Water-Cure Journal and Herald of Health* 27 (May 1859): 77.

Mumford, Prentice. "The Coming Woman." *Lippincott's Monthly Magazine* 9 (January 1872): 107.

[Neal, John]. "Gymnasium." *American Journal of Education* 1 (June 1826): 61.

[_____]. "Gymnasic Exercises in London." *American Journal of Education* 1 (June 1826): 75.

[_____]. "Gymnastic Schools in England." *American Journal of Education* 2 (January 1827): 55-56.

_____. *Wandering Recollections of a Somewhat Busy Life: An Autobiography.* Boston: Roberts Brothers, 1869.

"The Noyes School." *American Journal of Education* 1 (June 1826): 378-79.

Parkman, Francis. "The Woman Question." *North American Review* 129 (October 1879): 309.

"Physical Culture at Vassar College." *The Herald of Health and Journal of Physical Culture* 13 (February 1869): 83-84.

"The Physical Education of Girls." *The Journal of Health* 1 (9 September 1829): 15.

"The Physical Education of Girls." *The Lily* 4 (March 1852): 8-9.

"Physical Training." *Harpers Weekly* 4 (22 September 1860): 594.

Porter, James. "Female Independence." *The Mother's Assistant & Young Lady's Friend* 4 (April 1844): 94-95.

Powell, E. M. "Physical Culture at Vassar College." *The Herald of Health and Journal of Physical Culture* 13 (March 1869): 133-35.

"Preservation of Beauty." *The Journal of Health* 2 (24 November 1830): 89-90.

"Professor Fowler in England." *The Herald of Health and Journal of Physical Culture* 13 (June 1869): 281.

"Professor Voelker's Gymnasium, London." *American Journal of Education* 1 (July 1826): 430-32.

"Progress of Physical Education." *The American Journal of Education* 1 (January 1826): 19-23.

"Prospectus." *The American Journal of Education* 1 (January 1826): 3.

"Prospectus of the London Gymnastic Society." *American Journal of Education* 1 (August 1826): 502-503.

"Prospectus for the New Haven Gymnasium; A School for the Education of Boys, to be Established at New Haven, Conn.; by Sereno E. Dwight and Henry E. Dwight." *American Journal of Education* 3 (February 1828): 115-16.

"Review of Charles Londe's Medical Gymnastics; or Exercise Applied to the Organs of Man." *American Journal of Education* 1 (April 1826): 253-59.

"Reviews." *American Journal of Education* 1 (August 1827): 489.

"Round Hill School." *American Journal of Education* 1 (July 1826): 437-39.

"Rules for a Young Lady." *The Ladies Magazine and Literary Gazette* 3 (May 1830): 46-47.

"Russell T. Trall: Portrait, Character and Biography." *Herald of Health* 4 (July 1864): 2-4.

Seymour, Mary Alice. "Fern Grove Gymnasium." *The Herald of Health and Journal of Physical Culture* 15 (March 1870): 110-12.

"She Was Frail, and So She Died." *The Phrenological Journal and Life Illustrated* 51 (November 1870): 310-11.

[Stanton, Elizabeth Cady]. "Man Superior—Intellectually—Morally and Physically." *The Lily* 3 (June 1851): 31-32.

"Suggestions to Parents: Physical Education." *The American Journal of Education* 2 (May 1827): 289-92.

Swank, Emi B. "Importance of Physiological Knowledge." *The Lily* 17 (June 1855): 94.

Taylor, George H. "Body and Mind—In Two Chapters" *The Water-Cure Journal and Herald of Health* 16 (December 1853): 125-26; and 17 (January 1854): 22-23.

_____. "Consumption." *The Herald of Health and Journal of Physical Culture* 14 (August 1869): 68-71.

_____. "Efficacy of the Movement-Cure." *The Water-Cure Journal and Herald of Health* 27 (June 1859): 82-83.

_____. "The Movement-Cure." *The Water-Cure Journal and Herald of Health* 27 (May 1859): 65-66.

Taylor, Mrs. "Physical Training for Young Ladies." *Lewis's New Gymnastics for Ladies, Gentlemen and Children and Boston Journal of Physical Culture* 1 (February 1861): 54.

"Thoughts on the Education of Females." *The American Journal of Education* 1 (June 1826): 351-52.

Trall, Russell, T. "Exercise-pathy," *The Water-Cure Journal and Herald of Reforms* 24 (October 1857): 74-76.

"Treatise on Gymnastics." *American Journal of Education* 2 (October 1827): 629-30.

Tyler, Moses Coit. "Concerning a Muscular Christian." *The Herald of Health and Journal of Physical Culture* 8 (October 1866): 145-49.

_____. "Minutes of the Brawnville Athletic Club." *The Herald of Health and Journal of Physical Culture* 10 (August 1867): 50-54.

_____. "Muscular Christinity." *The Herald of Health and Journal of Physical Culture* 8 (September 1866): 97-99.

Vail, W. T., M.D. "Exercise a Remedial Measure." *The Water-Cure Journal and Herald of Reforms* 23 (May 1857): 104.

"Variety in Exercise." *The Journal of Health* 1 (28 April 1830): 243-44.

Vaughan, M. C. "Letter from Mrs. Vaughan to Amelia Bloomer." *The Lily* 4 (August 1852): 67.

*"Walking." The Mother's Assistant & Young Lady's Friend* 3 *(April 1843):* 87.

"The Wasp Waist." *Phrenological Journal and Life Illustrated* 50 (January 1870): 46-48.

"The Weaker Sex." *The Herald of Health and Journal of Physical Culture* 16 (May 1870): 227-28.

West, M. S. "Essentials to Right Government." *The Mother's Assistant* 3 (September 1843): 193-96.

"Western Female Institute." *American Annals of Education and Instruction* 3 (August 1833): 380-81.

"What Women are Doing." *The Laws of Life* 32 (June 1889): 168.

Willard, Emma. "Address." *Ladies Magazine and Literary Gazette* 6 (May 1833): 236-37.

"William Bentley Fowle." *The American Journal of Education* 10 (June 1861): 603.

Windship, George Barker, M.D. "Autobiographical Sketches of a Strength-Seeker." *The Atlantic Monthly* 9 (January 1862): 102-15.

_____. "Physical Culture," *The Massachusetts Teacher* 13 (April 1860): 128.

Wood, A. L., M.D. "Physical Development at Home." *The Herald of Health and Journal of Physical Culture* 16 (August 1870): 90.

Wymond, E. M. "Progress of Female Education." *The Mother's Assistant & Young Lady's Friend* 3 (April 1843): 92-94.

"Young Womanhood in America." *Phrenological Journal and Packard's Monthly* 50 (May 1870): 344-46.

### Secondary Sources

#### Books, Book Chapters, and Reports

Abram, Ruth J. *Send Us a Lady Physician: Women Doctors in America, 1835-1920.* New York: W. W. Norton and Co., 1985.

Abzug, Robert H. *Passionate Liberator: Theodore Dwight Weld and the Dilemma of Reform.* New York: Oxford University Press, 1980.

Adelman, Melvin L. *A Sporting Time: New York City and the Rise of Modern Athletics, 1820-1870.* Urbana: University of Illinois, 1986.

Ainsworth, Dorothy. *The History of Physical Education in Colleges for Women.* New York: A. S. Barnes and Company, 1930.

Albertson, Roxanne. "Sports and Games in Eastern Schools, 1780-1880." In *Sport in American Education: History and Perspective.* Wayne M. Ladd and Angela Lumpkin, eds. History of Sport and Physical Education Academy Symposia—24 March 1977 and 6 April 1978. Washington: American Alliance for Health, Physical Education, Recreation, and Dance, 1979.

Atkinson, Paul. "The Feminist Physique: Physical Education and the Medicalization of Women's Education." In J. A. Mangan and

Roberta J. Park, eds. *From Fair Sex to Feminism: Sport and the Socialization of Women in the Industrial and Post-Industrial Eras.* London: Frank Cass and Company, 1987.

Baker, Elizabeth Renwick. "Historical Perspectives of Research on Physical Activity and the Menstrual Cycle." In *The Menstrual Cycle and Physical Activity.* Jacqueline L. Puhl and C. Harmon Brown, M.D., eds. Chicago: Human Kinetics, 1986.

Banner, Lois. *American Beauty.* New York: Alfred A. Knopf, 1983.

Banta, Martha. *Imaging American Women: Idea and Ideas in Cultural History.* New York: Columbia University Press, 1987.

Barney, Robert K. "German Turners in America: Their Role in Nineteenth-Century Exercise Expression and Physical Education Legislation." In *A History of Physical Education and Sport in the United States and Canada.* Earle F. Ziegler, ed. Champaign, IL: Stites Publishing, 1975.

Bell, Linda A., ed. *Visions of Women: Being a Fascinating Anthology with Analysis of Philosophers's Views of Women from Ancient to Modern Times.* Clifton NJ: Humana Press, 1983.

Blake, John B. "Diseases and Medical Practice in Colonial America." In *History of American Medicine: A Symposium.* Felix Marti-Ibanez, M.D., ed. New York: MD Publications, Inc., 1958.

_____. "Health Reform." In *The Rise of Adventism: Religion and Society in Mid-Nineteenth-Century America.* Edwin S. Gaustad, ed. New York: Harper & Row, 1974.

Bledstein, Burton J. *The Culture of Professionalism: The Middle Class and the Development of Higher Education in America.* New York: W. W. Norton & Co., 1976.

Boydston, Jeanne, Mary Kelley and Anne Margolis. *The Limits of Sisterhood: The Beecher Sisters on Women's Rights and Woman's Sphere.* Chapel Hill: University of North Carolina Press, 1988.

Caskey, Marie. *Chariot of Fire: Religion and the Beecher Family.* New Haven: Yale University Press, 1978.

Cayleff, Susan E. *Wash and be Healed, The Water-Cure Movement and Women's Health.* Philadelphia: Temple University Press, 1987.

Clinton, Catharine. *The Other Civil War: American Women in the Nineteenth Century.* New York: Hill and Wang, 1984.

Cogan, Frances B. *All-American Girl: The Ideal of Real Womanhood in Mid-Nineteenth-Century America.* Athens: University of Georgia Press, 1989.

Cott, Nancy F. and Elizabeth H. Pleck. *A Heritage of Her Own: Toward a New Social History of American Women.* New York: Simon and Schuster, 1979.

Curti, Merle. *The Social Ideas of American Educators: With New Chapter on the Last Twenty-Five Years.* Totowa, NJ: Littlefield, Adams & Co., 1966.

Daniels, George H. *American Science in the Age of Jackson.* New York: Columbia University Press, 1968.

Davies, John D. *Phrenology: Fad and Science.* New Haven: Yale University Press, 1955.

Desbonnet, Edmund. *Les Rois de la Force.* Paris: Berger-Levrault, 1911.

Donnelly, Mabel Collins. *The American Victorian Woman: The Myth and the Reality.* New York: Greenwood Press, 1986.

Douglas, Ann. *The Feminization of American Culture.* New York: Avon Books, 1977.

Dufay, Pierre. *Le Pantalon Feminin.* Paris: 1906.

Ehrenreich, Barbara and Deidre English. *For Her Own Good: 150 Years of the Experts Advice to Women.* New York: Anchor Press, 1979.

Faust, Albert Bernhardt. *The German Element in the United States With Special Reference to its Political, Moral, Social and Educational Influence.* 2 vols. Boston: Houghton Mifflin, 1909.

Fellman, Anita Clair and Michael Fellman. *Making Sense of Self: Medical Advice Literature in Late Nineteenth-Century America.* Philadelphia: University of Pennsylvania Press, 1981.

Fishburn, Katherine. *Women in Popular Culture: A Reference Guide.* Westport, CT: Grenwood Press, 1982.

Flexner, Eleanor. *Century of Struggle: The Woman's Rights Movement in the United States.* rev. ed. Cambridge: Harvard University Press, 1975.

Gerber, Ellen. *Innovators and Institutions in Physical Education.* Philadelphia: Lea and Febiger, 1971.

Glassner, Barry. *Bodies: Why We Look the Way We Do (And How We Feel About It).* New York: G. P. Putman's Sons, 1988.

Goodman, Nathan G. *Benjamin Rush: Physician and Citizen, 1746-1813.* Philadelphia: University of Pennsylvania Press, 1934.

Goodsell, Willystine. *Pioneers of Women's Education in the United States.* New York: McGraw Hill, Inc., 1931.

Gorham, Deborah. *The Victorian Girl and the Feminine Ideal.* Bloomington: Indiana University Press, 1982.

Gould, Stephen Jay. *The Mismeasure of Man*. New York: W. W. Norton & Co., 1981.

Green, Elizabeth Alden. *Mary Lyon and Mount Holyoke: Opening the Gates*. Hanover NH: University Press of New England, 1979.

Green, Harvey. *Fit for America: Health, Fitness, Sport and American Society*. New York: Pantheon Books, 1986.

Guttmann, Allen. *From Ritual to Record: The Nature of Modern Sports*. New York: Columbia University Press, 1978.

_____. *Women's Sports: A History*. New York: Columbia University Press, 1991.

Hackensmith, C. W. *History of Physical Education*. New York: Harper & Row, 1967.

Hale, Sarah Josepha. *Biography of Distinguished Women; or, Woman's Record, from the Creation to A.D. 1869*. New York: Harper & Brothers, 1876.

Haley, Bruce. *The Healthy Body and Victorian Culture*. Cambridge, Massachusetts: Harvard University Press, 1978.

Haller, John S. and Robin M. Haller. *The Physician and Sexuality in Victorian America*. Urbana: University of Illinois, 1974.

Hartwell, Edward Mussey. *School Document No. 22: Report of the Director of Physical Training, December 1891*. Boston: Rockwell and Churchill, 1891.

Helsinger, Elizabeth K., Robin Lauterbach Sheets, and William Veeder. "The Woman Question: Social Issues, 1837-1883." In *The Woman Question: Soceity and Literature in Britain and America, 1837-1883*. vol. 2. New York: Graland Publishing, 1983.

Hill, Joseph A. *U.S. Department of Commerce: Women in Gainful Occupations, 1870-1920*. Census Monograph IX. Westport CT: Greenwood Press, [1929] 1978.

Hobson, Barbara Mill. *Uneasy Virtue: The Politics of Prostitution and the American Reform Tradition*. New York: Basic Books, Inc., 1987.

Holliman, Jennie. *American Sports: 1785-1835*. Durham, NC: The Seeman Press. 1931.

Hudson, Charles. *History of the Town of Lexington, Middlesex County, Massachusetts, From Its First Settlement to 1868, With a Genealogical Register of Lexington Families*. Boston: Wiggin & Lunt, 1868.

Hymowitz, Carol and Michaele Weissman. *A History of Women in America*. New York: Bantam Books, 1978.

Jenkyns, Richard. *The Victorians and Ancient Greece.* Cambridge: Harvard University Press, 1980.

Kelly, Mary, ed. *Woman's Being, Woman's Place: Female Identity and Vocation in American History.* Boston: G. K. Hall & Co., 1979.

Kennedy, Susan Eastbrook. *If All We Did Was Weep at Home: A History of White Working-Class Women in America.* Bloomington: Indiana University Press, 1979.

Kerber, Linda K. "The Republican Mother" In *Women's America: Refocusing the Past.* 2nd ed. Linda Kerber and Jane DeHart-Matthews, eds. New York: Oxford University Press, 1987.

Kern, Stephen. *Anatomy and Destiny: A Cultural History of the Human Body.* Indianapolis: Bobbs-Merrill Company, 1975.

L"Esperance, Jean. "Doctors and Women in Nineteenth-Century Society: Sexuality and Role." In *Health Care and Popular Medicine in Nineteenth Century England: Essays in the Social History of Medicine.* John Woodward and David Richards, eds. London: Croom Helm, 1977.

Leach, William. *True Love and Perfect Union: The Feminist Reform of Sex and Society.* New York: Basic Books, Inc. 1980.

Lenskyj, Helen. *Out of Bounds: Women, Sport and Sexuality.* Toronto: The Women's Press, 1988.

Leonard, Fred Eugene. *Pioneers of Modern Physical Training.* New York: Association Press, 1915.

_____. *A Guide to the History of Physical Education.* 2nd ed. R. Tait McKenzie, ed. Philadelphia: Lea & Febiger, 1927.

Lerner, Gerda. *The Grimke Sisters from South Carolina: Pioneers for Woman's Rights and Abolition.* New York: Schocken Books, 1974.

_____. *The Woman in American History.* Menlo Park CA: Addison-Wesley Publishing Co., 1971.

McCrone, Kathleen E. *Playing the Game: Sport and Physical Education of English Women: 1870-1914.* Lexington: University Press of Kentucky, 1981.

McIntosh, Peter C. *Physical Education in England Since 1800.* London: G. Bell & Sons, 1952.

Mandell, Richard D. *Sport: A Cultural History.* New York: Columbia University Press, 1984.

Marks, Patricia. *Bicycles, Bangs, and Bloomers: The New Woman in the Popular Press.* Lexington: University Press of Kentucky, 1990.

Marr, Harriet. *The Old New England Academies Founded Before 1826.* New York: E. P. Dutton, 1959.

Metzner, Henry. *A Brief History of the North American Gymnastic Union: In Commemoration of the One Hundredth Anniversary of the Opening of the First Gymnastic Field in Germany by Friedrich Ludwig Jahn.* Indianapolis: National Executive Committe of the North American Gymnastic Union, 1911.

Morantz-Sanchez, Regina M. *Sympathy and Science: Women Physicians in American Medicine.* New York: Oxford University Press, 1985.

Munrow, A. D. *Landmarks in the History of Physical Education.* London: Routledge and Kegan Paul, 1957.

Murray, Anne Wood. "The Bloomer Costume and Exercise Suits." In *Waffen-und Kostumkunde.* Munich: Deutscher Kunstverlad, 1982.

*National Cyclopaedia of American Biography: Being the History of the United States as Illustrated in the Lives of the Founders, Builders, and Defenders of the Republic and of the Men and Women who are Doing the Work and Moulding the Thought of the Present Time.* New York: James T. White, 1909.

Newman, Louise Michele. *Men's Ideas/Women's Realities: Popular Science, 1870-1915.* New York: Pergamon Press, 1985.

Newton, Stella Mary. *Health, Art and Reason: Dress Reformers of the Nineteenth Century.* London: John Murray, 1974.

Nissenbaum, Stephen. *Sex, Diet and Debility in Jacksonian America: Sylvester Graham and Health Reform.* Westport, CT: Greenwood Press, 1980.

Norton, Mary Beth. *Liberty's Daughters: the Revolutionary Experience of American Women.* Boston: Little, Brown and Co., 1980.

Norwood, William Frederick "Medicine in the Era of the American Revolution," In *History of American Medicine: A Symposium.* Felix Marti-Ibanez, M.D., ed. New York: MD Publications, Inc., 1958.

Park, Roberta J. "Biological Thought, Athletics and the Formation of a 'Man of Character': 1830-1900." In James Anthony Mangan and James Walvin, eds. *Manliness and Morality: Middle-class Masculinity in Britain and America: 1800-1940.* New York: St. Martin's Press, 1987.

Postell, William D. "Medical Education and Medical Schools in Colonial America." In *History of American Medicine: A Symposium.* Felix Marti-Ibanez, M.D., ed. New York: MD Publications, Inc., 1958.

Purcell, Mabelle. *Two Texas Female Seminaries.* Wichita Falls, TX: University Press, 1978.

Rice, Emmett A. *A Brief History of Physical Education.* New York: A. S. Barnes and Co., 1927.

Robinson, Josephine. *Circus Lady.* New York: Thomas Y. Crowell, 1926.

Rosenberg, Charles E. "The Therapeutic Revolution: Medicine, Meaning, and Social Change in Nineteenth Century America." In *The Therapeutic Revolution: Essays in the History of American Medicine.* Morris J. Vogel and Charles E. Rosenberg, eds. University of Pennsylvania Press, 1979.

Ross, Ishbel. *Child of Destiny: The Life Story of the First Woman Doctor.* New York: Harper & Brothers, 1949.

Rothstein, William G. *American Physicians in the Nineteenth Century: From Sects to Science.* Baltimore: John Hopkins University Press, 1972.

Rudofsky, Bernard. *The Unfashionable Human Body.* New York: Doubleday and Company, 1971.

Schlesinger, Arthur M. *The Age of Jackson.* Boston: Little, Brown & Co., 1953.

Schmidt, Albert-Marie. *John Calvin and the Calvinist Tradition.* Trans. Ronald Wallace. New York: Harper & Brothers, 1960.

Schwartz, Hillel. *Never Satisfied: A Cultural History of Diets, Fantasies and Fat.* New York: Doubleday-Anchor Books, 1986.

Scott, Gladys and Mary J. Hoferek eds. *Women as Leaders in Physical Education and Sports: A Lecture Series Sponsored by the University of Iowa Department of Physical Education and Dance.* Iowa City: University of Iowa, 1979.

Shaftel, Norman. "The Evolution of American Medical Literature." In *History of American Medicine: A Symposium.* Felix Marti-Ibanez, M.D., ed. New York: MD Publications, Inc., 1958,.

Sklar, Katherine Kish. *Catharine Beecher: A Study in American Domesticity.* New York: Norton and Company, 1973.

_____. "Catharine Beecher: Transforming the Teaching Profession." In *Women's America: Refocusing the Past.* 2nd ed. Linda Kerber and Jane De Hart-Matthews, eds. New York: Oxford University Press, 1987.

Smith, F[rancis]. B. *The People's Health 1830-1910.* London: Croom Helm, 1979.

Spears, Betty. "The Emergence of Women in Sport." In *Women's Athletics: Coping With Controversy.* Barbara J. Hoepner, ed. Published by the Division for Girls and Women's Sports of the American Association for Health, Physical Education, and Recreation, 1974.

_____. "Senda Berenson Abbott—New Woman, New Sport." In *A Century of Women's Basketball: From Frailty to Final Four*. Joan Hult and Marianna Trekell, eds. Reston, VA: American Alliance for Health, Physical Education, Recreation, and Dance, 1991.

_____ and Richard A. Swanson. *History of Sport and Physical Activity in the United States*. Dubuque, IA: William C. Brown, 1978.

Steele, Valerie. *Fashion and Eroticism: Ideals of Feminine Beauty from the Victorian Era to the Jazz Age*. New York: Oxford University Press, 1985.

Stern, Madeline. *Heads and Headlines: The Phrenological Fowlers*. Norman, OK: University of Oklahoma Press, 1971.

Stowe, Lyman Beecher. *Saints, Sinners and Beechers*. Indianapolis: Bobbs-Merill Company, 1934.

Struna, Nancy L. "'Good Wives and 'Gardeners, "Spinners and Fearless Riders: Middle and Upper-rank Women in the Early American Sporting Culture." In J. A. Mangan and Roberta J. Park, eds. *From Fair Sex to Feminism: Sport and the Socialization of Women in the Industrial and Post-Industrial Eras*. London: Frank Cass and Company, 1987.

Todd, Jan. "Bernarr Macfadden: Reformer of Feminine Form." In *Sport and Exercise Science: Essays in the History of Sports Medicine*. Jack Berryman and Roberta J. Park, eds. Urbana: University of Illinois Press, 1992.

Thomas, Benjamin P. *Theodore Weld: Crusader for Freedom*. New Brunswick, NJ: Rutgers University Press, 1950.

Van Dalen, Deobold, Elmer Mitchell and Bruce Bennett. *A World History of Physical Education*. Englewood Cliffs, NJ: Prentice Hall, 1963.

Verbrugge, Martha H. *Able-Bodied Womanhood: Personal Health and Social Change in Nineteenth-Century Boston*. New York: Oxford University Press, 1988.

Vertinsky, Patricia. "Body Shapes: The Role of the Medical Establishment in Informing Female Exercise and Physical Education in Nineteenth-Century North America." In *From Fair Sex to Feminism: Sport and the Socialization of Women in the Industrial and Post Industrial Eras*. J. A. Mangan and Roberta J. Park, eds. London: Frank Cass, Publishing, 1987.

_____. *The Eternally Wounded Woman: Women, Exercise and Doctors in the Late Nineteenth Century*. New York: Manchester University Press, 1990.

Walsh, Mary Ruth. *Doctors Wanted: No Women Need Apply: Sexual Barriers in the Medical Profession, 1835-1975.* New Haven: Yale University Press, 1977.

Walters, Ronald G. *American Reformers: 1815-1860.* New York: Hill and Wang, 1978.

Weatherford, Doris. *Foreign and Female: Immigrant Women in America, 1840-1930.* New York: Schocken Books, 1986.

Weiss, Harry B. and Howard R. Kemble. *The Great American Water-Cure Craze: A History of Hydropathy in the United States.* Trenton, NJ: The Past Times Press, 1967.

Weston, Arthur. *The Making of American Physical Education.* New York: Appleton-Century-Crofts, 1962.

White, Alain C. The History of the Town of Litchfield, Connecticut: 1720-1920. Litchfield: Enquirer Print, 1920.

White, Cynthia L. *Women's Magazines: 1693-1968.* London: Michael Joseph, 1983.

Whorton, James C. *Crusaders for Fitness: The History of American Health Reformers.* Princeton, NJ: Princeton University Press, 1982.

Wilder, Alex, M.D. *The History of Medicine.* New Sharon, ME: New England Eclectic Publishing Company, 1901.

Woloch, Nancy. *Women and the American Experience.* New York: Alfred A. Knopf, 1984.

Woodward, Helen. *The Lady Persuaders.* New York: Ivan Obolensky, 1960.

Woody, Thomas. *A History of Women's Education in the United States.* 2 vols. New York: Science Press, 1929.

Yates, Gayle Graham, ed. *Harriet Martineau on Women.* New Brunswick, NJ: Rutgers University Press, 1985.

## Serial Articles

Atkinson, Paul. "Strong Minds and Weak Bodies: Sports, Gymnastics and the Medicalization of Women's Education." *British Journal of Sport History* 2 (May 1985): 62-71.

Atwater, Edward C. and Lawrence A. Kohn. "Rochester and the Water-Cure: 1844-1854." *Rochester History* 32 (October 1970): 1-24.

Ballin, Hans. "Biographical Sketch of Friedrich Ludwig Jahn." *Mind and Body* 1 (October 1894): 1-7.

_____. "Johann Heinrich Pestalozzi." *Mind and Body* 2 (February 1896): 221-25.

Barney, Robert K. "Adele Parot: Beacon of the Dioclesian Lewis School of Gymnastic Expression in the American West." *Canadian Journal of the History of Sport* 5 (December 1974): 63-75.

_____. "Mary E. Allen: Thought and Practice in Nineteenth-Century American Gymnastics." *Journal of Health, Physical Education and Recreation* 51 (April 1980): 82-86.

Bassett, John S. "The Round Hill School." *American Antiquarian Society Proceedings* 27 (April 1917): 18-62.

Bennett, Bruce. "The Making of Round Hill School." *Quest* 4 (1963-1965): 58-59.

Berryman, Jack. "The Tradition of the Six Things Non-Natural: Exercise and Medicine from Hippocrates through Ante-Bellum America." *Exercise and Sport Sciences Reviews* 17 (1989): 518-19.

_____. "The Ladies' Department of the American Farmer, 1825-1830; A Locus for the Advocacy of Family Health and Exercise." *Associates National Agriculture Library Today* 2 (September 1977): 8-15.

Betts, John R. "American Medical Thought on Exercise as the Road to Health, 1820-1860." *Bulletin of the History of Medicine* 45 (1971): 138-52.

_____. "Mind and Body in Early American Thought." *Journal of American History* 54 (1968): 787-805.

_____. "The Technological Revolution and the Rise of Sport, 1850-1900." *The Mississippi Valley Historical Review* 40 (September 1953): 231-56.

Betz, Carl. "Swedish Versus German Gymnastics." *Mind and Body* 1 (March 1894): 10-13.

Ralph Billett. "Evidence of Play and Exercise in Early Pestalozzian and Lancasterian Elementary Schools in the United States, 1809-1845." *Research Quarterly* 23 (1952): 127-35.

Blake, John B. "Mary Gove Nichols, Prophetess of Health." *Proceedings of the American Philosophical Society* 106 (June 1962): 219-34.

Borish, Linda J. "The Robust Woman and the Muscular Christian: Catharine Beecher, Thomas Higginson and Their Vision of American Society, Health and Physical Activities." *International Journal of the History of Sport* 4 (Summer 1987): 139-54.

Bullough, Vern and Martha Voght. "Women, Menstruation and Nineteenth-Century Medicine." *Bulletin of the History of Medicine* 47 (1973): 66-82.

Burnham, John C. "Change in the Popularization of Health in the United States." *Bulletin of the History of Medicine* 59 (1984): 183-97.

Cole, Edith Walters. "Sylvester P. Graham, 'Father of the Graham Cracker.'" *Southern Speech Journal* 32 (1967): 206-14.

Coleman, W. "Health and Hygiene in the *Encyclopedie,* a Medical Doctrine for the Bourgeosie." *Journal of the History of Medicine* 29 (1974): 399-421.

_____. "The People's Health: Medical Themes in Eighteenth-Century French Popular Literature." *Bulletin of the History of Medicine* 51 (1977): 55-74.

Cyriax, Richard J. "A Short History of Mechano-Therapeutics in Europe Until the Time of Ling." *Janus* 19 (1914): 178-88.

Ellis, George E. "Recollections of Round Hill School." *Educational Review* 1 (April 1891): 337-44.

Fee, Elizabeth. "Nineteenth-Century Craniology: The Study of the Female Skull." *Bulletin of the History of Medicine* 53 (1979): 415-33.

Fletcher, Gerald F. "The History of Exercise in the Practice of Medicine." *Journal of the Medical Association of Georgia* 72 (January 1973): 34-36.

Haller, John S. "From Maidenhood to Menopause: Sex Education for Women in Victorian America." *Journal of Popular Culture* 6 (Summer 1972): 49-69.

Hildebrandt, Edith L. "The Historical Aspect of Physical Education." *Mind and Body* 26 (April 1919): 49-585.

Hoff, Hebbel E., M.D., and John F. Fulton, M.D. "The Centenary of the First American Physiological Society Founded at Boston by William A. Alcott and Sylvester Graham." *Bulletin of the Institute of the History of Medicine* 5 (October 1937): 687-734.

Holland, Judith R. and Carole Oglesby. "Women in Sport: The Synthesis Begins." *Annals of the American Academy of Political and Social Science.* No. 445 (1979): 80-90.

Howard, Mildred S. "A Century of Physical Education." *Mount Holyoke Alumnae Quarterly* 19 (February 1936).

Joseph, L. H. "Physical Education in the Early Middle Ages." *Ciba Symposia* 10 (March-April 1949): 1028-31.

Joynt, Robert J. "Phrenology in New York State." *New York State Journal of Medicine* 73 (1 October 1973): 2382-84.

Kelly-Gadol, Joan. "The Social Relation of the Sexes: Methodological Implications of Women's History." *Signs: Journal of Women in Culture and Society* 1 (1976): 809-23.

Kennard, June. "The History of Physical Education." *Signs: Journal of Women in Culture and Society* 2 (Summer 1977): 835-42.

Klein, Siegmund. "American Pioneers of Weightlifting." *Strength & Health* 10 (November, 1942): 15, 40-41.

Legan, Marshall Scott. "Hydropathy in America: A Nineteenth-Century Panacea." *Bulletin of the History of Medicine* 45 (May-June 1971): 267-80.

Leonard Fred Eugene. "Adolf Spiess, The Founder of School Gymnastics in Germany." *Mind and Body* 11 (November 1904): 217-23.

_____. "The Beginnings of Modern Physical Training in Europe." *Mind and Body* 11 (November 1904): 239-41.

_____. "Chapters from the Early History of Physical Training in America. Part I: Captain Alden Partridge, and His Military Academies." *Mind and Body* 13 (November 1906): 257-65.

_____. "Chapters from the Early History of Physical Training in America. Part II: The Introduction of 'Calisthenics' for Girls and Women (Dating From About 1830)." *Mind and Body* 13 (December 1906): 289-96.

_____. "The First Introduction of Jahn Gymnastics Into America (1825-1830)." 6 parts. *Mind and Body* 12 (September, October, November, December 1905) and 12 (January, February 1906): 193-98, 217-23, 248-54, 281-87, 313-19, 345-51.

_____. "Friedrich Ludwig Jahn, and the Development of Popular Gymnastics (Vereinsturnen) in Germany." 2 parts. *Mind and Body* 12 (July, August 1905): 133-39; 170-75.

_____. "German-American Gymnastic Societies and the North American Turnerbund." *American Physical Education Review* 15 (December 1910): 617-28.

_____. "Johann Christoph Friedrich GutsMuths, Teacher of Gymnastics at Schnepfenthal 1786-1835." *Mind and Body* 17 (January 1911): 321-26.

_____. "The Introduction of Manual Labor as a System of Exercise in Educational Institutions (1825-1835)." 3 parts. *Mind and Body* 13 (May, June, July 1906): 65-71, 97-103, 129-35.

_____. "The 'New Gymnastics" of Dio Lewis (1860-1868)." *American Physical Education Review* 11 (June, September 1906): 83-95, 187-98.

_____. "Per Henrik Ling and His Successors at the Stockholm Normal School of Gymnastics." 2 parts. *Mind and Body* 12 (May, June 1905): 74-79, 102-105.

Lewis, Guy. "The Muscular Christianity Movement." *Journal of Health, Physical Education and Recreation* 37 (May 1966): 27-28, 42.

McCall, Laura. "'The Reign of Brute Force is Now Over': A Content Analysis of Godey's Lady's Book, 1830-1860." *Journal of the Early Republic* 9 (Summer 1989): 217-36.

McClary, Charles. "Introducing a Classic: *Gunn's Domestic Medicine.*" *Tennessee Historical Quarterly* 45 (1986): 210-16.

McCoy, Raymond F. "Hygienic Recommendations of the *Ladies Library.*" *Bulletin of the History of Medicine* 4 (1936): 367-72.

McCurdy, Persis Harlow. "The History of Physical Training at Mount Holyoke College." *American Physical Education Review* 14 (1909): 138-50.

Morantz, Regina Markell and Sue Zschoche. "Professionalism, Feminism, and Gender Roles: A Comparative Study of Nineteenth-Century Medical Therapeutics. *Journal of American History* 67 (December 1980): 568-88.

Morantz, Regina Markell. "Making Women Modern: Middle Class Women and Health Reform in Nineteenth-Century America." *Journal of Social History* 10 (1977): 490-507.

Mosedale, Susan Sleeth. "Science Corrupted: Victorian Biologists Consider 'The Woman Question." *Journal of the History of Biology* 11 (1978): 1-55.

Naylor, Mildred V. "Sylvester Graham, 1794-1851." *Annals of Medical History* 4 (1942): 236-40.

Olivova, Vera. "From the Arts of Chivalry to Gymnastics." *Canadian Journal of History of Sport* 9 (December 1981): 29-55.

Park, Roberta J. "'The Advancement of Learning': Expressions of Concern for Health and Exercise in English Proposals for Educational Reform—1640-1660." *Canadian Journal for History of Sport and Physical Education* 8 (1977): 51-61.

_____. "The Attitudes of Leading New England Transcendentalists Toward Healthful Exercise, Active Recreations and Proper Care of the Body: 1830-1860." *Journal of Sport History* 4 (1977): 34-50.

_____. "Concern for Health and Exercise as Expressed in the Writings of 18th-Century Physicians and Informed Laymen." *Research Quarterly* 47 (1976): 756-67

_____. "Concern for the Physical Education of the Female Sex from 1675 to 1800 in France, England, and Spain." *Research Quarterly* 45 (1974): 104-19.

_____. "'Embodied Selves': The Rise and Development of Concern for Physical Education, Active Games, and Recreation for American Women, 1776-1865." *Journal of Sport History* 5 (Summer 1978): 5-41.

_____. "Harmony and Cooperation: Attitudes Toward Physical Education and Recreation in Utopian Social Thought and American Communitarian Experiments, 1825-1865." *Research Quarterly* 45 (October 1974): 276-92.

_____. "Physiologists, Physicians, and Physical Educators: Nineteenth-Century Biology and Exercise, Hygienic and Educative." *Journal of Sport History* 14 (Spring 1987): 28-60.

_____. "Strong Bodies, Healthful Regimens, and Playful Recreations as Viewed by Utopian Authors of the 16th and 17th Centuries." *The Research Quarterly* 49 (1978): 498-511.

Paul, Joan. "The Health Reformers: George Barker Windship and Boston's Strength Seekers." *Journal of Sport History* 10 (Winter 1983): 41-57.

Putnam, Granville B. "The Introduction of Gymnastics in New England." *New England Magazine* 3 (September 1890): 111-13.

Rader, Benjamin G. "The Quest for Subcommunities and the Rise of American Sport. *American Quarterly* 29 (Fall 1977): 355-69.

Reimer, Bernhard. "The Grandfather of German Gymnastics." *Mind and Body* 1 (May 1894): 1-3

Rogers, F. B. "Shadrach Ricketson (1768-1839): Quaker Hygienist." *Journal of the History of Medicine* 20 (1965): 140-50.

Rogers, James F. "Too Early But Right—Our First School Hygienist." *School Board Journal* 114 (June 1947): 29-30.

Rosenberg, Charles E. "Medical Text and Social Context: Explaining William Buchan's *Domestic Medicine.*" *Bulletin of the History of Medicine* 57 (1983).

Salomon, Louis B. "The Least Remembered Alcott." *New England Quarterly* 34 (March 1961): 87-92.

Schatzman, Morton, M.D. "Paranoia or Persecution: The Case of Schreber." *History of Childhood Quarterly* 1 (Summer 1973): 62-88.

Shattuck, George. "Centenary of Round Hill School." *Proceedings of the Massachusetts Historical Society* 57 (December 1923): 205-209.

Shryock, Richard H. "Sylvester Graham and the Popular Health Movement, 1830-1870." *The Mississippi Valley Historical Review* 18 (June 1931-March 1932): 172-83.

Showalter, Elaine. "Victorian Women and Menstruation." *Victorian Studies* 14 (1970): 83-89.

Sklar, Kathryn Kish. "All Hail to Pure Cold Water!" *American Heritage* 26 (December 1974): 64-70.

Smith-Rosenberg, Carroll and Charles Rosenberg. "The Female Animal: Medical and Biological Views of Woman and Her Role in Nineteenth-Century America." *Journal of American History* 60 (September 1973): 332-56.

Stearns, Bertha-Monica. "Before Godeys." *American Literature* 2 (1930): 248-55.

Stocking, George W. "Lamarckianism in American Social Science, 1890-1915." *Journal of the History of Ideas* 23 (1962): 239-56.

Struna, Nancy and Mary L. Remley. "Physical Education for Women at The University of Wisconsin, 1863-1913." *Canadian Journal of History of Sport and Physical Education* 4 (1973): 8-21.

Struna, Nancy. "Puritans and Sport, The Irretrievable Tide of Change." *Journal of Sport History* 4 (Spring 1977): 15-30.

Temkin, Owsei. "Gall and the Phrenological Movement." *Bulletin of the History of Medicine* 21 (May-June 1947): 275-317.

Thomas, John L. "Romantic Reform in America, 1815-1865." *American Quarterly* 17 (1965): 656-81.

Todd, Jan. "Against All Odds: The Origins of Weight Training for Female Athletes in North America." *Iron Game History* 2 (April 1992): 4-14.

_____. "Minerva," Empress of Strength." *Iron Game History* 1 (April 1990): 14-15.

_____. "Strength is Health: George Barker Windship and the First American Weight Training Boom." *Iron Game History* 3 (September 1993): 3-14.

Turner, Bryan S. "The Government of the Body: Medical Regimens and the Rationalization of Diet." *The British Journal of Sociology* 33 (June 1982): 254-69.

Verbrugge, Martha H. "Healthy Animals and Civic Life: Sylvester Graham's Physiology of Subsistence." *Reviews in American History* 9 (1981): 359-64.

_____. "Women and Medicine in Nineteenth-Century America." *Signs: Journal of Women in Culture and Society* 1 (1976): 957-72.

Vertinsky, Patricia. "The Effect of Changing Attitudes Toward Sexual Morality Upon the Promotion of Physical Education for Women in Nineteenth-Century America. *The Canadian Journal of the History of Sport and Physical Education* 7 (December 1976): 26-38.

_____. "Rhythmics—A Sort of Physical Jubilee: A New Look at the Contributions of Dio Lewis." *The Canadian Journal of the History of Sport and Physical Education* 9 (May 1978): 31-42.

_____. "Sexual Equality and the Legacy of Catharine Beecher." *Journal of Sport History* 6 (Spring 1979): 38-49.

Walker, William B. "Luigi Cornaro: A Renaissance Writer on Personal Hygiene." *Bulletin of the History of Medicine* 28 (1954): 525-34.

Walsh, Anthony A. "The American Tour of Dr. Spurzheim. *Journal of the History of Medicine* 27 (1972): 187-205.

Welter, Barbara. "The Cult of True Womanhood, 1820-1860." *American Quarterly* 18 (Summer 1966): 151-74.

Wood, Ann Douglas "'The Fashionable Diseases': Women's Complaints and Their Treatment in Nineteenth-Century America." *Journal of Interdisciplinary History* 4 (Summer 1973): 25-52.

Wosh, Peter J. "Sound Minds and Unsound Bodies: Massachusetts Schools and Mandatory Physical Training." *New England Quarterly* 55 (March-December 1982): 40-59.

Wrobel, Arthur. "Orthodoxy and Respectability in Nineteenth-Century Phrenology." *Journal of Popular Culture* 9 (1975): 38-50.

Young, Dwight L. "Orson Squire Fowler: To Form a More Perfect Human." *Wilson Quarterly* 14 (Spring 1976): 120-27.

Zirkle, Conway. "The Early History of the Inheritance of Acquired Characteristics and of Pangenesis." *Transactions of the American Philosophical Society* 35 (Part 2, 1946): 110-21.

# Index

Abbott Academy, 284

Adams, Abigail, 18

Adams, John Quincy, 79

Agassiz, Louis, 268

Albertson, Roxanne, 21

Alcott, A. Bronson, 227-228

Alcott, Louisa, 221

Allen, Mrs. Joseph, 220

Allen, Nathaniel T., 217, 219-221, 250, 252

American Alliance for Health, Physical Education, Recreation, and Dance, 293

American Association for the Advancement of Physical Education, 293

American Institute of Instruction, 211, 221-222, 225, 239, 240

American Women's Educational Association, 151

Amoros, Colonel, 71

Andry, Nicholas, 93

*Orthopaedia*, 21 fig., 22, 22 fig.

Anonymous, 58

*Calisthénie ou Gymnastique des Jeunes Filles, Traité...lémentaire Des*

*Differéns Exercises, Propes A Fortifier*

*Le Corp, A Entretnir La Sante, Et A*

*Preparer Un Bon Tempérament,* 54,

57 fig., 69 fig.

Apparatus training: involving use of,

Arm Pull Device, 248

bars, 49, 50 fig., 51 fig., 54, 69 fig.

bells, 106, 109, 109 fig.

Blow Gun, 223, 240

Column of Pegs, 39 fig.

dumbbells, 98, 98 fig., 101, 185, 186, 188, 192-193, 242-244, 242 fig., 243 fig., 249, 251, 253, 289

Flying Course, 38, 50, 52 fig., 54, 57 fig.

Gymnastic Crown, 248, 248 fig.

Gymnastic Polymachinon, 186, 186 fig.

Health Lift, 173, 184-185, 189, 191, 191 fig., 192, 192 fig., 194-195

hoops/rings, 95, 95 fig., 242, 243 fig., 253

Indian club, 22, 90, 186, 193, 210, 242, 243 fig., 250, 251, 253, 289

Indian scepter, 97-98, 97 fig., 99, 100, 101

jump rope, 45 fig.

oscillator, 106, 110, 111 fig.

Pangymnastikon, 244-247, 244 fig., 246 fig., 249, 267

Patent Spring, 106, 108 fig.

Shoulder Pusher, 248-249

side lift machines, 195, 195 fig.

Spirometer, 223

Triangle, 89, 91, 93, 94 fig., 101,
    106, 107 fig., 244. *See also*
    Flying
Course
wands/canes, 22, 93, 94 fig., 98,
    101, 106, 107 fig., 124, 242,
    243 fig.
weighted bags, 157, 108 fig., 248
Weighted helmet, 40 fig., 248
Ashley, Sarah, 225, 247
Austin, Harriet, 178, 179, 183,
    288, 290
Backus, Miss, 128
Bacon, Mary, 19, 20
Bancroft, George, 76-77
Banner, Lois, 161
Barnett, S.M., 196
Basedow, Johann Berhard, 18
*Philanthropinum,* 18-19
Batcheldor, Anny, 125
Beach, Wooster, *Family Physician
    and Home Guide,* 181, 181
    fig.
Beaujeu, J.A.
gymnastic movement, 33, 45-52,
    53, 81
strength and health, 46, 47, 49, 50
*A Treatise on Gymnastic Exercises,
    Or Calisthenics For the Use of
    Young Ladies,* 31 fig., 46, 48
    fig., 50 fig., 51 fig., 52 fig., 56
    fig.
Beaujeu-Hawley, Madame
gymnastic school, 33
gymnastics movement, 45, 52-53
Beck, Carl, 36, 76, 78
Beecher, Catharine Esther, 138
    fig.
American Women's Educational
Association, 150, 151

association with Blackwell, 142-
    145
calisthenics, 112, 120, 130, 137-
    140, 147, 151, 152-162, 222
Hartford Seminary, 139-140, 152
health reformer, 150
idea of female form, 17
Laws of Health, 140, 142, 148,
    149, 265
Litchfield Academy, 24, 138
personal movement cure, 145-
    148, 148 fig., 154 fig., 157,
    157 fig., 179
promoter of teacher profession,
    140
promoter of women's exercise,
    149, 150, 157-158, 159, 162
questioned authorship, 104, 105
teaching at Lewis' school, 265,
    287
water cure, 141-142, 159
Works:
*Calisthenic Exercises for Schools,
    Families and Health
    Establishments,* 154, 154 fig.,
    155
*Calisthenics Exercises for Home,
    Schools and Families,* 136 fig.,
    155 fig., 156 fig., 157 fig., 160
*Domestic Economy,* 152
*Educational Reminiscences and
    Suggestions,* 104, 158, 162
*Letters to the People on Health
    and Happiness,* 16 fig., 141,
    142, 143, 147, 148, 149, 150,
    151, 154, 161
*Physiology and Calisthenics for
    Schools and Families,* 150,
    151, 152, 154, 239

*Suggestions Respecting
    Improvements in Education,*
    149
*Treatise on Domestic Economy,*
    153
*A Treatise on Domestic Economy
    for the Use of Young Ladies at
    Home and at School,* 149
Beecher, Edward (brother), 139
Beecher, Lyman (father), 138
Bell, John, *The Journal of Health,*
    55, 58
Bennett, Bruce, 76
Bentham, Jeremy, 44
Berenson, Senda
Boston Normal School of
    Gymnastics, 293
Smith College, 292-293
Berkely, Marion, literary heroine,
    272-273
Bicycle riding, as exercise, 290-
    291
Blackwell, Dr. Elizabeth
supporter of exercise, 137, 142-
    145, 143 fig., 153, 154, 159
ideal womanhood, 183
*The Laws of Life With Special
    Reference to the Physical
    Education of Girls,* 144
Blaikie, William, *How to Get
    Strong and How to Stay So,*
    294
Blanchard, Miss, 270
Bloomer, Amelia, 159
Borish, Linda, 160
Boston Monitorial School for
    Girls gymnastics program,
    54, 72-76, 81
Boston Normal School of
    Gymnastics, 290

Branson, Caroline, 194
Branson, Elizabeth, 194
Brinhilda, strongwoman, 183
Broca, Paul, 218
Brooks, John, 290
Brown, Charles Brockden
*Alcuin: A Dialogue,* 19
genderless exercise, 11, 19
Brown, Love, 129, 228, 265
Bryn Mawr College, 292
Burrage, J.C., 226
Butler Health Lift Company, 194
Butler's Lifting Cure, 173
Butler, David P., 189-195, 251
*Butler's System of Physical
    Training: The Lifting Cure,*
    189
Caledonian clubs, strength con-
    tests, 185
Calisthenics
American system, 119
Beecher, 112, 120, 130, 137, 149,
    152-162, 222
Clias, 43, 90
exercises, 37, 43, 49, 53, 88 fig.,
    106, 155-157, 155 fig., 156
    fig., 157, 242
exercises with implements, 90,
    106, 136 fig., 156 fig., 157
Fairchild, 121
grace and decorum, 89
Gove, 53, 119
Grant, 120
Hartford Female Seminary, 120,
    139, 158
in schools, 90, 104, 152-153, 222,
    294
Lewis, 223
Lieber, 54
Litchfield Academy, 21, 23

Lyon, 120, 123-125, 128, 131
"M", 104-112
Madame Beaujeu, 52
Mount Holyoke, 123-129, 250
movement, 33, 42, 59, 81, 89-112,
    119-131, 162
Riofrey, 103
Roper, 81
Spurzheim, 129
teacher preparation, 128
Tenney, 121
Titcomb, 127
Voarino, 91-96
White, 121

Camp, Walter, 294
Capron, George, 177
Casey, James K., oscillator, 110
Channing, Walter, 227
Chapin, Mary, 125, 128-129
Chester, Caroline, 20, 21
Chiosso, Captain James, 190
Gymnastic Polymachinon, 186,
    186 fig.
The Gymnastic Polymachinon,
    186 fig.
Circuses, strength acts, 185
Clapp, Cornelia
Manual of Gymnastics Prepared
    for the Use of the Students of
    Mt. Holyoke Seminary, 271
Clapp, Otis, 226
Clarke, Edward H.
Sex in Education, 292
Classical ideals, 38, 46, 112. 188
of womanhood, 15 fig.,16-17, 16
    fig., 161, 172, 180 fig., 273
Clias, Captain Phokion Heinrich,
    37-44
calisthenics, 43, 90

Works:
An Elementary Course of
    Gymnastic Exercises; Intended
    to Improve The Physical
    Powers of Man, 37
Callisthénie, ou Somascétique
    Naturelle, Appropriée A
    L'Education Phyisique Des
    Jeunes Filles, 42, 44 fig., 45
    fig.
Kalisthenie oder Uebungen zur
    Schoenheit und Kraft fuer
    Maedchen, 38 fig., 39 fig., 40
    fig., 40, 43 fig.
Anfrangsgrunde der Gymnastik
    oder Turnkunst, 37
Principes de gymnastique, 37
Coffin, John G.
Boston Medical Intelligencer, 56,
    58
gymnastics/physical education,
    73-75, 78, 81
Cogswell, Joseph C., 76-77
Coles, L.B., 25
Combe, Andrew, 174
Combe, George
classical statuary, 17, 55
Constitution of Man, 174, 175
Constantia. See Murray, Judith S.
Costume
"American", 288, 289
Beaujeu, 51-52
Butler, 195
Lewis, 215, 219, 225, 241, 241 fig.,
    246, 262 fig
Mount Holyoke, 124
reform, 240
Riofrey, 101 fig., 102
Warner, 51
Watson, 253

Cymburga, strongwoman, 183
Dance
as exercise, 12, 81, 99, 109
Beaujeu, 47
Litchfield Academy, 19, 23
Mount Holyoke, 125
Riofrey, 102, 103
student diaries, 19
Davies, John, 173
Dickinson, Emily, 123
Dioclesian Institute, 214
Dodge, Emeline, 289
Domestic work, 34, 89, 99-100
Beecher, 144, 153, 159, 160, 162
Coffin, 74, 81
Fowle, 75, 81
Fowler, 184
Lyon, 122-123
Mount Holyoke, 122-123, 282
Dowd, David L., 294
Dufay, Pierre, 23
Dunton, Delos
Home of the Free, 183
Dwight, Henry (brother), 80
Dwight, Sereno (brother), 80
Dwight, Timothy (father), 13, 19,
    80
Eastman, Mary F., 216, 219, 269,
    272
Education
movement, Berhard, 18
opportunities for women, 20, 24,
    57, 73
Educational system
denying rights, 11, 73
for men, 12, 71, 76
Emerson, Dr. Sarah, 269
Emerson, Ralph Waldo, 173
Erenhoff, C., 143
Evans, Miss, 270, 271

Fairchild, Augusta, 182
Fairchild, Harriet, 121
Family School for Young Ladies,
    254, 263-267, 270
Farnham, Eliza, 178
Felton, Cornelius C., 78-79
Livingston County High School,
    79-80
Normal College, 226
Fisher, Alexander Metcalf, 139
Fitzgerald, P.A.
Exhibition Speaker, 251, 251 fig.,
    252 fig.
Fletcher, J.H., 274
Flying Course, 38, 38 fig, 42., 50,
    91
Follen, Charles, 36, 76, 78
Fowle, William Bentley, 54, 56, 73
    fig., 81, 89
Boston Monitorial School, 71-76,
    81
first gymnastics program, 77-78
purposive exercise intro, 71-72
Fowler, Jonathan, 182
Fowler, Lorenzo and Orson
Phrenological Almanac, 175
The American Phrenological
    Journal, 175
Fowler, Lorenzo Nelson
Fowler Brothers Phrenological
    Cabinet, 175
Fowler, Orson Squire, 174 fig.,
    189, 190
phrenology and exercise, 173-
    185, 196-197
Works:
Creative and Sexual Science, 172,
    179 fig.
Maternity, or the Bearing and
    Nursing of Children, 184

*Private Lectures on Perfect Men,*
*Women and Children,* 174
fig., 176, 180 fig.
Franklin, Benjamin, 17
French, Lydia, 122
Fuller, Margaret, 255
Gage, Frances D., 291
Garrison, William Lloyd, 252,
269
Gender equity, 159-160
Beaujeu, 51, 54
Bell, 55-56
Blackwell, 144
Coffin, 74
Lewis, 211, 256, 269, 271, 290
Pierce, 20
Wollstonecraft, 13, 17
Georgii, Professor
Swedish Central Gymnastic
Institute, 143-144
Swedish Movement Cure, 143
German-style gymnastics. *See*
Gymnastics, European
Gilman, Charlotte Perkins, 290
Gleason, Mrs. R.B., 150, 183
Glenwood Ladies Seminary, 268
Goodale, Lucy, 123
Goodyear Company
"Pocket Gymnasium or Health
Pull", 196
Gove, Mary, 53, 119
Grant, Zilpah, 24, 152, 159
purposive exercise, 120
Gray, Asa, 23
Green, Harvey
*Fit for America,* 161, 196
Grigg, William, 58-59, 129
Grimke, Angelina, 140
Grimke, Sarah, 265
Guilford, L.T., 120

Gulick, Luther Halsey, 212, 240,
267, 271, 272
GutsMuths, Johann Friedrich
Schnepfenthal Philanthropic
School, 33-34, 35
Works:
*Gymnastics for Youth or a*
*Practical Guide to Healthful*
*and Amusing Exercises for the*
*Use of Schools. An Essay*
*Toward the Necessary*
*Improvement of Education;*
*Chiefly as it relates to the*
*Body.,* 34, 71
*Gymnastik fur die Jugen:*
*Enthaltend eine Praktische*
*Anwisung zu Leibesubungen.*
*Ein Beytraq zur Nothigsten*
*Verbesserung der Korperlichen*
*Erziehung.,* 34
Gymnasiums
Beaujeu, 45, 52-53
Clias, 37, 71
Dwight, 80
first in US?, 72
Follen, 78-79
Fowle, 77-78
Hall, 289
Hamilton, 91
Hubbard, 80
Jacques103 fig.
Lewis, 223, 224 fig., 226
Nachtegall, 36
Neal, 80
Plumb, 289
Riofrey, 101 fig.
Roper, 80
Völker, 36, 44, 71
Gymnastics, 25, 33-59, 71-81,
146, 222, 293

American, 52-53, 55-59
Beaujeu, J.A., 44-52
Beaujeu, Madame, 45, 52-53
British, Clias, 37-44
European movement, 33-37, 119
Fowle, 71-76
Fowler, 184
French schools, 42
German-style. *See also*
    European, 78-79, 89, 177
GutsMuths, 33-34
in the media, 55-58
Lewis, 218-229, 239-257, 266,
    269, 273, 285
New England, 71-81
programs in colleges, high
    schools, 79-80, 221
programs/exercises, 34, 43, 46-47,
    53-54
remedial, therapeutic, 36, 37, 39,
    40-44, 46, 57, 144
Riofrey, 100, 102
Round Hill School for Boys, 71-
    72, 76-77
Swedish, Ling, 36-37, 143-144,
    154, 218-219
Swedish, Nissen, 290
teachers, 225-229
*Turnen and Turners*, 35
Völker, 36, 44-45
Welch, 267-268
Gymnastique De Tronchin, 99-
    100. *See also* domestic work
Hale, Sarah Josepha, 151, 178
Works:
*Biography of Distinguished
    Women*, 138 fig.
*Godey's Ladies Book*, 129
*The Ladies' Magazine*, 104, 129
Hall, Mary, 289

Hamilton, Gustavus
*Elements of Gymnastics for Boys
    and Calisthenics for Young
    Ladies*, 90-91
Hanaford, J.H., 295
Hanna, Delphine, 268
Hartford Female Seminary, 120,
    139, 152, 158
Hartwell, Edward Mussey, 72,
    222
Hawley, Alanson, 226
Hawley, Mrs.. *See* Beaujeu-
    Hawley
Hawthorne, Una, 221
Health, 18, 34, 46, 47, 49, 55, 57,
    71, 80, 81, 89, 102, 105-106,
    161, 289
as women's profession, 149, 160,
    227
Hale, 130
Lewis, 198, 217, 226, 269, 272,
    274
Lewis, Helen, 240
Litchfield Academy, 19
Lyon, 121
Taylor, 145-148
Health Lift
Fowler, 173, 184-185, 196, 197
Windship, 187-189, 197
Health Lift machines, Butler,
    189-192, 191 fig., 194
Health Lift movement, 197-198
Health Lift Company of New
    York, 194
Health reform
Austin, 290
Beecher, 150
Jackson, 291
Lewis, 214, 217, 218, 220
Hemenway, Mary, 290

Henry, Patrick, 177
Higginson, Thomas Wentworth, 160, 211, 229
Hitchcock, Edward, 223, 270
Hitchcock, Edward, Jr.
  A Manual of the Gymnastic Exercises as Practiced by the Junior Class in Amherst College, 271
Holbrook, Dio Lewis (son), 270
Holbrook, M.L. (father), 270
Hollister, Gideon, 23
Homeopathy
Lewis, 214
Welch, 267
Homer, Miss, 283
Horseback riding
as exercise, 288, 289
Beecher, 139-140
Morley, 285
Hubbard, L.V., 80
Hunt, Lucy B.
  Hand-Book of Light Gymnastics, 270
Huntting, Margaret, 123, 124, 125
Hydropathy
Lewis, 264
Beecher, 141-142.
See also Water cure
Indebetou, Govert, 143
Intercollegiate sport, for women, 294
Ipswitch Female Seminary, 120
Jackson, James C., 291
Jacques, Daniel H., 17, 103-104
  Hints Toward Physical Perfection: Or the Philosophy of Human Beauty, 103, 103 fig., 180
Jahn, Friedrich Ludwig
Graue Kloster, 34

gymnastics, 34-36, 76, 79, 80
Works:
  Deutches Volksthum, 35
  Die Deutsche Turnkunst, 35, 77
Janes, Lewis
Butler Health Lift Company-NY, 194-196
  Health-Exercise: The Rationale and Practice of the Lifting-Cure or Health Lift, 191 fig., 192 fig., 198
Jefferson, Thomas, 79, 80
Jenkins, Eliza, 122
Johnson, Fanny, 288
Kehoe, Sim D.
  The Indian Club Exercise, 210
Kellerman, Annette, 294
Kellogg, John Harvey
  Ladies Guide in Health and Disease, 198
King, Anna Benton, 127
Kloss, Maurice
  The Dumb Bell Instructor for Parlor Gymnasts, 242, 243 fig., 244, 250-251
LaLanne, Jack, 294
Lamarck, J.B., 24-25
Lamarckianism, 24-25
Fowler, 178, 197
GutsMuths, 34
Lasell Seminary for Young Women, 221, 240
Lawrence, Lizzie, 288
Laws of Health, 289, 294
Beecher, 140, 148, 149, 160
Lewis, 219
Leavitt, John W., 194
Leigh, Mrs., 105
Leiter, Frances W., 291
Leonard, Fred Eugene, 54, 104

*A Guide to the History of Physical Education*, 270fig.

Leonard, T.E., 228

Lewis, Dioclesian, 162, 212

Adelphi Academy, 293

exercises in schools, 128, 198

Family School for Young Ladies, 254, 263-267, 264 fig., 270, 292

female shape, 179, 255

Morley, 281, 284-287

movement cure sanitarium, 263, 266-267

New Gymnastics, 124, 173, 193-194, 198, 211-229, 239, 241-241, 250, 252, 253, 265, 273, 285, 287

Normal College, 78, 224 fig., 225-229, 266, 267-268, 271

Works:

*Chastity*, 269

*Chats With Young Women*, 269

*Curious Fashions*, 269

*Dio Lewis's Monthly*, 269

*Gypsies: Or Three Year's Camp Life in the Mountains of California*, 269

*In a Nutshell: Suggestions to American College Students*, 212 fig., 247, 269

*Lewis's New Gymnastics for Ladies, Gentlemen and Children and Boston Journal of Physical Culture*, 241 fig., 251

*Lewis's Gymnastic Monthly and Journal of Physical Culture*, 224, 226, 238 fig., 240

*Lewis's New Gymnastics for Men, Women and Children and*

*Boston Journal of Physical Culture*, 239

*Nuggets*, 269

*Our Digestion*, 269

*Our Girls*, 239, 254-255, 269

*Prohibition a Failure*, 269

*The Dio Lewis Treasury*, 269

*The Homeopathist*, 214

*The New Gymnastics for Men, Women and Children(10th)*, 250-254, 254 fig., 271

*The New Gymnastics for Men, Women and Children(1st)*, 229, 239, 240-250, 242 fig., 243 fig., 246 fig., 248 fig., 262 fig.

*Weak Lungs, and How to Make Them Strong*, 215, 244 fig.

Lewis, Delecta Barbour, 212-213, 216

Lewis, Helen Cecelia Clarke, 212, 219, 220, 224, 240, 274

personal health214-216, 217, 218

Family School for Young Ladies, 264, 267

Lewis, Loran (brother), 212, 213, 214

Lieber, Franz, 36, 54, 58, 79

Lincoln, Mrs. W.O.,

Ling, Pehr Henrik, 143-144, 272

Swedish gymnastics, 36, 159, 162, 218-219

Litchfield Academy, 19-24, 72, 138

Mary Bacon, 19, 20

Chester, Caroline, 20, 21.

*See also* Pierce

Locke, John

*Some Thoughts Concerning Education*, 12

Lyon, Mary, 24, 112, 131, 159, 288

American calisthenics, 119-125, 121 fig

*Book of Duties*, 122, 124

"M", 104-112

*A Course of Calisthenics for Young Ladies in Schools and Families*, 90, 104, 105, 107 fig., 108

fig., 109, 109 fig., 111 fig, 159

Macauley, James William, 53

Majestic Womanhood, 11, 13, 16, 17, 173, 197, 239, 291

Mann's Reactionary Lifter, 194-196, 195 fig.

Mann, Horace, 222

*Common School Journal*, 33, 53, 73 fig.

*Sixth Annual Report as Secretary of the Massachusetts board of Education*, 174

Mann, Mary, 239-240

Mansfield, E.D., 20

Manual labor. *See* Domestic work

Martineau, Harriet, 174

May, Abigail, 268

McCarthy, Lewis,

McCurdy, Persis Harlow, 120

McFadden, Bernarr

*Woman's Physical Development*, 294

McLean Asylum, 221

McRae, Reverend David, 182

Mendell, Miss and Hosmer, Miss, *Notes of Travel and Life*, 185

Michigan University, 270

Mills College, 182

Milo, William

*Notes on Beauty, Vigor and Development; or How to Acquire Plumpness of Form , Strength of Limb, and Beauty of Complexion, With Rules for Diet and bathing, and a Series of Improved Physical Exercises*, 180-181

Milwaukee Female College, 158

Morley, Anna Clarissa Treat (mother), 281, 287

Morley, Anna Elizabeth "Lizzie"

Abbott Academy, 284

Family School for Young Ladies, 281, 284-288

health problems, 282-284

Mount Holyoke, 123, 128-129, 281-285

Morley, Edward William (brother), 281-288

Morley, Sardis Brewster (father), 281

Mount Holyoke Female Seminary, 118 fig.

Batcheldor, Anny, 125

Blanchard, Miss, 270

Brown, Love, 129, 228, 265

calisthenics,112, 121-128,

Chapin, Mary, 125, 128-129

Dickinson, Emily, 123

Evans, Miss, 270, 271

exhibition calisthenics, 124, 125, 250

French, Lydia, 122

Goodale, Lucy, 123

hallway exercises, 123, 282

Homer, Miss, 283

Huntting, 123,124, 125

Jenkins, Eliza, 122

King, Anna Benton, 127

Morley, Anna Elizabeth "Lizzie", 281-285
phys. ed. teacher preparation, 128, 228
Stillman, Julia, 288
Walker, Annie, 125
Ware, Mary, 125
See also Lyon; Titcomb
Movement Cure, 36, 137, 142, 145, 148, 159, 161, 162, 179, 289
exercises, 146 fig., 147, 147 fig.
Swedish, Taylor, 145-148
Lewis, 215, 218, 224-225, 227, 285
Lewis sanitarium, 263, 266-267
Mumford, Prentice, 274
Murray, Judith Sargeant, 18
Nachtegall, Franz, 36
National Cyclopaedia of American Biography, 73 fig, 118 fig., 121 fig., 143 fig., 145 fig.
Neal, John, 45, 80
New Gymnastics, 268, 269, 270, 273, 287
New Gymnastics, Lewis, 211, 221-229, 239-257, 265, 290
Nichols, Reverend Howard Stanley, 288
Nissen, Dr. Hartwig
Boston Normal School of Gymnastics, 290
Swedish Gymnastics, 290
Normal Institute for Physical Educators, 225-229, 249, 266, 267-268, 270, 286
Normal Institute for the Training of Teachers in Dio Lewis's New Gymnastics, 268

Northup, Reverend Bridey G., 222
Norton, Mary Beth, 13
Orcutt, Mary T.
Manual of Gymnastics, 268
Parot, Adele, 269
Paul, J. Fletcher, 196
Philbrick, John D., 223, 226, 239
Phillips, Wendell 220
Phrenology, 190, 256, 291
Fowler, 173-185, 196-197
Physical anthropometry, 291
Physical appeal
and calisthenics, 89, 91, 97, 100, 109
for women, 12, 16, 19, 24, 57-58, 71, 75, 102, 111, 180, 273
upperclass, 14-16
Physical education
begins in United States schools, 71-72
Berenson, 293
college for females teaching, 119, 270
first college exclusively for, 226, 271
first professional society for, 293
first teacher in, 76
first textbook for and by women, 104
Hale, 129-130
Hamilton, 90-91
Lewis, 218, 225-229, 250,267, 269, 270
Litchfield Academy, 21
mandantory in public schools, 269
Mount Holyoke, 122, 228
new definition, 130
Riofrey, 101, 102

school programs, 160, 174, 198
support for, 55-57
Welch, 268
Wollstonecraft theories, 12, 17, 97
women's profession, 268, 289
women's, 11, 43, 72, 96, 111, 144, 240, 249, 271, 290, 291, 294
Physical fitness, 11, 34, 49, 58, 71, 144, 224
and calisthenics, 89-90
Lyon, 121
movement, 25
upper class woman, 14-15
Physical nature, woman's, 11, 14
Physical potential,woman's, 12, 33, 46, 54, 58, 81, 96, 183
Lewis, 239, 254, 255, 294
McFadden, 294
Physical training
Beaujeu, 45, 48
Beecher, 139, 151
cardiovascular, 294
Clias, 38-39
Follen, 78-79
for men, 12
in schools, 11, 36, 218, 219, 239-240, 292
Jahn, 35
Lamarck, 24
Lewis, 218, 219, 221, 249, 271
Mount Holyoke, 127
Pierce, 20, 23, 24
Plumb, 289
Round Hill School for Boys, 76
Royal Hibernian Military School, 46
Schnepfenthal Philanthropic School, 34
to women's rights, 291

Walker, 96, 100
Webster, Noah, 19
Pierce, Sarah, 12, 19-24, 72, 137-138, 158
Plumb, Mrs. Z.R., Academy of Physical Culture, 289
Porter, William T.
Power, Hiram, 180 fig.
Progressive resistance
Butler, 190-192
Lewis, 246-247
Prudden, Bonnie, 294
Purposive exercise, 17, 24, 80, 89, 107, 112, 130, 281, 288, 295
at Harvard, 78
Beaujeu, 47
Beecher, 137, 138, 153, 160
Clarke, 292
Fowle, 71, 74, 81
Gage, 291
gender separation, 90-91, 129, 131
GutsMuths, 33-34
in college curriculum, 293
Lewis, 211, 214, 219, 228, 263, 266, 269, 292
Litchfield Academy, 19-20, 23, 72
Lyon, 119
Nissen, 290
Riofrey, 102
Rousseau, 11
Sargent , 290
Walker, 96, 100
water cure, 141
Watson, 253
Putnam, Granville B., 77
Quincy, Edmund, 78-79
Raymond, Mary, 289
Reeves, Judge Tappan, 19
Ricketson, Shadrach, 17

Rights, womens, 13, 14, 16, 18, 197, 211, 220, 239, 255, 269, 291
Norton, 13
to health, 11
to physical strength, 11
Riofrey, Bureaud, 58, 105
*Physical Education Especially Adapted to Young Ladies*, 100, 101
utilitarian fitness, 100-104
Rodgers, Eliza, 288
Roper, Mr., 80-81
Roth, Mathias
*The Free Gymnastic Exercises of P. H. Ling, Arranged by H. Rothstein*, 154
Round Hill School for Boys, 71-72, 76-77, 139
Bancroft, 76-77
Cogswell, 76-77
*See also* Beck, Charles
Rousseau, Jean Jacques, 15, 17, 18, 89, 111
*Emile*, 11, 12
gender based exercise, 11-13, 91
Roland, Helen, 295
Royal Hibernian Military School, Beaujeu, 46, 53
Royce, Charles S.,
Rush, Benjamin, 18, 215
Salzmann, Christian Gotthilf, 34, 80
Sandow, Eugen, 294
Sargeant, Dudley Allen, 198, 211-212
Sargeant, Dudley Allen
Sargent System, 290, 292
Sargent's School of Physical Education, 290, 292

Savage, Helen, 228
Schnepfenthal Philanthropic School. *See* GutsMuths
Schools
for physical educators, first normal, 211
starting gymnastics programs, 79-80, 222
women's, 11, 18, 23, 80, 197, 198, 292
Schreber, Daniel, 242, 249
Schreber, Daniel Gottlieb Moritz
*The Pangymnastikon; or, All Gymnastic Exercises Brought Within the Compass of a Single Piece of Apparatus, as the Simplest Means for the Complete Development of Muscular Strength and Endurance*, 244-245
Sedgwick, Catharine, American Women's Educational Association, 151
Severance, T.C., 226
Sewell, S.E., 226
Seymour, Mary Alice, 272-273
Sheldon, Lucy
dance, 19
walking vs. exercise, 23
Shew, Dr. Joel, 142
Shew, Mrs. M.L., 142
Sigourney, Lydia, American Women's Educational Association, 151
Silliman, Benjamin, 174
Skinner, John Stuart
*American Farmer*, 57-58
Sklar, Katherine, 104, 137, 139, 140, 158
Smith, Hattie, 289

Smith College, 270, 292
Spears and Swanson
*History of Sport and Physical
    Activity in the United States,*
    104
Spears, Betty, 293
Springfield College, 211-212
Spurzheim, Johann Caspar
calisthenics, 129
phrenology and education, 173-
    174, 175
Stanton, Elizabeth Cady, 179
gender equity, 159, 183-184
on women's exercise, 290-291
Stillman, Julia, 288
Stone, Lucy, 159
Stowe, Harriet Beecher, 139, 143,
    151
Strength, 11, 90, 289, 290
for men, 12, 89, 112, 182
for women, 16, 17, 47, 50, 54-55,
    57, 89, 95-96, 99, 109, 112,
    144, 155, 183, 196, 197
health lift, 184-185
Lewis, 198, 212, 218, 288
Strongmen, 182, 197
Struna, Nancy, 161
Taylor, Dr. George H.
movement cure, 137, 142, 145-
    148, 145 fig., 153, 154, 159,
    250
Works:
*Health by Exercise,* 147 fig.
*Illustrated Sketch of the Movement
    Cure,* 146, 146 fig., 148 fig.
Taylor, Mrs. M.L., 221, 240
Tenney, Abigail, 121
Thomas, Martha Carey, 292
Ticknor, George, 76, 78
Tilden Ladies Seminary, 268

*Tom Brown's School Days,* 96
Titcomb, Mary, 125-127
Trall, Russell, 288, 289
exercises in schools, 250, 251
*Illustrated Family Gymnasium,*
    251 fig.
Triat, Hippolyte, 185
Trine, Miss, 270
Tronchin, 99-100
Troy Female Seminary, 120, 139
*Turnen*
gymnastics, 35
Beck, 76
societies, 36, 185
Tyler, Moses Coit
*The Brawnville Papers,* 269
Valentine, Thomas W., 221-222
Van Dalen, Mitchell, and Bennett
*A World History of Physical
    Education,* 104
Vanderpoel, Emily Noyes
*Chronicles of a Pioneer School,* 21
*More Chronicles of a Pioneer
    School,* 21
Vassar College, 270, 270 fig.
Vertinsky, Patricia, on gender
    specific programs, 160
on Gilman, 290
Vitalism, 177
Voarino, Signor G.P., 91-96
*A Second Course of Calisthenic
    Exercises; With A Course of
    Private Gymnastics for
    Gentlemen,* 88 fig., 94-95, 95
    fig.
*A Treatise on Calisthenic
    Exercises, Arranged for the
    Private Tuition of Young
    Ladies,* 91, 92 fig., 92, 94 fig.
Völker, Carl, 80, 91

gymnastics, 36, 44-45
Walker, Alexander
*Beauty: Analysis and Classification of Beauty in Women*, 15 fig., 157
Walker, Annie, 125
Walker, Donald, 96-100
Works:
*British Manly Exercises*, 96, 250
*Exercises for Ladies*, 96, 97 fig., 98 fig.
*Walker's Manly Exercises*, 96
Walking, as exercise, 144, 184, 193, 215, 288, 289
Coffin, 74
Fowle, 75
Lewis, 248, 265
Litchfield Academy, 20-24
Mount Holyoke, 122
Walker, 98-99
water cure, 141, 142
Ware, Mary, 125
Warner, Patricia, 51
Water cure, 289
Shew, Joel, 142
therapeutic, 141-142, 159.
*See also* Hydropathy
Watson, J. Madison
*Handbook of Calisthenics and Gymnastics: A Complete Drill-Book for Schools, Families and Gymnasiums with Music to Accompany the Exercises*, 247 fig., 252-253, 253 fig.
*Watson's Manual of Calisthenics: A Systematic Drill-Book Without Apparatus for Schools, Families and Gymnasiums, With Music to Accompany the Exercises*, 253, 280 fig.
Webster, Daniel, 79
Weightlifting, Fowler, 185
Weir, Elizabeth, 221
Welch, Folansbee Goodrich, Normal College, 267-268
*Moral, Intellectual and Physical Culture*, 268
Weld, Angelina Grimke, 265
Weld, Theodore, 265
Wellness, 294
Wells, Samuel, "vital fluid", 176
West Newton Normal School, 149
Western Female Institute, 153
White, Alain, 23
White, Hannah, 121
Whorton, James, 137, 255
*Crusaders for Fitness*, 130
Willard, Emma, 120, 139
Willard, Frances, 291
Windship, George Barker
"Autobiographical Sketches of a Strength-Seeker", 187
gymnastic training, 187
weight lifting, 186-189, 190, 191, 196, 198, 251-252
women's exercise, 128, 162, 196
Wollstonecraft, Mary, 13-17, 25, 75
*A Vindication of the Rights of Women*, 11, 12
comparison to Pierce, 20
ideal body, 16
Young, Caroline E., 194

Index prepared by Kimberly Ayn Beckwith, Austin, Texas.